UCLA Symposia on Molecular and Cellular Biology, New Series

Series Editor, C. Fred Fox

RECENT TITLES

Volume 50
Interferons as Cell Growth Inhibitors and Antitumor Factors, Robert M. Friedman, Thomas Merigan, and T. Sreevalsan, *Editors*

Volume 51
Molecular Approaches to Developmental Biology, Richard A. Firtel and Eric H. Davidson, *Editors*

Volume 52
Transcriptional Control Mechanisms, Daryl Granner, Michael G. Rosenfeld, and Shing Chang, *Editors*

Volume 53
Progress in Bone Marrow Transplantation, Robert Peter Gale and Richard Champlin, *Editors*

Volume 54
Positive Strand RNA Viruses, Margo A. Brinton and Roland R. Rueckert, *Editors*

Volume 55
Amino Acids in Health and Disease: New Perspectives, Seymour Kaufman, *Editor*

Volume 56
Cellular and Molecular Biology of Tumors and Potential Clinical Applications, John Minna and W. Michael Kuehl, *Editors*

Volume 57
Proteases in Biological Control and Biotechnology, Dennis D. Cunningham and George L. Long, *Editors*

Volume 58
Growth Factors, Tumor Promoters, and Cancer Genes, Nancy H. Colburn, Harold L. Moses, and Eric J. Stanbridge, *Editors*

Volume 59
Chronic Lymphocytic Leukemia: Recent Progress and Future Direction, Robert Peter Gale and Kanti R. Rai, *Editors*

Volume 60
Molecular Paradigms for Eradicating Helminthic Parasites, Austin J. MacInnis, *Editor*

Volume 61
Recent Advances in Leukemia and Lymphoma, Robert Peter Gale and David W. Golde, *Editors*

Volume 62
Plant Gene Systems and Their Biology, Joe L. Key and Lee McIntosh, *Editors*

Volume 63
Plant Membranes: Structure, Function, Biogenesis, Christopher Leaver and Heven Sze, *Editors*

Volume 64
Bacteria–Host Cell Interaction, Marcus A. Horwitz, *Editor*

Volume 65
The Pharmacology and Toxicology of Proteins, John S. Holcenberg and Jeffrey L. Winkelhake, *Editors*

Volume 66
Molecular Biology of Invertebrate Development, John D. O'Connor, *Editor*

Volume 67
Mechanisms of Control of Gene Expression, Bryan Cullen, L. Patrick Gage, M.A.Q. Siddiqui, Anna Marie Skalka, and Herbert Weissbach, *Editors*

Volume 68
Protein Purification: Micro to Macro, Richard Burgess, *Editor*

Volume 69
Protein Structure, Folding, and Design 2, Dale L. Oxender, *Editor*

Volume 70
Hepadna Viruses, William Robinson, Katsuro Koike, and Hans Will, *Editors*

Volume 71
Human Retroviruses, Cancer, and AIDS: Approaches to Prevention and Therapy, Dani Bolognesi, *Editor*

Volume 72
Molecular Biology of the Human Brain, Edward G. Jones, *Editor*

Volume 73
The T-Cell Receptor, Mark M. Davis and John Kappler, *Editors*

Please contact the publisher for information about previous titles in this series.

UCLA Symposia Board

Human Retroviruses, Cancer, and AIDS

Approaches to Prevention and Therapy

Human Retroviruses, Cancer, and AIDS

Approaches to Prevention and Therapy

Proceedings of an Abbott-UCLA
Symposium Held at Keystone, Colorado
April 1–6, 1987

Editor

Dani Bolognesi
Department of Surgery
Duke University Medical Center
Durham, North Carolina

Alan R. Liss, Inc. • New York

Address all Inquiries to the Publisher
Alan R. Liss, Inc., 41 East 11th Street, New York, NY 10003

Printed in the United States of America

Library of Congress Cataloging-in-Publication Data

Abbott-UCLA Symposium on Human Retroviruses, Cancer, and AIDS: Approaches to Prevention and Therapy (1987 : Keystone, Colo.)
Human retroviruses, cancer and AIDS : approaches to prevention and therapy : proceedings of an Abbott-UCLA Symposium held at Keystone, Colorado, April 1–6, 1987 / editor, Dani Bolognesi.
p. cm. — (UCLA symposia on molecular and cellular biology ; new ser., v. 71)
"The 1987 Abbott-UCLA Symposium on Human Retroviruses, Cancer, and AIDS: Approaches to Prevention and Therapy was held at Keystone, Colorado, April 1–6, 1987"—Pref.
Includes bibliographies and index.
ISBN 0-8451-2670-9
1. Retrovirus infections—Congresses. 2. Human immunodeficiency viruses—Congresses. 3. AIDS (Disease)—Etiology—Congresses. 4. Cancer—Etiology—Congresses. I. Bolognesi, Dani. II. Abbott Laboratories. III. University of California, Los Angeles. IV. Title. V. Series.
[DNLM: 1. Acquired Immunodeficiency Syndrome—microbiology—congresses. 2. HTLV-III—congresses. 3. Neoplasms—microbiology—congresses. 4. Retroviridae—congresses. W3 U17N new ser. v. 71 / QW 166 A134h 1987]
QR201.R47A23 1987
616.97'90194—dc19
DNLM/DLC
for Library of Congress 87-29322
CIP

Contents

Contributors

Stuart A. Aaronson, Laboratory of Cellular and Molecular Biology, National Cancer Institute, Bethesda, MD 20892 **[407]**

M. Alizon, Unité d'Oncologie Virale, CNRS EA 1157, Institut Pasteur, 75724 Paris Cedex 15, France **[31]**

Jonathan S. Allan, Department of Cancer Biology, Harvard School of Public Health, Boston, MA 02115 **[341]**

Harvey Alter, Department of Transfusion Medicine, National Institutes of Health, Bethesda, MD 20892 **[327]**

Janet Andersen, Dana-Farber Cancer Institute, Boston, MA 02115 **[447]**

Suresh K. Arya, Laboratory of Tumor Cell Biology, National Cancer Institute, National Institutes of Health, Bethesda, MD 20892 **[43,57]**

R. Axel, College of Physicians and Surgeons, Columbia University, New York, NY 10032 **[283]**

Margreet Bakker, Department of Virology, Academic Medical Center, University of Amsterdam, 1105 AZ Amsterdam, The Netherlands **[241]**

David Baltimore, Whitehead Institute for Biomedical Research, Cambridge, MA 02142 **[477]**

H. Bannert, Institute of Virus Research, German Cancer Research Center, 6900 Heidelberg, Federal Republic of Germany **[75]**

Joan E. Barton, Wyeth Laboratories, Inc., Microbiology Division, Philadelphia, PA 19101 **[349]**

Jay H. Beckstead, AIDS Immunobiology Research Laboratory, Department of Medicine, San Francisco General Hospital, San Francisco, CA 94143; present address: Department of Pathology, University of California, San Francisco, San Francisco, CA 94143 **[213]**

Gary Berg, Department of Nuclear Medicine, National Institutes of Health Clinical Center, NIH, Bethesda, MD 20892 **[393]**

Phillip Berman, Department of Molecular Biology and Immunology, Genentech, Inc., South San Francisco, CA 94080 **[257]**

P. Beverley, U.C.H.M.S., London, United Kingdom **[283]**

William A. Blattner, Environmental Epidemiology Branch, National Cancer Institute, Bethesda, MD 20892 **[123]**

The numbers in brackets are the opening page numbers of the contributors' articles.

Dani P. Bolognesi, Department of Surgery, Duke University Medical Center, Durham, NC 27710 **[149,161,229,313]**

Samuel Broder, The Clinical Oncology Program, Division of Cancer Treatment, National Cancer Institute, Bethesda, MD 20892 **[365,393,407]**

Pim Brouwers, National Institute of Mental Health, NIH, Bethesda, MD 20892 **[393]**

Claudine Bruck, Department of Genetics, Smith Kline - RIT, 1330 Rixensart, Belgium **[241]**

Arturo Brunetti, Department of Nuclear Medicine, National Institutes of Health Clinical Center, NIH, Bethesda, MD 20892 **[393]**

Daniel Capon, Department of Molecular Biology and Immunology, Genentech, Inc., South San Francisco, CA 94080 **[257]**

Helen Carson, Repligen Corporation, Cambridge, MA 02139 **[149]**

Tran C. Chanh, Department of Virology and Immunology, Southwest Foundation for Biomedical Research, San Antonio, TX 78284 **[283,341]**

Cecilia Cheng-Mayer, Department of Medicine and Cancer Research Institute, University of California, School of Medicine, San Francisco, CA 94143 **[91]**

George J. Cianciolo, Howard Hughes Medical Institute, Durham, NC 27710 **[161]**

Michael E. Clark, Duke University Medical Center, Durham, NC 27710 **[161]**

Steven C. Clarke, Genetics Institute, Inc., Cambridge, MA 02140 and Division of Medical Oncology, Dana-Farber Cancer Institute, Harvard Medical School, Boston, MA 02215 **[197]**

F. Clavel, Unité d'Oncologie Virale, CNRS EA 1157, Institut Pasteur, 75724 Paris Cedex 15, France **[31]**

Jerry M. Collins, Clinical Pharmacology Branch, National Cancer Institute, NIH, Bethesda, MD 20892 **[393]**

Anthony J. Conley, Wyeth Laboratories, Inc., Microbiology Division, Philadelphia, PA 19101 **[349]**

Terry D. Copeland, Laboratory of Molecular Virology and Carcinogenesis, BRI-Basic Research Program, NCI-Frederick Cancer Research Facility, Frederick, MD 21701 **[135]**

S.P. Cort, Immunology Branch, Division of Host Factors, Center for Infectious Diseases, Centers for Disease Control, Atlanta, GA 30333 **[269]**

W.L. Cosand, Genetic Systems Corporation, Seattle, WA 98121 **[269]**

G.D. Cross, Immunology Branch, Division of Host Factors, Center for Infectious Diseases, Centers for Disease Control, Atlanta, GA 30333 **[269]**

Michael J. Currens, The Clinical Oncology Program, National Cancer Institute, Bethesda, MD 20892 **[407]**

John E. Dahlberg, Laboratory of Cellular and Molecular Biology, National Cancer Institute, Bethesda, MD 20892 **[407]**

Marinos Dalakas, National Institute of Neurological and Communicative Disorders and Stroke, NIH, Bethesda, MD 20892 **[393]**

A.G. Dalgleish, Clinical Research Center, Harrow, United Kingdom **[283]**

G. Darai, Institute of Medical Virology, University of Heidelberg, 6900 Heidelberg, Federal Republic of Germany **[75]**

Alan R. Davis, Wyeth Laboratories, Inc., Microbiology Division, Philadelphia, PA 19101 **[349]**

Frank de Wolf, Department of Virology, Academic Medical Center, University of Amsterdam, 1105 AZ Amsterdam, The Netherlands **[241]**

Surendra K. Dheer, Wyeth Laboratories, Inc., Microbiology Division, Philadelphia, PA 19101 **[349]**

Robert E. Donahue, Genetics Institute, Inc., Cambridge, MA 02140 and Division of Medical Oncology, Dana-Farber Cancer Institute, Harvard Medical School, Boston, MA 02215 **[197]**

Gordon R. Dreesman, Department of Virology and Immunology, Southwest Foundation for Biomedical Research, San Antonio, TX 78284 **[341]**

Jorg W. Eichberg, Department of Virology and Immunology, Southwest Foundation for Biomedical Research, San Antonio, TX 78284 **[327,341]**

M. Emerman, Unité d'Oncologie Virale, CNRS EA 1157, Institut Pasteur, 75724 Paris Cedex 15, France **[31]**

Myron Essex, Department of Cancer Biology, Harvard School of Public Health, Boston, MA 02115 **[341]**

Louise A. Evans, Department of Medicine and Cancer Research Institute, University of California, School of Medicine, San Francisco, CA 94143 **[91]**

Kathleen Fargnoli, Department of Molecular Genetics, Roche Research Center, Hoffmann-La Roche, Inc., Nutley, NJ 07052 **[175]**

Anthony S. Fauci, National Institute of Allergy and Infectious Diseases, Bethesda, MD 20892 **[187]**

Ellen G. Feigal, AIDS Immunobiology Research Laboratory, Department of Medicine, San Francisco General Hospital, San Francisco, CA 94143 **[213]**

Barbara K. Felber, NCI-Frederick Cancer Research Facility, BRI-Basic Research Program, Frederick, MD 21701 **[439]**

Christopher Fennie, Department of Molecular Biology and Immunology, Genentech, Inc., South San Francisco, CA 94080 **[257]**

Margaret A. Fischl, Department of Medicine, Jackson Memorial Hospital, Miami, FL 33136 **[393]**

R.M. Flügel, Institute of Virus Research, German Cancer Research Center, 6900 Heidelberg, Federal Republic of Germany **[75]**

Robert C. Gallo, Laboratory of Tumor Cell Biology, National Cancer Institute, NIH, Bethesda, MD 20205 **[149,175,313]**

Suzanne Gartner, Laboratory of Tumor Cell Biology, National Cancer Institute, Bethesda, MD 20892 **[123]**

Joseph Gibbons, Departments of Internal Medicine and Biochemistry, University of Alabama at Birmingham, Comprehensive Cancer Center, BHS 288, Birmingham, AL 35294 **[101]**

Livia Giurgia, Institut Pasteur du Brabant, 1040 Brussels, Belgium **[241]**

J. Goodchild, Worcester Foundation for Experimental Biology, Shrewsbury, MA 01545 **[423]**

Michael S. Gottlieb, 4849 Van Nuys Blvd., Suite 101, Sherman Oaks, CA 91403, **[463]**

Jaap Goudsmit, Department of Virology, Academic Medical Center, University of Amsterdam, 1105 AZ Amsterdam, The Netherlands **[241]**

Jordan Grafman, National Institute of Neurological and Communicative Disorders and Stroke, NIH, Bethesda, MD 20892 **[393]**

Timothy Gregory, Department of Molecular Biology and Immunology, Genentech, Inc., South San Francisco, CA 94080 **[257]**

Jerome E. Groopman, Division of Hematology/Oncology, Department of Medicine, New England Deaconess Hospital, Cambridge, MA 02140 **[197]**

M. Guyader, Unité d'Oncologie Virale, CNRS EA 1157, Institut Pasteur, 75724 Paris Cedex 15, France **[31]**

Beatrice H. Hahn, Departments of Internal Medicine and Biochemistry, University of Alabama at Birmingham, Comprehensive Cancer Center, BHS 288, Birmingham, AL 35294 **[57,101]**

Barton F. Haynes, Duke University Medical Center, Durham, NC 27710 **[161]**

Louis E. Henderson, Laboratory of Molecular Virology and Carcinogenesis, BRI-Basic Research Program, NCI-Frederick Cancer Research Facility, Frederick, MD 21701 **[135]**

Maurice R. Hilleman, Merck Institute for Therapeutic Research, Merck Sharp & Dohme Research Laboratories, West Point, PA 19486 **[291]**

Jacques Homsy, Department of Medicine and Cancer Research Institute, University of California, School of Medicine, San Francisco, CA 94143 **[91]**

Shiu-Lok Hu, ONCOGEN, Seattle, WA 98121 **[327]**

Paul P. Hung, Wyeth Laboratories, Inc., Microbiology Division, Philadelphia, PA 19101 **[349]**

Jennifer Jackson, Repligen Corporation, Cambridge, MA 02139 **[149]**

Freda K. Jacobsen, National Cancer Institute, NIH, Bethesda, MD 20892 **[393]**

Rudolf Jaenisch, Whitehead Institute, Cambridge, MA 02142 **[447]**

Valentina Jarocki-Witek, Wyeth Laboratories, Inc., Microbiology Division, Philadelphia, PA 19101 **[349]**

Ruth F. Jarrett, Laboratory of Tumor Cell Biology, National Cancer Institute, Bethesda, MD 20892 **[407]**

Margaret M. Johnson, Division of Hematology/Oncology, Department of Medicine, New England Deaconess Hospital, Cambridge, MA 02140 **[197]**

Patrick Kanda, Department of Virology and Immunology, Southwest Foundation for Biomedical Research, San Antonio, TX 78284 **[341]**

Lawrence Kaplan, AIDS Immunobiology Research Laboratory, Department of Medicine, San Francisco General Hospital, San Francisco, CA 94143; present address: AIDS Activities, San Francisco General Hospital, San Francisco, CA 94110 **[213]**

M.S. Kennedy, Immunology Branch, Division of Host Factors, Center for Infectious Diseases, Centers for Disease Control, Atlanta, GA 30333 **[269]**

Ronald C. Kennedy, Department of Virology and Immunology, Southwest Foundation for Biomedical Research, San Antonio, TX 78284 **[283,341]**

Raymond W. Klecker, Clinical Pharmacology Branch, National Cancer Institute, NIH, Bethesda, MD 20892 **[393]**

Beverley Kostek, Wyeth Laboratories, Inc., Microbiology Division, Philadelphia, PA 19101 **[349]**

Richard Kramer, Department of Molecular Genetics, Roche Research Center, Hoffmann-La Roche, Inc., Nutley, NJ 07052 **[175]**

Kai Krohn, Laboratory of Tumor Cell Biology, Bethesda, MD 20205 **[149]**

Willy J.A. Krone, Department of Virology, Academic Medical Center, University of Amsterdam, 1105 AZ Amsterdam, The Netherlands **[241]**

Prasanna Kumar, Division of Hematology-Oncology, University of Alabama at Birmingham, Birmingham, AL 35294 **[57]**

Joep Lange, Department of Virology, Academic Medical Center, University of Amsterdam, 1105 AZ Amsterdam, The Netherlands **[241]**

Alphonse J. Langlois, Department of Surgery, Duke University Medical Center, Durham, NC 27710 **[161,229,313]**

Steven M. Larson, National Institutes of Health Clinical Center, NIH, Bethesda, MD 20892 **[393]**

Laurence Lasky, Department of Molecular Biology and Immunology, Genentech, Inc., South San Francisco, CA 94080 **[257]**

Patricia Lekas, AIDS Immunobiology Research Laboratory, Department of Medicine, San Francisco General Hospital, San Francisco, CA 94143 **[213]**

Frances LeSane, Laboratory of Human Carcinogenesis, National Cancer Institute, Bethesda, MD 20892 **[123]**

R.L. Letsinger, Worcester Foundation for Experimental Biology, Shrewsbury, MA 01545; present address: Northwestern University, Evanston, IL 60201 **[423]**

Jay A. Levy, Department of Medicine and Cancer Research Institute, University of California, School of Medicine, San Francisco, CA 94143 **[91]**

Michael D. Lubeck, Wyeth Laboratories, Inc., Microbiology Division, Philadelphia, PA 19101 **[349]**

Paul A. Luciw, Department of Medical Pathology, University of California, Davis, Davis, CA 95616 **[115]**

H. Kim Lyerly, The Department of Surgery, Duke University Medical Center, Durham, NC 27710 **[229,313]**

Debra Lynn, Repligen Corporation, Cambridge, MA 02139 **[149]**

P. Maddon, College of Physicians and Surgeons, Columbia University, New York, NY 10032 **[283]**

M. Malkovsky, Clinical Research Center, Harrow, United Kingdom **[283]**

Dean L. Mann, Laboratory of Human Carcinogenesis, National Cancer Institute, Bethesda, MD 20892 **[123]**

Bruce B. Mason, Wyeth Laboratories, Inc., Microbiology Division, Philadelphia, PA 19101 **[349]**

Makoto Matsukura, The Clinical Oncology Program, National Cancer Institute, Bethesda, MD 20892 **[407]**

Shuzo Matsushita, The Clinical Oncology Program, National Cancer Institute, Bethesda, MD 20892 **[407]**

Thomas J. Matthews, Department of Surgery, Duke University Medical Center, Durham, NC 27710 **[149,161,229,313]**

B. Maurer, Institute of Virus Research, German Cancer Research Center, 6900 Heidelberg, Federal Republic of Germany **[75]**

A.C. Mawle, Immunology Branch, Division of Host Factors, Center for Infectious Diseases, Centers for Disease Control, Atlanta, GA 30333 **[269]**

Nanette McAtee, Clinical Pharmacology Branch, National Cancer Institute, NIH, Bethesda, MD 20892 **[393]**

Ronald S. McCaffrey, Section of Medical Oncology, Boston University Medical School, Boston, MA 02118 **[407]**

Jan McClure, Genetic Systems, Seattle, WA 98121 **[327]**

J.S. McDougal, Immunology Branch, Division of Host Factors, Center for Infectious Diseases, Centers for Disease Control, Atlanta, GA 30333 **[269]**

Michael S. McGrath, AIDS Immunobiology Research Laboratory, Department of Medicine, San Francisco General Hospital, San Francisco, CA 94143 **[213]**

Hiroaki Mitsuya, The Clinical Oncology Program, National Cancer Institute, Bethesda, MD 20892 **[407]**

Katherine L. Molnar-Kimber, Wyeth Laboratories, Inc., Microbiology Division, Philadelphia, PA 19101 **[349]**

L. Montagnier, Unité d'Oncologie Virale, CNRS EA 1157, Institut Pasteur, 75724 Paris Cedex 15, France **[31]**

Patricia A. Moran, Southwest Foundation for Biomedical Research, San Antonio, TX 78284 **[327]**

John E. Morin, Wyeth Laboratories, Inc., Microbiology Division, Philadelphia, PA 19101 **[349]**

William Morton, Regional Primate Center, University of Washington, Seattle, WA 98195 **[327]**

Charles E. Myers, Clinical Pharmacology Branch, National Cancer Institute, NIH, Bethesda, MD 20892 **[393]**

Gerald Nakamura, Department of Molecular Biology and Immunology, Genentech, Inc., South San Francisco, CA 94080 **[257]**

J.K.A. Nicholson, Immunology Branch, Division of Host Factors, Center for Infectious Diseases, Centers for Disease Control, Atlanta, GA 30333 **[269]**

Stephen Oroszlan, Laboratory of Molecular Virology and Carcinogenesis, BRI-Basic Research Program, NCI-Frederick Cancer Research Facility, Frederick, MD 21701 **[135]**

Thomas J. Palker, Duke University Medical Center, Durham, NC 27710 **[161]**

Elizabeth S. Parks, Department of Pediatrics, University of Miami School of Medicine, Miami, FL 33101 **[101]**

Wade P. Parks, Department of Pediatrics, University of Miami School of Medicine, Miami, FL 33101 **[101]**

Eric Patzer, Department of Molecular Biology and Immunology, Genentech, Inc., South San Francisco, CA 94080 **[257]**

George N. Pavlakis, NCI-Frederick Cancer Research Facility, BRI-Basic Research Program, Frederick, MD 21701 **[439]**

Carlo Federico Perno, Clinical Oncology Program, National Cancer Institute, NIH, Bethesda, MD 20892 **[393]**

B. Matija Peterlin, Howard Hughes Medical Institute, University of California, San Francisco, San Francisco, CA 94143 **[115]**

Mikulas Popovic, Laboratory of Tumor Cell Biology, National Cancer Institute, Bethesda, MD 20892 **[123]**

Scott D. Putney, Repligen Corporation, Cambridge, MA 02139 **[149,313]**

Richard R. Randall, Howard Hughes Medical Institute, Durham, NC 27710 **[161]**

Annamari Ranki, Laboratory of Tumor Cell Biology NCI/NIH, Bethesda, MD 20205 **[149]**

E.P. Reddy, Department of Molecular Biology, Hoffmann-La Roche, Inc., Nutley, NJ 07052; present address: Wistar Institute, Philadelphia, PA 19104 **[175]**

Marvin S. Reitz, Laboratory of Tumor Cell Biology, National Cancer Institute, Bethesda, MD 20892 **[407]**

A. Rethwilm, Institute of Virus Research, German Cancer Research Center, 6900 Heidelberg, Federal Republic of Germany **[75]**

Gregory Reyes, AIDS Immunobiology Research Laboratory, Department of Medicine, San Francisco General Hospital, San Francisco, CA 94143; present address: GeneLabs, Inc., Redwood City, CA 94063 **[213]**

Marjorie Robert-Guroff, Laboratory of Tumor Cell Biology NCI-NIH, Bethesda, MD 20205 **[149]**

W. Gerard Robey, National Cancer Institute, FCRF Frederick, MD 21701 **[149]**

Ruth M. Ruprecht, Dana-Farber Cancer Institute, Boston, MA 02115 **[447]**

James Rusche, Repligen Corporation, Cambridge, MA 02139 **[149,313]**

Michael S. Saag, Departments of Internal Medicine and Biochemistry, University of Alabama at Birmingham, Comprehensive Cancer Center, BHS 288, Birmingham, AL 35294 **[101]**

Bijan Safai, Department of Dermatology, Memorial Sloan-Kettering Hospital, New York, NY 10021 **[161,393]**

P.S. Sarin, Worcester Foundation for Experimental Biology, Shrewsbury, MA 01545; present address: National Cancer Institute, Bethesda, MD 20892 **[423]**

Q. Sattentau, U.C.H.M.S., London, United Kingdom **[283]**

Michael Schaber, Department of Molecular Genetics, Roche Research Center, Hoffmann-La Roche, Inc., Nutley, NJ 07052 **[175]**

Peter J. Schmidt, National Institute of Mental Health, NIH, Bethesda, MD 20892 **[393]**

Alan M. Schultz, Laboratory of Molecular Virology and Carcinogenesis, BRI-Basic Research Program, NCI-Frederick Cancer Research Facility, Frederick, MD 21701 **[135]**

Arlene H. Sharpe, Whitehead Institute, Cambridge, MA 02142 **[447]**

George M. Shaw, Departments of Internal Medicine and Biochemistry, University of Alabama at Birmingham, Comprehensive Cancer Center, BHS 288, Birmingham, AL 35294 **[57,101]**

Craig Shimasaki, Department of Molecular Biology and Immunology, Genentech, Inc., South San Francisco, CA 94080 **[257]**

Lia Smit, Department of Virology, Academic Medical Center, University of Amsterdam, 1105 AZ Amsterdam, The Netherlands **[241]**

Douglas Smith, Department of Molecular Biology and Immunology, Genentech, Inc., South San Francisco, CA 94080 **[257]**

Ralph Snyderman, Duke University Medical Center, Durham, NC 27710 **[161]**

P. Sonigo, UREG, INSERM U 163 and CNRS UA 271, Institut Pasteur, 75724 Paris Cedex 15, France **[31]**

Raymond C. Sowder, Laboratory of Molecular Virology and Carcinogenesis, BRI-Basic Research Program, NCI-Frederick Cancer Research Facility, Frederick, MD 21701 **[135]**

Zachary Spigelman, Section of Medical Oncology, Boston University Medical School, Boston, MA 02118 **[407]**

A. Robert Spitzer, National Institute of Neurological and Communicative Diseases and Stroke, NIH, Bethesda, MD 20892 **[393]**

Masatoshi Tateno, Department of Medicine and Cancer Research Institute, University of California, School of Medicine, San Francisco, CA 94143 **[91]**

Marie E. Taylor, Division of Hematology-Oncology, University of Alabama at Birmingham, Birmingham, AL 35294 **[57]**

Howard M. Temin, McArdle Laboratory, University of Wisconsin, Madison, WI 53706 **[1]**

Rose V. Thomas, Clinical Pharmacology Branch, National Cancer Institute, NIH, Bethesda, MD 20892 **[393]**

Sandra Tong-Starksen, Howard Hughes Medical Institute, University of California, San Francisco, San Francisco, CA 94143 **[115]**

Paul A. Volberding, Medical Oncology, AIDS Activities Division, San Francisco General Hospital, San Francisco, CA 94110; present address: San Francisco General Hospital, Ward 84, San Francisco, CA 94110 **[381]**

Christopher Walker, Department of Medicine and Cancer Research Institute, University of California, School of Medicine, San Francisco, CA 94143 **[91]**

Kent J. Weinhold, Department of Surgery, Duke University Medical Center, Durham, NC 27710 **[229,313]**

Gilbert C. White, Department of Medicine, University of North Carolina, Chapel Hill, NC 27514 **[161]**

Alison Wichman, National Institute of Neurological and Communicative Disorders and Stroke, NIH, Bethesda, MD 20892 **[393]**

Flossie Wong-Staal, Laboratory of Tumor Cell Biology, National Cancer Institute, Bethesda, MD 20205 **[175]**

Connie M. Wright, NCI-Frederick Cancer Research Facility, BRI-Basic Research Program, Frederick, MD 21701 **[439]**

Robert Yarchoan, Clinical Oncology Program, National Cancer Institute, NIH, Bethesda, MD 20892 **[393]**

M. Zamecnik, Worcester Foundation for Experimental Biology, Shrewsbury, MA 01545 **[423]**

P.C. Zamecnik, Worcester Foundation for Experimental Biology, Shrewsbury, MA 01545 **[423]**

Gordon Zandle, Wyeth Laboratories, Inc., Microbiology Division, Philadelphia, PA 19101 **[349]**

Joyce M. Zarling, ONCOGEN, Seattle, WA 98121 **[327]**

Leonard I. Zon, Division of Hematology/Oncology, Department of Medicine, New England Deaconess Hospital, Cambridge, MA 02140 and Division of Medical Oncology, Dana-Farber Cancer Institute, Harvard Medical School, Boston, MA 02215 **[197]**

Preface

The 1987 Abbott-UCLA Symposium on **Human Retroviruses, Cancer and AIDS: Approaches to Prevention and Therapy** was held at Keystone, Colorado, April 1–6, 1987. This conference, attended by approximately 300 scientists, dealt with the properties of human retroviruses and their relationship to disease, focusing mainly on AIDS, but including also leukemias, lymphomas and degenerative diseases. It is apparent from progress over the past two years that the potential impact of these agents on human health is far greater than could ever be anticipated since their discovery by Gallo and colleagues in 1978.

Indeed, the Symposium featured discussions of a new class of human immunodeficiency virus (HIV) originating from West Africa. New agents with properties of retroviruses also were reported in association with nervous system disorders and Kawasaki's disease. A new human foamy virus also was described, as was HBLV—a new human herpes virus possibly related to B-cell lymphomas in man.

A detailed analysis of their genuine structures and translation products was updated along with the identification of an eighth gene for HIV. Insights not only as to how HIV's and HTLV's control expression of their genes, but also as to how they influence cellular processes possibly related to their pathogenic effect received attention.

While the mechanism of HIV pathogenesis is not definitive, some of its elements are beginning to be understood. There are both direct and indirect consequences of HIV infections in the host that lead to impairment and destruction of the immune system. It was evident from the discussions that the virus infects many different types of cells in addition to its primary target, the T4 lymphocyte. Most notable among these are cells of the macrophage lineage that appear to be much more resistant to the cytopathic effects of the virus and thus may represent long-lived reservoirs of virus infection. The issue of virus latency and the nature of the signals that activate its expression also were discussed in relation to pathogenesis.

One session was devoted to the relationship of the virus to its receptor, a select portion of the T4 cell surface marker. Considerable advances have been made in identifying the molecular nature of the binding site on the virus glycoprotein (gp120) to T4 receptors and the requirements for optimal binding to occur. The importance of understanding this interaction in relation to pathogenesis, as well as preventive and interventive strategies, was discussed.

Steady progress also has occurred in the area of vaccine development for AIDS. The depth of knowledge about the functional and immunologic domain of the virus envelope components is leading the way to a better understanding of the key targets for immune attacks on the virus and the infected cell. In that regard both humoral and cell-mediated processes with potential for inhibition of virus infectivity and destruction of infected cells have been defined. The challenge remains as to how these can best be induced in a naive host so as to constitute a protective response against transmission of HIV.

The final topic of the Symposium was an update on the status of treatment strategies for AIDS. This included not only current drugs in clinical trials, particularly AZT, but also new approaches involving other targets of opportunity. The early and continuing success with AZT provides an important base on which to build what one hopes is an effective armamentarium to conquer the disease.

This Symposium was attended by a rich mixture of an international group of scientists and clinicians from academia, government, and the private sector. The meeting was opened by a Keynote Address by Howard Temin and David Baltimore summarized the meeting at its closure. I would personally like to thank them for graciously accepting these roles and for their thoughtful and insightful remarks which are documented in this volume.

Special thanks are due to Abbott Laboratories for their generous sponsorship of this meeting. We also gratefully acknowledge additional contributions from Burroughs Wellcome Co., Glaxo, Inc., Hoffmann-LaRoche, Inc., Merck and Company, Pfizer Central Research, Pfizer, Inc. and E.I. du Pont de Nemours & Co. For their wonderful organizational skills, their graciousness and patience, heartfelt thanks go to Fred Fox and his staff, particularly Robin Yeaton and Betty Handy.

Dani Bolognesi

**Human Retroviruses, Cancer, and AIDS:
Approaches to Prevention and Therapy, pages 1–28**

EVOLUTION OF RETROVIRUSES AND OTHER RETROTRANSCRIPTS

(Keynote address for Meeting on Human Retroviruses, Cancer, and AIDS, Keystone, Colorado, April 1,1987)[1]

Howard M. Temin

McArdle Laboratory, University of Wisconsin, Madison, Wisconsin 53706

ABSTRACT HIV is a newly appearing virus. Its evolution involved mechanisms of variation like those used in other retrovirus evolution and selection for increased replication. The mechanisms of variation for all retroviruses include mutation, gene conversion, and recombination. All of these processes occur at relatively high rates. Recombination can involve cellular sequences as well as unrelated retroviruses, resulting in complex virus lineages. Thus, retrovirus evolution in general and HIV evolution in particular involved many different kinds of genetic variation and can have involved multiple different lineages of descent.

INTRODUCTION

One of the most frequently asked questions about AIDS and HIV is where did HIV come from. A similar question has been raised for the HTLVs and adult T-cell leukemia. The answers to these questions may be important in understanding and controlling the epidemics caused by these viruses. Three answers have been proposed to the question of origins for HIV: 1.) HIV has existed for a long time in isolated villages in Africa, but it was only recognized recently when it was transmitted into populations in the cities; 2.) HIV was created in a genetic engineering laboratory, probably in the USA but

[1]The work in my laboratory was supported by Public Health Service research grants CA-22443 and CA-07175.

perhaps in Haiti; and 3.) HIV is a newly appearing virus derived from some viral precursor probably from infected monkeys.

To differentiate among these answers we need to know some African history and some molecular virology. Historians of Africa report that there was wide diffusion of cultural artefacts in Africa and that villages were not isolated from each other (1). Therefore, answer 1.) is ruled out because of the absence of the required isolation. The molecular structure and organization of the HIV genome are much more complex than that of any previously known retrovirus, and thus, no earthly scientist could have constructed HIV before the time it first appeared (2). Therefore, answer 2.) is also ruled out. Thus, we are left with answer 3.): HIV is a newly appearing virus derived from some viral precursor.

A similar question about origins has been discussed for years with regards to retroviruses in general (3). Since there are more data relevant to this question and similar mechanisms are probably involved in the evolution of all elements that use reverse transcription, consideration of the more general question should help us to understand the origin of HIV.

Possible answers to the general question of the origin of retroviruses include: 1.) retroviruses existed from the beginning of life, that is, were the first living entities; 2.) retroviruses evolved from the cellular genome, esp. cellular movable genetic elements; or 3.) retroviruses evolved from DNA viruses. (I do not consider the fourth possibility that retroviruses evolved from RNA viruses, because their replications are too different.) Perhaps the only statement that now can be definitively made concerning the origin of retroviruses is that retroviruses and some cellular movable genetic elements are evolutionarily homologous, that is, the similarities between retroviruses and some cellular movable genetic elements represent an evolutionary relationship.

What kinds of experiments can we do to help determine evolutionary relationships? In classical evolutionary studies, fossils are used to determine common ancestors, and evolutionary relationships are inferred from the pattern of ancestors, assuming only vertical transfer of genetic characters. Obviously this modality dependent upon fossils cannot be applied to retroviruses or to any other viruses. Recently, molecular evolutionists have developed methods using nucleotide sequence data to create evolutionary trees based entirely on the properties of molecules present in living organisms (4). Such evolutionary trees depend upon extensive nuleotide sequence data and assume only classical (vertical) transfer of genetic information.

One major concern with interpretation of sequence data, as well as morphological data, is the need to separate convergent and divergent evolution. In other words, when there is similarity between two sequences does this similarity indicate descent from a common ancestor. In this case there is homology and divergent evolution. Alternatively, does the similarity represent only functional similarity without indicating descent from a common ancestor. In this case there is analogy and convergent evolution. In morphological evolution, finding fossils linking two groups allows separation of these processes. In molecular evolution, use of more classical evolutionary data allows separation of the two alternatives, although infrequently horizontal transfer of certain genetic information has been proposed.

What kind of data do retrovirologists have to approach the question of origins? One is knowledge of the different kinds of retroviruses and their sequence organization; two is knowledge of the genetic processes used by retroviruses; and three is knowledge of the selective factors involved in retrovirus replication.

HISTORY OF RETROVIROLOGY

Apparently, the first retrovirus, equine infectious anemia virus was discovered by two French scientists, Valee and Carre, in 1904 (5). This report was followed in 1908 by the demonstration of viral transmission of chicken leukemia by Ellerman and Bang (6) and of chicken sarcoma by Rous (7). The first mammalian retrovirus, mouse mammary tumor virus, was described in the middle 1930s, while murine leukemia virus was not described until 1951 (8). Now probably hundreds of different retroviruses have been described, although still only a fraction of these have been sequenced and their genes well characterized.

Even more recently, cellular movable genetic elements with sequence, organizational, and functional homologies to retroviruses have been discovered (see reviews in 9,10). These and other sequences generated by reverse transcription make up perhaps as much as 20% of the avian and mammalian genomes. In addition, it has been shown that both hepadnavirus (hepatitis B virus and its relatives) and cauliflower mosaic virus replication involves reverse transcription (11).

ORGANIZATION OF RETROVIRUS GENOMES

All retroviruses and the homologous retrotransposons have a relatively similar genetic organization. In the DNA form of the genome, directly repeated sequences with signals for RNA transcription and 3' RNA processing surround protein coding sequences (Figure 1). However, within this overall organization there are significant differences in the number and arrangement of the coding sequences (12,13).

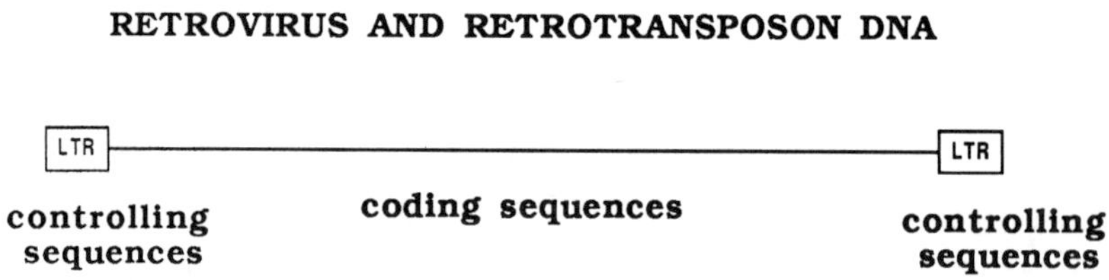

FIGURE 1. Structure of retrovirus and retrotransposon DNAs. LTR is long terminal repeat. The LTR contains sequences controlling RNA transcription, 3' RNA end processing, and integration.

Perhaps the genome of the C-type oncoretrovirus is the best studied. In particular, there are three major coding sequences, gag, pol, and env, with no intergene sequences between them; only a small distance between env and the 3' LTR; and clustering of most cis-acting sequences at the ends of the genome (Figure 2). C-type oncoretroviruses differ from one another in what tRNA is used as a primer for minus strand DNA synthesis, in whether the protease is coded in the gag or pol gene or both, in the mechanism of synthesis of the gag-pol precursor, and in the specific nucleotide sequences of the viruses.

ONCORETROVIRUS DNA

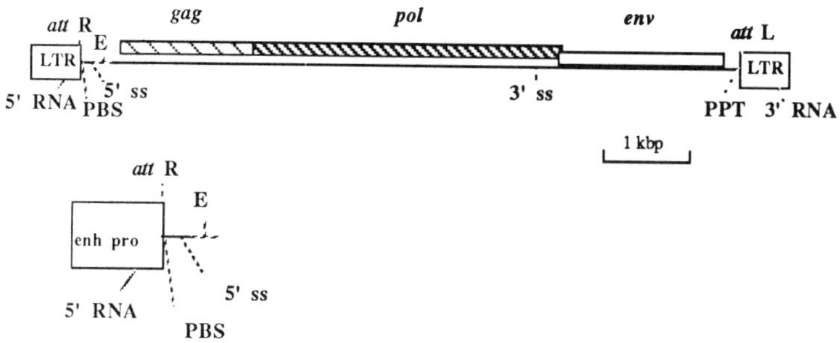

FIGURE 2. Structure of oncoretrovirus DNA. gag, pol, and env are genes for virion proteins, and LTR is long terminal repeat. The LTRs contain controlling sequences for RNA synthesis. 5' RNA is the position of the 5' end of viral RNA, and 3' RNA is the position of the 3' end of viral RNA. attR and attL form the attachment site for viral DNA integration. E is the encapsidation (packaging) sequence for viral RNA. PBS and PPT, primer binding site and polypurine track, respectively, are locations of the primers for minus and plus strand viral DNA synthesis, respectively. 5' and 3' ss are the 5' and 3' splice sites for formation of viral env mRNA. With the exception of 3' ss, all of the viral cis-acting control sequences are at the ends of the genome. Avian leukosis and mammalian leukemia viruses differ in whether the viral protease is encoded in the gag (avian) or pol (mammalian) gene and whether the pol gene is expressed as the result of a frame shift or by suppression. An enlargement of the 5' portion of the genome is shown below the whole genome.

D-type oncoretroviruses differ in organization from C-type viruses only in having a separate gene for the viral protease (Figure 3)(13). This difference involves only a few base pair differences from a C-type oncoretrovirus. That is, only a few mutations introducing start and stop codons and frame shifts could change a C-type viral genome to a D-type viral genome. B-type oncoretroviruses (MMTV) differ from D-type viruses only in having the env gene overlap the 3' LTR and in having a large U3 region of the LTRs containing another open reading frame (Figure 3)(14).

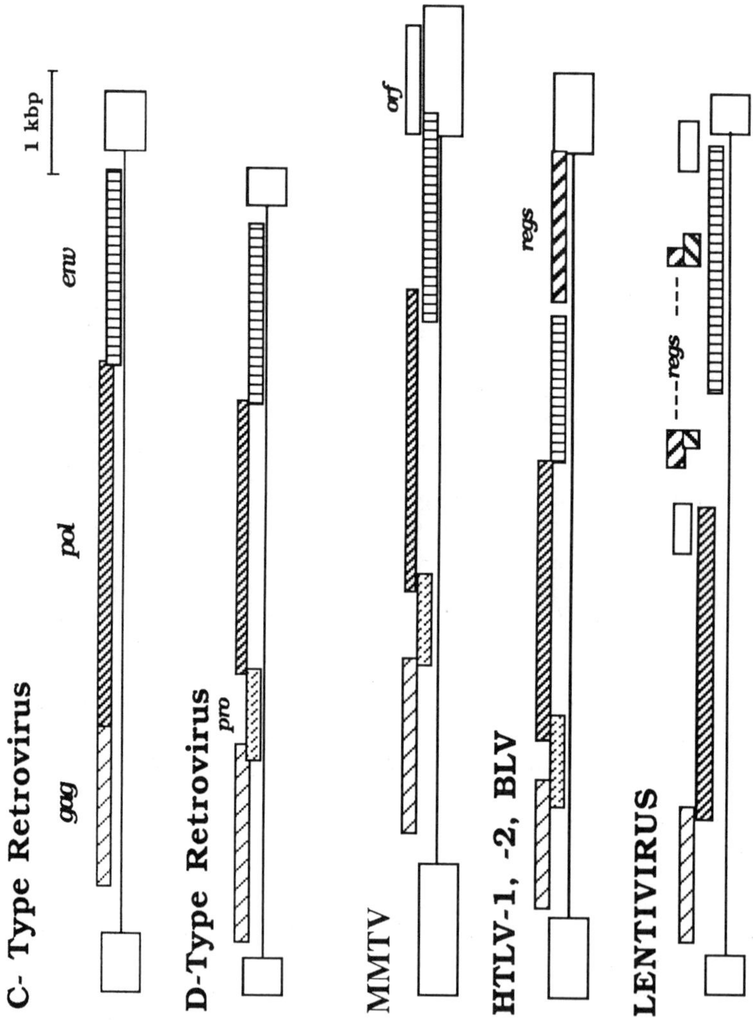

FIGURE 3. Structure of retrovirus DNAs and their coding sequences. Open box is LTR; line is internal viral sequences; filled boxes are open reading frames

(continued)

with different shadings representing different genes; gag, pol, and env are genes for major viral proteins; pro is viral protease; orf is open reading frame of unknown function; regs are genes for regulatory proteins with many different names; MMTV is mouse mammary tumor virus, a B-type oncoretrovirus; HTLV-1 and -2 are human T-cell lymphotropic viruses; BLV is bovine leukemia virus; lentiviruses include HIV and Visna virus.

HTLV-1, HTLV-2, and bovine leukemia virus (BLV) have a more complex genome containing, in addition to gag, pro, pol, and env, genes coding for regulatory proteins between env and the 3' LTR, regs (Figure 3)(15). Lentiviruses like HIV and Visna virus have a still more complex genome with genes coding for nonstructural, presumably regulatory, proteins between pol and env, overlapping with env, and perhaps 3' to env overlapping the 3' LTR (Figure 3)(16-18).

Hepadnavirus and cauliflower mosaic virus genomes have some additional genes involved in other aspects of their viral life cycles (19,11).

RETROVIRUS REPLICATION

The life cycle of oncoretroviruses is fairly well described, although new facets continue to be discovered (Figure 4) (20). Virions attach to specific cell-surface receptors and enter cells by receptor-mediated endocytosis. The viral genome is released into the cytoplasm, presumably by low pH-mediated fusion with intracellular membranes. Reverse transcription takes place in the cytoplasm to form unintegrated viral DNA. The linear unintegrated viral DNA is transported to the nucleus where it is ligated to form a circle with two juxtaposed LTRs. The viral DNA is integrated into cellular DNA with loss of 4 bp at the junction of the two LTRs and duplication of 4 to 6 bp of cellular DNA at the site of integration (depending on the virus species) to form the provirus. Viral RNA is transcribed, processed, transported, and translated by cellular machinery to form progeny viral RNA genomes and proteins. Full length viral RNA is encapsidated by viral proteins either in the cisternae or at the plasma membrane, and progeny virus is formed by budding from the cell at modified portions of the plasma membrane. Virion maturation is completed by proteolytic processing in the released virions.

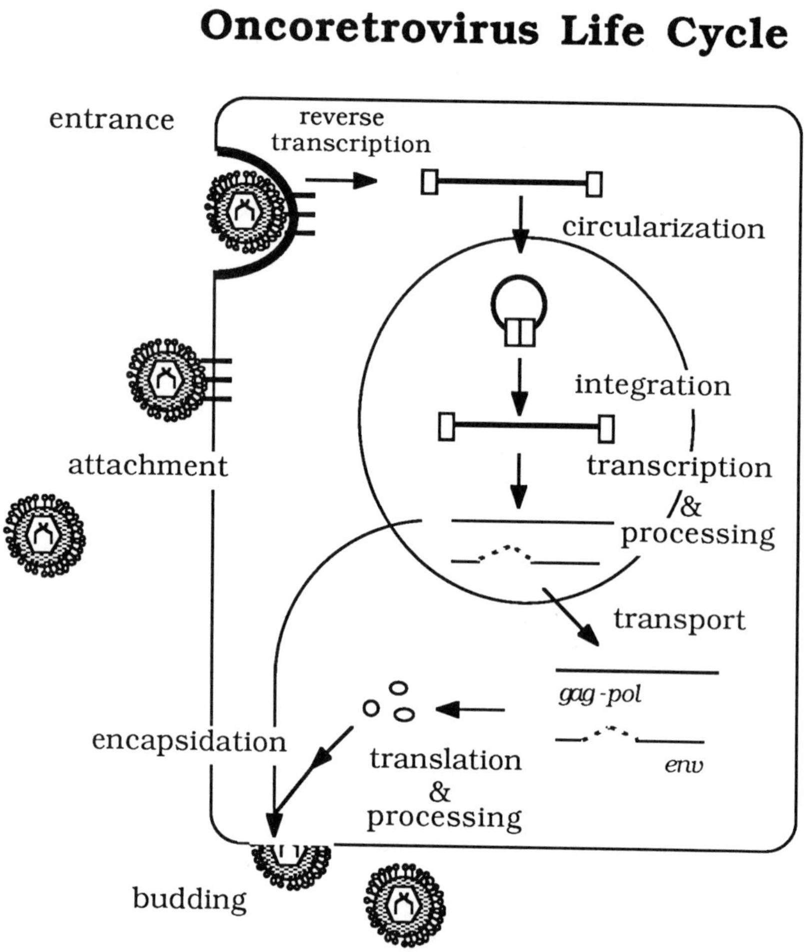

FIGURE 4. Life cycle of oncoretrovirus. Infection and virus production from one cell are shown. Open box is LTR; lines are internal viral sequences. DNA is represented with a heavier line; RNA, with a lighter line. Dashed line is cellular DNA. The peaked dashed line represents intervening sequence. Circles are proteins.

Replication of B- and D-type oncoretroviruses is probably very similar to replication of C-type oncoretroviruses.

Replication of HTLV-1-type viruses is more complicated than that of C-type viruses as a result of the action of the viral regulatory proteins (Figure 5)(2). After provirus formation, a low basal level of viral proteins are made. A high level of transcription of viral RNA requires the presence of the viral regulatory protein(s). A latent state consisting of a provirus with no viral RNA or protein can perhaps be maintained in the absence of the viral regulatory protein(s).

Replication of lentiviruses is even more complex with apparent controls at the levels of transcription, RNA processing, and translation (see reference 2). Thus, the lentiviruses could have latent states controlled at many different levels. (It is possible or even likely that future work will uncover similar types of controls in oncoretrovirus replication.)

OTHER RETROTRANSCRIPTS

All other retrotranscripts (DNA sequences resulting from reverse transcription) exist primarily as DNA sequences and not as RNA-containing particles (Figure 6). Endogenous retroviruses have sequences very similar to oncoretroviruses but are only maintained in the cellular genome (21). A few endogenous retroviruses are infectious and can produce virions. Thus, these endogenous retroviruses are latent replication-competent retroviruses. However, the great majority of endogenous retroviruses are pseudo-oncoretroviruses. That is, like pseudogenes they have mutations that render the endogenous retroviruses noninfectious. These mutations include both base pair changes and large deletions. Because of their close sequence homology with known infectious retroviruses, these non-infectious endogenous retroviruses are considered defective retroviruses. For example, most chickens have endogenous defective avian leukosis virus genomes; mice have endogenous defective murine leukemia and mammary tumor virus genomes; cats have endogenous defective feline leukemia virus genomes; etc.

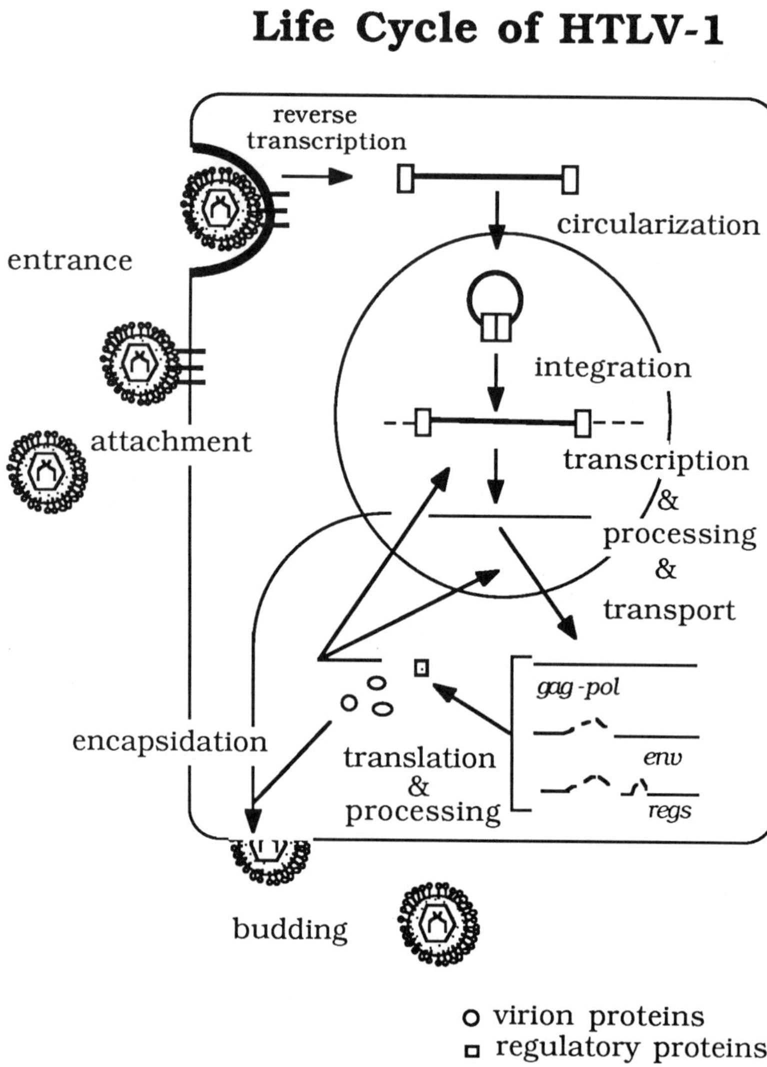

FIGURE 5. Life cycle of HTLV-1 and HTLV-2. Infection and virus production from one cell are shown. Symbols are as described in the legend to Figure 4. regs represents regulatory proteins (squares).

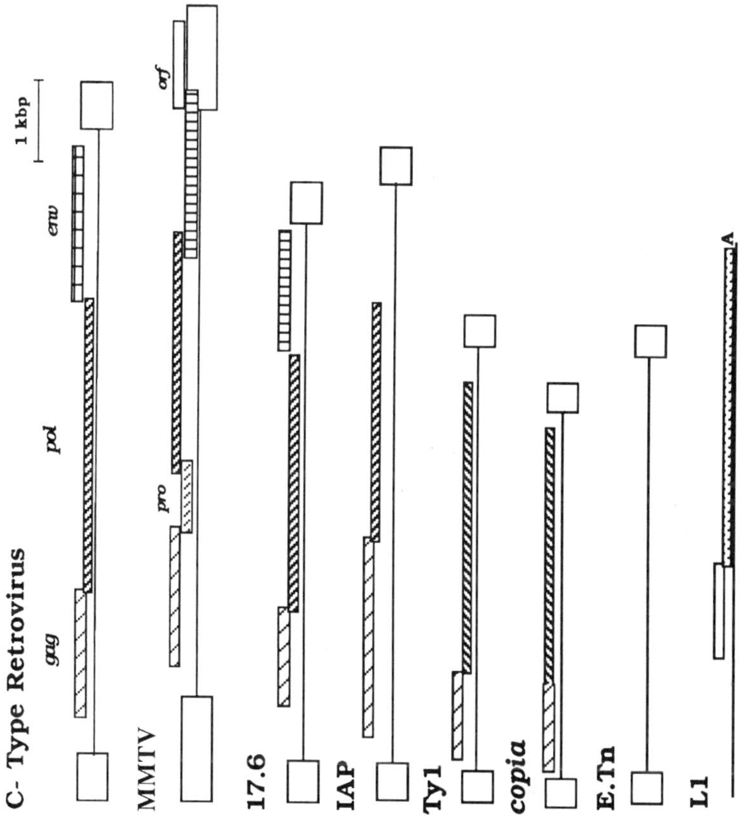

FIGURE 6. Structure of retrotransposon and other retrotranscript DNAs. Endogenous DNA sequences are shown. Symbols are as described in the legend of Figure 3. C-type oncoretrovirus and MMTV DNAs are like those shown in Figure 3 with the exception that the C-type retrovirus expresses its <u>pol</u> gene as a result of a frame shift and the <u>env</u> gene has a different strain-specific sequence. IAP is intracisternal A-particle sequence (22); 17.6 is a <u>Drosophila</u> cellular movable genetic element (23); Tyl

(continued)

Fig. 6 (continued)
is a yeast cellular movable genetic element (24); *copia* is another *Drosophila* cellular movable genetic element (25); E.Tn is a mouse cellular movable genetic element with LTRs, but no internal coding sequences (26); L1 is a mouse long interspersed repeat element (28). The A in L1 stands for a 3' A-rich sequence. All genomes are surrounded by a small direct repeat of cellular DNA with the exception of some L1 elements.

17.6, a *Drosophila* cellular movable genetic element, has a genome like that of an endogenous retrovirus, and circular DNA of 17.6 has been found (Figure 6)(23). However, no exogenous retroviruses are known in *Drosophila*.

Another group of retrotranscripts also shares the sequence organization of retroviruses, but they do not have any very closely related infectious retrovirus relatives nor do they have a complete retrovirus genome. All but L1 have TG/AC...CA/GT dinucleotide termini. These retrotranscripts are called retrovirus-like sequences. For example, the genome of an intracisternal A-particle (IAP) has *gag* and *pol* sequences, but no *env* coding sequences. There is, however, a nonsense stretch of nucleotides between *pol* and the 3' LTR which might represent the remnants of a completely mutated *env* gene or the insertion of non-coding DNA (Figure 6)(22). IAP genomes code for proteins which form intracellular particles containing IAP RNA. Some of these particles are probably able to mediate accurate reverse transcription and integration because IAP genes have been found in historical time to integrate into new positions in the cellular genome. Other retrovirus-like sequences also must have integrated into new positions in the cellular genome during evolutionary times since they are amplified and dispersed in the cellular genome. Some of these other retrovirus-like sequences may use retrovirus proteins in their dispersion, for example, VL30 RNA is found encapsidated in murine leukemia virus proteins (21). VL30 sequences form another family of cellular movable genetic elements. VL30 DNA has retrovirus-like LTRs and PBS. Recent sequencing reveals a VL30 endonuclease domain abuts the 3' LTR (29). Thus, VL30 DNA is simpler than IAP DNA.

A similar group of retrotranscripts includes other cellular movable genetic elements of *Drosophila* and yeast, that is, *copia* and Ty elements. These elements share much of the sequence organization of oncoretroviruses, with the major exception that they, like VL30 DNA, lack any _env_ gene, even a remnant (Figure 6) (24,25). Thus, it is not surprising that these elements lack exogenous particles and an infectious cycle. These retrotranscripts, like IAP, form intracellular particles and can transpose their genomes in cells by reverse transcription. Interestingly, in the coding portion of these sequences with similarity to the retrovirus _pol_ gene, the relative locations of the reverse transcriptase and endonuclease domains of the _pol_ gene are switched. In retroviruses, IAP, and VL30, the order is reverse transcriptase-endonuclease, while in Tyl and _copia_ it is endonuclease-reverse transcriptase. Tyl and _copia_ differ from each other in the mechanism of expression of the _pol_ domains. In Tyl a frame shift is required to express these sequences; in _copia_ there is no stop codon at the end of the _gag_-like sequence, so a gag-pol fusion polyprotein apparently is the primary translation product. (In retroviruses there is either a stop codon or a frame shift between the _gag_ and _pol_ sequences.) Elements like 17.6 are more similar to retroviruses than _copia_ in that 17.6 has a third large open reading frame, a putative _env_-like gene, and the reverse transcriptase domain of its _pol_ gene is 5' to an endonuclease-like domain.

Another LTR-containing group of cellular movable genetic elements is the E.Tn sequences of mice (Figure 6) (26,27). Although the LTR, PBS, and PPT sequences of E.Tn elements resemble those of retroviruses, there are no open reading frames in the E.Tn internal nucleotides. Thus, these elements may have only _cis_-acting sequences acted upon by retrovirus and retrotransposon proteins.

A complementary major group of cellular movable genetic elements in mammals has been variously called the BamHl, Kpnl, LINES 1, or Ll family (28). A similar group of sequences in _Drosophila_ is called the I factors and is responsible for some hybrid dysgenesis (30). These sequences do not have LTRs (Figure 6). However, they do have some sequence homology to retrovirus _pol_ genes; they also have an A-rich region at their 3' ends; and they are usually surrounded by a small direct repeat. These characteristics indicate transposition through an RNA intermediate. There are also smaller dispersed repeated sequences that appear to be 5' truncated copies of the Ll elements. The large copy number of these Ll and I elements and the existence of open reading frames in their sequences suggest that among them are functional elements which can transpose. Such functional elements might code for proteins involved in reverse transcription, for example, RNA binding proteins, reverse transcriptase, and integrase. The elements also might have some _cis_-acting sequences for these proteins to act upon during encapsidation, reverse transcription, and integration. Action of these sequences would result in new dispersed DNA copies of these elements. These elements could be thought of either as primitive or degenerate retroviruses. One might also propose that retroviruses resulted from recombination between L1 and E.Tn elements.

Finally, there are many sequences that show signs of being products of reverse transcription but which do not have any coding sequences for reverse transcription and integration functions. These retrosequences include cDNA or processed pseudogenes and Alu sequences. It is not known how these sequences were formed. They could contain sequences analogous to retrotransposon or retrovirus _cis_-acting sequences. Alternatively or additionally, retrotransposon and retrovirus proteins could act with low probability on any RNA sequences to form cDNA copies and then to integrate those DNA copies in the cellular genome. However, the absence of retrovirus-like coding sequences in these cDNA retrosequences indicates that the cDNA sequences are not genetically related to retrotranscripts. However, they are probably related in the sense that the proteins encoded by retrotranscripts were necessary for the formation of these other retrosequences.

RETROVIRUS VARIATIONAL PROCESSES

We now consider the types of genetic processes that modify retroviruses to understand the types of processes that were involved in the evolution of retrotranscripts.

Mutation

Retroviruses undergo mutation as shown by comparison between sequences of viruses of one species or strain and by direct study of mutations. The different types of mutations found include small and large deletions, duplications, base pair changes, insertions, inversions, and translocations. Although it is commonly asserted that retroviruses mutate unusually rapidly, there has been relatively little direct measurement of the rates of any retrovirus mutations. The closest approach to a quantitative measurement of retrovirus mutation was made by Coffin et al. (31) who measured the frequency of base changes in viral RNA during successive passages of a retrovirus. O'Rear and Temin (32) and Shimotohno and Temin (33) sequenced some cloned retrovirus DNAs from a cloned virus stock (unspecified number of passages) and found a high frequency of variants. Darlix and Spahr (34) sequenced Rous sarcoma virus RNA fragments from a cloned virus stock (unspecified number of passages) and also found a very high frequency of variants.

Recent studies have looked carefully at mutation frequencies in vesicular stomatitis virus, poliovirus, and influenza virus. For vesicular stomatitis virus, Steinhauer and Holland (35) measured the substitution frequency of a specific 5' nucleotide in the viral genome and found a mutation frequency of $2x10^{-4}$. They argue that since the nucleotide studied represents a conserved nucleotide in different virus strains, substitutions at this nucleotide must be lethal. If this assumption is true and the lethality is at the level of RNA replication, then the frequency of $2x10^{-4}$ mutations/site is also the mutation rate. However, there was no direct test of these assumptions. Parvin et al. (36) directly sequenced portions of progeny of an influenza virus clone after growth in a single plaque from one to 10^6 pfu. They found a frequency of $7.5x10^{-5}$ substitutions per nucleotide. They did the same experiment with poliovirus after growth from one to $5x10^6$ pfu and found a frequency of altered nucleotides of less than $1x10^{-5}$ per nucleotide. Since there must have been several infectious cycles (they estimate five) and there must have been several (unknown) rounds of nucleic acid synthesis per infectious cycle, they argue that the mutation rates must have been even lower than these frequencies. At face value these data indicate large differences in the mutation rates per replication cycle among these RNA viruses. In any case, these rates appear to be lower than the rate of 10^{-3} to 10^{-4} substitutions/site/replication for uncorrected polymerase synthesis (37,38; but see 39).

We recently described a protocol for measuring mutation rates in a single cycle of retrovirus replication.

We have so far applied this protocol to reversion of a splicing mutation and to reversion of an amber mutation (Figure 7)(40,41). A single cycle of retrovirus replication requires both a step of RNA transcription and a step of reverse transcription. The rate of reversion of the splicing mutant was $5x10^{-3}$/genome/replication and of the amber mutant was $5x10^{-4}$/base pair/replication (40,41). Reversion of the splicing mutant apparently occurred by formation of large deletions or by small deletions or insertions. Approximately equal frequencies of each type of reversion apparently occurred. In a related study, two reversions without large deletions were sequenced. One had a deletion of one copy of a 9 bp tandem repeat; the other had a 330 bp insertion (42).

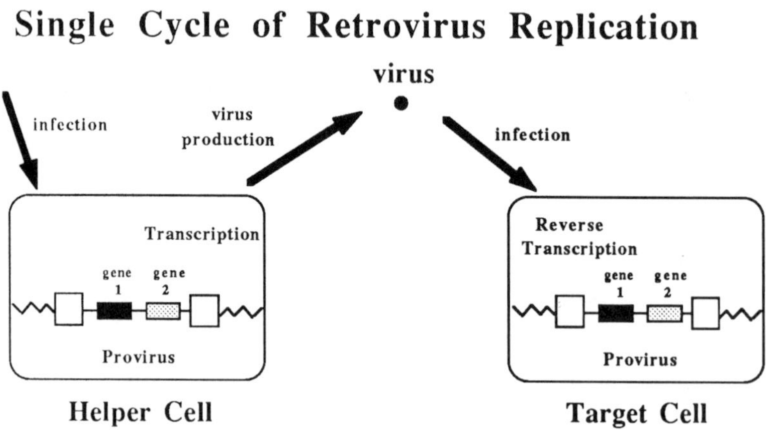

FIGURE 7. Protocol for measurement of mutation rate in a single cycle of retrovirus replication. A helper cell is infected with parental helper virus-free vector containing two genes whose functions can be separately assayed. Helper-free virus produced by this helper cell is used to infect a target cell where the functions of the two genes are measured. Since no helper virus is present and the vector is replication-defective, only a single cycle of viral replication can occur.

The rate of reversion of the retrovirus amber mutation per virus replication cycle is lower than those reported for substitutions in vesicular stomatitis virus and influenza virus and higher than that reported for poliovirus. Biologically it may be the whole virus life cycle rather than one polymerization cycle that is significant for the evolution of a virus. In any case, this result may indicate that the retrovirus reverse transcription and RNA transcription processes include error-correcting mechanisms, since they may be lower than uncorrected polymerase rates. In addition, these results indicate that retrovirus replication does not vary more than the replication of other single stranded RNA viruses and that relative to them retrovirus replication is not unusually error-prone. The high frequency of variation observed in different retrovirus isolates, for example, HIV, thus reflects strong selection of variants or many cycles of viral replication or both.

Recombination

Another common mode of retrovirus variation is recombination. In mixed infections, 50% of the progeny virus can be recombinant (43). A rate of recombination per virus replication cannot yet be derived from these experiments. However, since probably only a few cycles of virus replication occurred in these experiments, the rate of recombination per virus replication is probably very high. The mechanism of recombination is not yet known. It may involve copy-choice in reverse transcription, DNA displacement-assimilation, or abnormal splicing (44). Recombination itself does not appear to be mutagenic. However, recombination may be important in creating new viruses with novel properties as a result of insertions and deletions. HIV may be an example of this process. The evolution of MCF viruses from endogenous ecotropic and xenotropic viruses in AKR mice is a good example of this process (45).

Recombination can make simple evolutionary trees impossible. For example, recombination may be an explanation for the fact that although RSV is similar to murine leukemia retroviruses on the basis of overall organization, it is usually classified apart from MLVs on the basis of DNA sequence analysis. It is important to remember both that unrelated viruses can be packaged in the same virion proteins and that encapsidation sequence minus RNAs can be packaged in virion proteins (see 46,47).

As just mentioned, insertion and deletion of sequences in retrovirus genomes may be a result of recombination, for example, in the evolution of highly oncogenic retroviruses (Figure 8) (1). In addition, insertions, deletions, and translocations may be the results of reverse transcription errors and abnormal splicing.

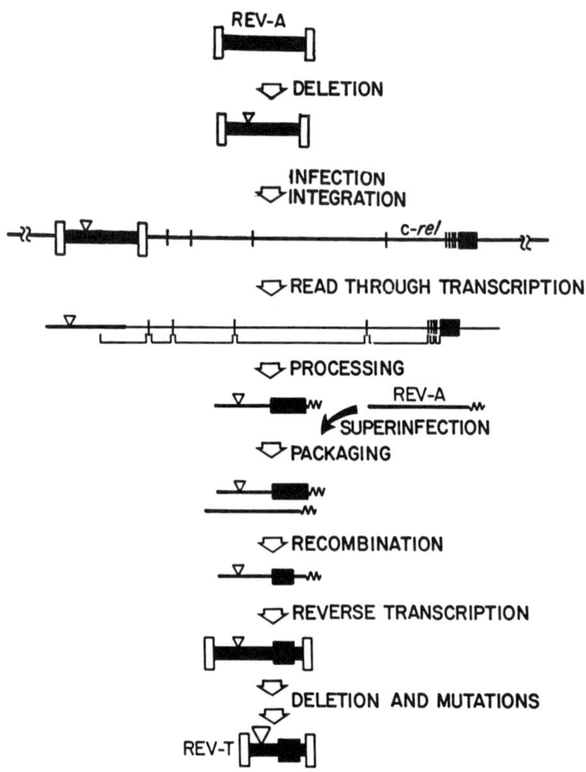

FIGURE 8. Possible pathway of evolution of a highly oncogenic retrovirus. See description in (51).

Gene conversion also appears to occur at a high rate in retrovirus replication. We have found what appears to be a high frequency of gene conversion using the following protocol (Figure 9) (41). Gene conversion may not be important for purely exogenous retroviruses, but it would be important when there are any homologous sequences in cells and infecting retroviruses and in cells with more than one provirus.

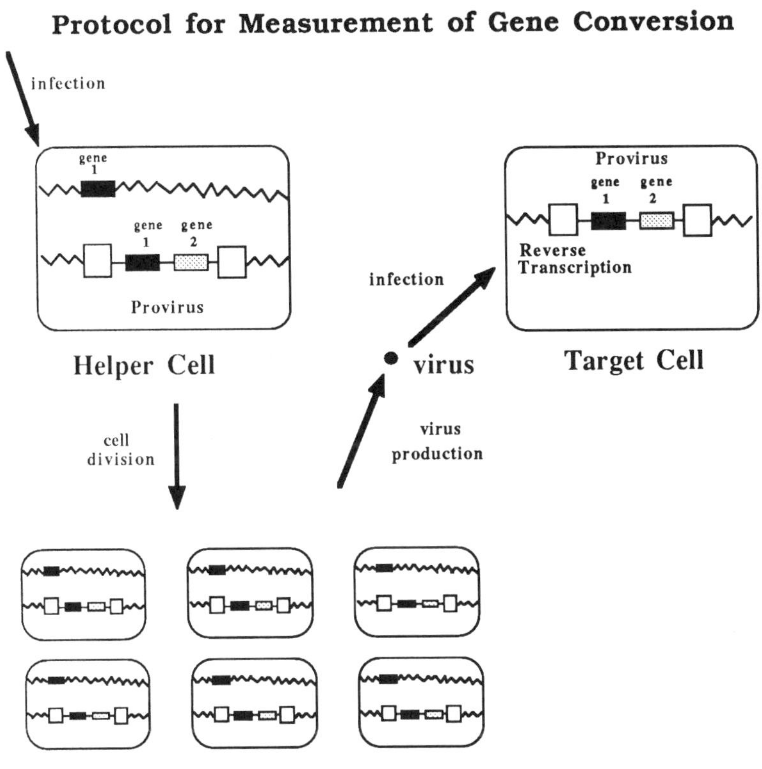

FIGURE 9. Protocol for measurement of gene conversion rate. The same general protocol is used as described in the legend of Figure 7 with the exception that the helper cell has an endogenous copy of a mutant gene in the retrovirus vector. Gene conversion probably occurs during growth of the infected helper cell.

EVOLUTION OF RETROVIRUSES

In the evolution of retroviruses the genetic processes discussed above supplied the variants for evolution. However, in contrast to most other evolution, retrovirus evolution involved horizontal as well as vertical information transfer. That is, progeny retroviruses differed from the parental retrovirus(es) not only by mutation, but also by incorporation of genetic information from wholly separate lineages (different retrovirus species or subfamilies or even cells). Thus, retrovirus evolution almost certainly did not involve only a single linear lineage, but rather involved several different lineages connected by recombination.

What Factors Acted to Select For or Against These Variants in Retrovirus Evolution?

The major factor resulting in increased numbers of retrotranscripts probably was selection for increased autonomy of replication both intracellular and intercellular. Cellular sequences usually replicate only at the same time and to the same extent as do other cellular sequences, and they are vertically transmitted as single or a small number of copies. However, the number of cellular movable genetic elements can increase in one cell or germ-line lineage relative to other sequences. (In contrast to gene amplification, for example, the increase in dihydrofolate reductase sequences in several conditions (49), the increase of retrovirus-like sequences is inherited and more stable.) Increased RNA transcription, reverse transcription, and integration would have been selected for since these processes together form additional proviruses. However, in contrast to cellular movable genetic elements which are limited to a single cell or organism lineage, retroviruses can spread by horizontal and/or vertical transmission. Thus, there was selection for extracellular forms of these elements which involved development of the ability to bud efficiently from one cell, attach to another cell, and enter into the second cell. There also would have been selection for the ability to spread in an organism, to avoid host defenses, and to spread to other organisms. Disease would also have been selected for if it resulted in more progeny virus by making any of these steps of replication and spread more efficient.

Now we shall consider retrovirus-induced cancer and cell killing by retroviruses in terms of these selective factors. We shall ask if a.) cancer and cell killing are processes that would result in greater virus replication and so would have been selected directly or if b.) they are phenomena that are unavoidable byproducts of retrovirus replication, that is, they are properties that exist because of linkage with another selected property.

Retroviruses and Cancer

There are five fairly well established mechanisms of cancer induction by retroviruses: 1.) addition of an oncogene; 2.) insertional activation of a proto-oncogene; 3.) cellular hyperplasia caused by a mutant env protein; 4.) cellular hyperplasia caused by transactivation of cellular genes; and 5.) suppression of immunosurveillance (50,51). Mechanisms 2.) to 5.) are only partial mechanisms of cancer induction and require other carcinogenic steps. Mechanism 4.) is still hypothetical (but see 52).

Now we shall consider retrovirus evolution in light of these mechanisms of cancer induction by retroviruses. Highly oncogenic retroviruses (mechanism 1.) are not transmitted naturally from animal to animal but are an evolutionary dead end except for passage by scientists. Thus, there is strong negative selection against highly oncogenic retroviruses. The low efficiency and long latent period for cancer induction by weakly oncogenic retroviruses (mechanism 2.) indicate that these replication-competent retroviruses are not selected either positively or negatively for their ability to cause cancer, again except for scientists. The insertional activation of proto-oncogenes by weakly oncogenic retroviruses (mechanism 2.) results from the existence of essentially random integration of retroviruses and the presence of promoters and enhancers in the retrovirus LTRs. Hyperplasia of infected cells (mechanisms 3. and 4.) increases the number of retrovirus infected cells and therefore of retrovirus genomes, proviruses. Hyperplasia is probably just as effective as infection of fresh uninfected cells in increasing numbers of progeny viruses and certainly is less likely to be abrogated by host defenses. Therefore, there would be strong positive selection for viral processes that result in hyperplasia of infected cells. If these processes also resulted in more virus replication in any one infected cell, they also would be selected on that basis. Suppression of immunosurveillance (mechanism 5.) would also be strongly positively selected since it would allow viruses to replicate for a longer time and to higher titers resulting in more progeny viruses.

Thus, most retrovirus cancer is not positively selected. Only retrovirus-induced hyperplasia and suppression of immunosurveillance would be positively selected.

Retroviruses and Cell Killing

Now we shall look at retrovirus-induced cell killing and ask whether there would have been selection for this property or if it is selected with some other property. Unfortunately, there are no clearly established mechanisms for retrovirus cell killing. However, several hypotheses have been proposed to explain retrovirus cell killing: 1.) expression of env proteins resulting in cell fusion; 2.) expression of other viral gene products resulting in cell death (direct or indirect effects); and 3.) superinfection resulting in abnormal endocytosis leading to cell death (53).

To evaluate the selective effect of each of these mechanisms, it would be useful to know what are the limiting steps in retrovirus production. Unfortunately, it is not really known what the limiting steps are in retrovirus production. In one case (47), the amount of viral proteins appears to be limiting for virus production. If it is generally true that the amounts of viral proteins are limiting for retrovirus production, increased expression of env and other viral proteins would tend to be selected positively when increased virus production is selected. However, if viral proteins kill cells, resulting in a shorter period of virus production, there would be both strong negative selection against virus production and strong positive selection for mechanisms to limit production of the toxic proteins or to render the viral proteins non-toxic. Thus, mechanisms 1.) and 2.) would not select for increased virus production.

Mechanism 3.) depends upon which receptor is used for superinfection and is based upon the observations that cytopathic and non-cytopathic viruses use different receptors. For example, cytopathic and non-cytopathic avian leukosis viruses have different envelope subgroups, as do cytopathic and non-cytopathic feline leukemia viruses. However, again, if the cell killing resulted in a shortened time of virus production, there would be selection against a high level of superinfection. This aim might be accomplished by earlier establishment of superinfection interference. Thus, cell killing by abnormal endocytosis could be controlled by this mechanism while still allowing positive selection for virus growth.

Evolution of Human Retroviruses

Now we shall apply these criteria to evolution of human retroviruses. What can we say about their evolution? We see a gradient in retrovirus and retrotransposon structures from only _cis_-acting sequences and only _trans_-acting sequences to _gag_ and _pol_, to _gag_, _pol_, and _env_, to _gag_, _pol_, _env_, and _regs_. Finally, there are the hepadna and cauliflower mosaic viruses with still more genes. This gradient suggests that the direction of evolution of these retrotranscripts was from simpler to more complex rather than the reverse. Thus, the HTLV-1-subfamily and lentiviruses would have evolved from simpler retroviruses by incorporation of other genes or by duplication and mutation. In these subfamilies, further evolution would have involved the variational processes I have described.

I shall defer further comment at this time, because undoubtedly the data to be presented at this meeting about the properties of human retroviruses and their simian relatives will fill in more of the information needed in reconstructing this evolution. I cannot guess what the new data will be. However, the factors I have discussed will remain central to any consideration of the evolution of retroviruses and their diseases.

In conclusion, retrovirus evolution involved many different kinds of genetic variation which occur at high rates and can involve multiple lineages of descent.

ACKNOWLEDGEMENTS

I thank Janet Embretson, Cindy Miller, Tom Gilmore, Celine Gelinas, Ralph Dornburg, and Joe Dougherty for useful comments on this manuscript. I am an American Cancer Scoiety Research Professor.

REFERENCES

1. Feierman S (1986). Personal communication.
2. Chen ISY (1986). Regulation of AIDS virus expression. Cell 47:1.
3. Temin HM (1970). Malignant transformation of cells by viruses. Perspect Biol Med 14:11.
4. Temin HM (1980). Origin of retroviruses from cellular moveable genetic elements. Cell 21:599.
5. Buonagurio DA, Nakada S, Parvin JD, Krystal M, Palese P, Fitch WM (1986). Evolution of human influenza A viruses over 50 years: rapid, uniform rate of change in NS gene. Science 232:980.
6. Vallee, Carre (1904). Sur la nature infectieuse de l' anemie du cheval. Comptes rendus hebdomadaires des seances academie des sciences 139:331.
7. Ellermann V, Bang O (1908). Experimentelle leukamie bei huhnern. Centralblatt fur Bakteriologie, Parasitenkunde und Infektionskrankheiten, Abt 1, (orig) 46:595.
8. Rous P (1911). A sarcoma of the fowl transmissible by an agent separable from the tumor cells. J Exp Med 13:397.
9. Gross L (1951). Spontaneous leukemia developing in C3H mice following inoculation, in infancy, with AK-leukemic extracts, or AK-embryos. Proc Soc Exp Biol Med 76:27.
10. Temin HM (1985). Reverse transcription in the eukaryotic genome: Retroviruses, pararetroviruses, retrotransposons, and retrotranscripts. Mol Biol Evol 2:455.
11. Rogers JH (1985). The origin and evolution of retroposons. Int Rev Cytol 93:187.
12. Mason W, Taylor J, Covey (1987). Retroid elements. Adv Virus Res, in press.
13. Coffin J (1982). Structure of the retroviral genome. In Weiss R, Teich N, Varmus H, Coffin J (eds): "RNA Tumor Viruses, Molecular Biology of Tumor Viruses, 2nd ed," New York: Cold Spring Harbor, pp. 261.
14. Coffin J (1985). Genome structure. In Weiss R, Teich N, Varmus H, Coffin J (eds): "RNA Tumor Viruses, Molecular Biology of Tumor Viruses, 2nd ed, 2/Supplements and Appendixes," New York: Cold Spring Harbor, pp. 17.
15. Sonigo P, Barker C, Hunter E, Wain-Hobson S (1986). Nucleotide sequence of Mason-Pfizer monkey virus: An immunosuppressive D-type retrovirus. Cell 45:375.

16. Moore R, Dixon M, Smith R, Peters G, Dickson C, (1987). Complete nucleotide sequence of a milk-transmitted mouse mammary tumor virus: Two frame-shift suppression events are required for translation of gag and pol. J Virol 61:480.
17. Seiki M, Hattori S, Hirayama Y, Yoshida M, (1983). Human adult T-cell leukemia virus: Complete nucleotide sequence of the provirus genome integrated in leukemia cell DNA. Proc Natl Acad Sci USA 80:3618.
18. Ratner L, Haseltine W, Patarca R, Livak KJ, Starcich B, Josephs SF, Doran ER, Rafalski JA, Whitehorn EA, Baumeister K, Ivanoff L, Petteway SR Jr, Pearson ML, Lautenberger JA, Papas TS, Ghrayeb J, Chang NT, Gallo RC, Wong-Stall F (1985). Complete nucleotide sequence of AIDS virus, HTLV-III. Nature 313:277.
19. Sonigo P, Alizon M, Staskus K, Klatzmann D, Cole S, Danos O, Retzel E, Tiollais P, Haase A, Wain-Hobson S (1985). Nucleotide sequence of the Visna lentivirus: Relationship to the AIDS virus. Cell 42:396.
20. Wain-Hobson S, Sonigo P, Danos O, Cole S, Alizon M (1985). Nucleotide sequence of the AIDS virus, LAV. Cell 40:9.
21. Hull R, Covey SN (1986). Genome organization and expression of reverse transcribing elements: Variations and a theme. J Gen Virol 67:1751.
22. Varmus H, Swanstrom R (1985). Replication of retroviruses. In Weiss R, Teich N, Varmus H, Coffin J (eds): "RNA Tumor Viruses, Molecular Biology of Tumor Viruses, 2nd ed, 2/Supplements and Appendixes," New York: Cold Spring Harbor, pp. 75.
23. Stoye J, Coffin J (1985). Endogenous viruses. In Weiss R, Teich N, Varmus H, Coffin J (eds): "RNA Tumor Viruses Molecular Biology of Tumor Viruses 2nd ed, 2/Supplements and Appendixes," New York: Cold Spring Harbor, pp. 357.
24. Ono M, Toh H, Miyata T, Awaya T (1985). Nucleotide sequence of the Syrian hamster intracisternal A-particle gene: Close evolutionary relationship of type A particle gene to types B and D oncovirus genes. J Virol 55:387.
25. Saigo K, Kugimiya W, Matsuo Y, Inouye S, Yoshioka K, Yuki S (1984). Identification of the coding sequence for a reverse transcriptase-like enzyme in a transposable genetic element in *Drosophila melanogaster*. Nature 312:659.
26. Clare J, Farabaugh P (1985). Nucleotide sequence of a yeast Ty element: Evidence for an ususual mech-

anism of gene expression. Proc Natl Acad Sci USA 82:2829.

27. Mount SM, Rubin GM (1985). Complete nucleotide sequence of the Drosophila transposable element copia: Homology between copia and retroviral proteins. Mol Cell Biol 5:1630.
28. Sonigo P, Wain-Hobson S, Bougueleret L, Tollais P, Jacob F, Brulet P (1987). Nucleotide sequence and evolution of E.Tn elements. Proc Natl Acad Sci USA, in press.
29. Kaghad M, Maillet L, Brulet P (1985). Retroviral characteristics of the long terminal repeat of murine E.Tn sequences. EMBO J 4:2911.
30. Loeb DD, Padgett RW, Hardies SC, Shehee WR, Comer MB, Edgell MH, Hutchison CA III (1986). The sequence of a large L1Md element reveals a tandemly repeated 5' end and several features found in retrotransposons. Mol Cell Biol 6:168.
31. Keshet E (1987). Personal communication.
32. Fawcett DH, Lister CK, Kellett E, Finnegan, DJ (1986). Transposable elements controlling I-R hybrid dysgenesis in D. melanogaster are similar to mammalian LINEs. Cell 47:1007.
33. Coffin JM, Tsichlis PN, Barker CS, Voynow S, (1980). Variation in avian retrovirus genomes. Ann NY Acad Sci 354:410.
34. O'Rear JJ, Temin HM (1982). Spontaneous changes in nucleotide sequence in proviruses of spleen necrosis virus, an avian retrovirus. Proc Natl Acad Sci USA 79:1230.
35. Shimotohno K, Temin HM (1982). Spontaneous variation and synthesis in the U3 region of the long terminal repeat of an avian retrovirus. J Virol 41:163.
36. Darlix J-L, Spahr P-F (1983). High spontaneous mutation rate of Rous sarcoma virus demonstrated by direct sequencing of the RNA genome. Nucl Acids Res 11:5953.
37. Steinhauer DA, Holland JJ (1986). Direct method for quantitation of extreme polymerase error frequencies at selected single base sites in viral RNA. J Virol 57:219.
38. Parvin JD, Moscona A, Pan WT, Leider JM, Palese P (1986). Measurement of the mutation rates of animal viruses: Influenza A virus and poliovirus type 1. J Virol 59:377.
39. Reanney D (1984). Genetic noise in evolution? Nature 307:318.

40. Kunkel TA, Loeb LA (1981). Fidelity of mammalian DNA polymerases. Science 213:765.
41. Topal MD, Fresco JR (1976). Complementary base pairing and the origin of substitution mutations Nature 263:285.
42. Dougherty JP, Temin HM (1986). High mutation rate of a spleen encrosis virus-based retrovirus vector. Mol Cell Biol 6:4387.
43. Dougherty J, Temin HM (1987). In preparation.
44. Miller C, Temin HM (1987). In preparation.
45. Linial M, Blair D (1982). Genetics of retroviruses. In Weiss R, Teich N, Varmus H, Coffin J (eds): "RNA Tumor Viruses, Molecular Biology of Tumor Viruses, 2nd ed," New York: Cold Spring Harbor, pp. 649.
46. Skalka AM, Boone L, Junghans R, Luk D (1982). Genetic recombination in avian retroviruses. J Cell Biochem 19:293.
47. Thomas CY, Khiroya R, Schwartz RS, Coffin JM (1984). Role of recombinant ecotropic and polytropic viruses in the development of spontaneous thymic lymphomas in HRS/J mice. J Virol 50:397.
48. Embretson JE, Temin HM (1986). Pseudotyped retroviral vectors reveal restrictions to reticuloendotheliosis virus replication in rat cells. J Virol 60:662.
49. Embretson JE, Temin HM (1987). Packaging of encapsidation minus retroviral RNAs in the Rev helper cell. Submitted.
50. Bishop JM, Varmus H (1985). Functions and origins of retroviral transforming genes. In Weiss R, Teich N, Varmus H, Coffin J (eds): "RNA Tumor Viruses Molecular Biology of Tumor Viruses, 2nd ed, 2/Supplements and Appendixes," New York: Cold Spring Harbor, pp. 249.
51. Johnston RN, Feder J, Hill AB, Sherwood SW, Schimke RT (1986). Transient inhibition of DNA synthesis results in increased dihydrofolate reductase synthesis and subsequent increased DNA content per cell. Mol Cell Biol 6:3373.
52. Teich N, Wyke J, Kaplan P (1985). Pathogenesis of retrovirus-induced disease. In Weiss R, Teich N, Varmus H, Coffin J (eds): "RNA Tumor Viruses, Molecular Biology of Tumor Viruses, 2nd ed, 2/Supplements and Appendixes," New York: Cold Spring Harbor, pp. 187.
53. Temin HM (1987). Retroviruses and the genetic basis of cancer. Revue du Practicien, in press.

54. Maruyama M, Shibuya H, Harada H, Hatkeyama M, Seiki M, Fujita T, Inoue J-i, Yoshida M, Taniguchi T (1987). Evidence for aberrant activation of the interleukin-2 autocrine loop by HTLV-1-encoded p40x and T3/Ti complex triggering. Cell 48:343.
55. Temin HM (1987). Mechanisms of cell killing and cytopathic effects by retroviruses. Submitted.

I. NEW HUMAN RETROVIRUSES AND THEIR PROPERTIES

Human Retroviruses, Cancer, and AIDS:
Approaches to Prevention and Therapy, pages 31–42

SEQUENCE ANALYSIS OF THE HUMAN IMMUNE DEFICIENCY VIRUS TYPE 2

M. Guyader[1], M. Emerman[1], P. Sonigo[2], F. Clavel[1], L. Montagnier[1], and M. Alizon[1]

1 : Unité d'Oncologie Virale (CNRS EA 1157)
2 : UREG (INSERM U 163 and CNRS UA 271)
Institut Pasteur, 25 rue du Dr. Roux,
75724 Paris CEDEX 15, France

ABSTRACT : HIV-2, the human retrovirus associated with AIDS in West Africa, and HIV-1, previously shown to be the agent of AIDS in the USA and Central Africa, share many of their biological properties : they both are cytopathic _in vitro_, and have a tropism for the T4 cells. However, the molecular cloning and sequencing of the HIV-2 proviral DNA revealed major genetic differences with HIV-1 (the homology ranges from 60 % for the more conserved _gag_ and _pol_ genes to 30-40 % for other genes), indicating that these retroviruses have diverged long before the actual AIDS epidemics.

INTRODUCTION

The acquired immune deficiency syndrome (AIDS) is caused by a retrovirus designated "human immune deficiency virus" (HIV), but previously known as LAV, HTLV-3 or ARV (for review, see ref. 1). Isolates from the North America, Western Europe, and Central Africa have the same biological properties, and antigenically cross-reactive proteins with the same molecular weights. Therefore, the same virus was assumed to cause AIDS and related conditions in these different areas (1). If the central Africa appeared as highly afflicted by AIDS (2), the western part of the continent seemed to be relatively spared. Recently, however, several typical cases were found in a survey of patients from Guinea Bissau and other countries of West Africa, but unexpectedly, most of these patients had a negative HIV serology (3-5). They were nevertheless found to be infected by a retrovirus related to HIV by its ultrastructure and biological properties, such as cytopathogenicity and tropism for the T4 positive cells (3). Anti-HIV antibodies could immunoprecipitate the viral proteins of these isolates that were corresponding to gag and pol products (because having molecular weights similar but not identical to these antigens of HIV) ; in contrast, the env products could not be immunoprecipitated, and the genome of this new retrovirus cross-hybridized only poorly in very low stringency conditions with HIV-specific DNA probes (3). This was in contrast with the wide cross-antigenicity at the envelope level, and the overall cross-hybridization in stringent conditions, that were previously observed among HIV isolates. These West African AIDS virus isolates were therefore designated as HIV type 2, while HIV-1 is now referring to the AIDS retrovirus previously identified in Central Africa, North-America and Europe.

Studies conducted in African patients visiting Portugal allowed us to to detect HIV-2 infection in some 30 individuals, originating from Guinea Bissaü and neighbouring areas (5). Among these, 14 were presenting with AIDS, according to the CDC criteria, and 8 with AIDS related complex (ARC). None of the AIDS and ARC patients appeared to be co-infected by HIV-1 and HIV-2, and therefore, HIV-2 must be considered as the etiological agent of AIDS in West Africa.

HIV-2 appears to be closely related to the simian immune deficiency viruses (SIV) a group of cytopathic retroviruses whose prototype, STLV-3_{mac}, was identified in captive rhesus monkeys (Macaca mulatta) with an AIDS-like disease, and later found to infect other primate species, either wild caught or in captivity (6-9). Indeed antigenic cross-reactivity is observed for all the proteins of HIV-2 and SIV, including the envelope glycoproteins, whereas sera from HIV-1 infected patients only immune precipitate the gag and maybe pol products of SIV (3). Genetic comparisons of SIV, HIV-1 and HIV-2 may elucidate the phylogeny of these viruses and the origins of the recent AIDS epidemics. As these retroviruses share most of their biological properties, the identification of conserved sequences is important to localize the functional domains of the viral proteins and regulating elements, and design new diagnostic and therapeutic tools. We have cloned the genome of one HIV-2 isolate and determined its complete nucleotide sequence, therefore allowing the comparison of its proteins with those of HIV-1. We also report preliminary studies on the regulation of HIV-2 expression.

RESULTS

Molecular Cloning of the HIV-2 Genome.

Because of the extremely low level of cross-hybridization of the HIV-1 and HIV-2 genomes, even with HIV-1 probes derived from domains of the gag and pol genes that were expected to be well-conserved, given the antigenical cross-reactivity of these proteins, we have decided to derive a HIV-2 specific probe by molecular cloning of a complementary DNA (cDNA). A library of some 10^4 recombinant M13 clones was obtained starting from cDNAs made from HIV-2 purified virions by the endogenous detergent-activated reaction, with oligo (dT) priming at the 3' end of the viral RNA. Probably because of the highly lytic nature of the virus, the viral specific cDNA only represented a minor fraction of the library (retrospectively found to be under 1 %) and direct detection of the HIV-2 cDNA was impossible. We could fortunately detect HIV-2 specific clones by a very low stringency screening using a HIV-1 LTR probe, probably because M13 plaque screening in situ is more sensitive and more specific in low stringencies (TM -42°C.) than Southern blot or even dot blot of genomic RNA. Several cDNA were analyzed and found to correspond to the 3' end of a retroviral RNA very distantly homologous to HIV-1 (10). Alignment of the sequences was only possible with a lot of insertions and deletions. HIV-2 specificity was demonstrated by using the cDNA clones to detect material in HIV-2 infected cells by Southern hybridization, corresponding both to integrated and unintegrated viral DNA. No signal was found in HIV-1 infected and uninfected cells.

A preliminary study of different HIV-2 isolates propagated in continuous cell lines or in normal lymphocytes, has revealed a genetic polymorphism similar to that observed among HIV-1 isolates. Similarly, the genome of SIV (isolate Mm 142 from STLV-3_{mac}, gift of Dr. R. Desrosiers) can be detected by the HIV-2 probes under conditions of medium stringency (Tm -25°C.), and has a distinct restriction map. In the same conditions, HIV-1 probes do not detect any material in SIV-infected cells. Therefore, it is confirmed that HIV-2 is more closely related to SIV than it is to HIV-1.

Using these cloned HIV-2 probes we were able to screen a genomic library made from a T4 cell line (CEM) infected with the ROD. isolate of HIV-2 obtained in 1985 by Dr. F. Brun-Vézinet and colleagues from an AIDS patient from Cape verde Islands (offshore Senegal, ref.3,4). Lambda clones containing proviral DNA were characterized by restriction mapping, and then used to determine the complete nucleotide sequence of the genome.

Nucleotide Sequence and LTR Analysis.

The genome of HIV-2 is 9,671 nucleotides long (in its RNA

form), whereas HIV-1 isolates are about 9,200 nucleotides long. This difference is partly explained by the respective sizes of the long terminal repeats (LTR, see below). The genetic organization of HIV-2 is analogous to that of HIV-1, that is, 5'LTR - gag -pol - central region -env - orf F -3'LTR. The "central region", also identified in the ovine lentivirus visna (11), contains five major open reading frames (ORF), four being clearly related to the ORF of HIV-1 that encode the Q (or sor), R, tat and art (or trs) genes of HIV-1 (1,12,13 for reviews). The fifth, which we designate ORF X, has no evident counterpart in HIV-1. Alignments of the nucleotide sequences of HIV-1 and 2 show their distant homology (from about 60 % for the more conserved gag and pol genes, to 30-40 % for the other viral genes and LTR, not shown). To allow these alignments to be made many insertions and deletions must be introduced into the sequences. We do not observe that insertions represent small duplications that would be indicative the of the recent divergence of retroviral sequences, as it was noticed among isolates of HIV-1 (14).

The limits of the LTR, and of their internal U3, R and U5 elements, were determined by sequence analysis and some complementary experiments, such as synthesis of cDNA using the endogenous reverse transcriptase activity and the endogenous $tRNA^{lys}$ primer ("strong-stop cDNA"). The U5 element is 125bp. long, U3 is 556 bp. and R 173 bp. (respectively 82, 456 and 97 bp. in HIV-1). All of the elements of the HIV-2 LTR are larger than in HIV-1, and alignment by computer programs shows large insertions and overall very distant homology for the aligned regions (10). However, the three Sp1 binding sites the core enhancers identified in HIV-1 (13,15), are also present and relatively well-conserved in the U3 element of HIV-2.

The analysis of the viral-specific $polyA^+$ RNA (not shown) from a T4 cell line infected and continuously producing HIV-2 revealed a pattern of transcription reminiscent of what is observed in HIV-1 infected cells : an over 9 Kb. species corresponding to full-length transcripts, and three types of spliced mRNA of 5, 4.5, and 2 Kb. also observed in HIV-1 (1).

Gag and Pol Proteins.

The gag precursor of HIV-2 has a calculated molecular weight (MW) of 57.1 kilodalton (KD), consistent with the p55 antigen seen by immunoprecipitation with patient sera , and is probably processed, by analogy with HIV-1, into the proteins designated p16, p26, and p12 (3,4). The HIV-2 pol ORF could encode for the p64 and p36 antigens of HIV-2 which by analogy correspond to the p68 and p34 (reverse transcriptase and endonuclease, respectively) of HIV-1.

The gag and pol proteins of HIV-1 and 2 were expected to share important conserved domains, since these HIV-2 proteins can be immune precipitated by HIV-1 sera. However, we found that only 58% and 59.4% of the amino-acids of respectively gag and pol are identical to the corresponding HIV-1 products, whereas the more distant isolates of HIV-1 (Zairian and US) show 90 to 95 % amino acid identity in these proteins. Several insertions and deletions have to be introduced in the alignments (data not shown), whereas they are rare in the comparisons of gag and pol genes between HIV-1 isolates. The gag and pol proteins of HIV-2 are no closer to those of the Zairian isolates than to the prototype HIV-1 (BRU isolate) isolated in 1983 from a French patient probably infected in the USA.

Alignments of different retroviral pol proteins confirm that the HIVs form a subgroup which is more related to the lentiviruses visna and equine infectious anemia virus (EIAV) than to any other human or animal retrovirus .

The Envelope Glycoproteins Share Punctual Homologous Domains.

The envelope gene of HIV-2, as in other retroviruses, gives rise to a large external glycoprotein (EGP), responsible of the interaction with the cell surface receptor, and a transmembrane glycoprotein (TMP) anchored through the lipid bilayer. The N-terminus of env contains a relatively hydrophobic stretch that is probably the signal peptide of the leader sequence ; no homology with HIV-1 envelope leader is found. A potential cleavage site between the external envelope glycoprotein (120 kD) and the transmembrane protein, previously thought to be the 36 KD antigen, and now putatively identified as a 40 KD antigen (4) is found at amino-acid 505 immediately after the Lys-Glu-Lys-Arg sequence. This cleavage site aligns partly to one (Lys-Ala-Lys-Arg) of the two potential cleavage sites found in HIV-1 (the other being located after the Arg-Glu-Lys-Arg stretch). The calculated MW of the extracellular glycoprotein (EGP) and of the transmembrane protein (TMP) of HIV-2 would be 57 KD and 41.7 KD respectively ; the discrepancy with the apparent MW of the EGP is explained by glycosylation (30 sites in HIV-2, about half of which are conserved with respect to HIV-1).

In an alignment of the envelopes of the two HIV , these two proteins are found overall very distantly related (41.7 % identity in the entire envelope, 39.4% in the EGP, 44.8% in the TMP). Even whithin divergent isolates of HIV-1, about 75 to 80 % identity is seen in the envelope (14). Large and numerous insertions have to be introduced, especially to allow the aligments of the EGP where only punctual domains are found to be conserved between the HIV-1 and 2. These domains are clustered into the conserved regions of the EGP of HIV-1 (identified by comparison of different isolates), and, generally fall around cysteine residues. Among the HIV-1 isolates, all of the Cys residues could be aligned in spite of overall important genetic variation, especially in the gp110. Twenty two of the twenty three Cys residues of HIV-1 can also be aligned to HIV-2, but the latter contains seven additional Cys, often in the regions representing insertions relatively to HIV-1. Thus, the folding of the HIV-2 EGP could be different from what exists in HIV-1, and some regions, therefore, might be exposed in a different manner.

Other Viral Proteins

The HIV-1 genome contains several other genes encoding proteins of small MW (10 to 27 kD), two of which (tat and art/trs) have an identified function : the positive regulation of viral expression (ref. 13 for review). No role has yet been identified for the p23 encoded by the ORF Q (or sor, or A), nor for the p27 encoded by the ORF F (or 3'ORF) and for the potential gene, which we designated R (14). All these elements are found in HIV-2, but the correspondind proteins are only distantly homologous. In the F protein, most of the difference between HIV-1 and 2 is due to a large insertion in the N terminus of HIV-2. The second half of the protein, encoded by the U3 element of the LTR, shows a higher conservation.

Based upon sequence homologies with HIV-1, the tat and art genes of HIV-2 are probably organized as split genes transcribed into a 2 kb. mRNA made of three exons : the 5' leader, a first coding exon located in the central region and a last exon colinear to the end of env. The tat protein of HIV-2 would be longer than that of HIV-1 (130 versus 86 AA), having two large insertions in the N terminus and in the second exon. The main domain of homology of the tat proteins corresponds to a region very rich in Cys residues whose structure is reminiscent of that of the "Cys fingers" of some transcription regulating elements that interact with nucleic acids. This region is followed by an Arg-Lys rich stretch that could also interact with DNA or RNA. No significant homology is seen in the second coding exon, which has been shown to be dispensible to the function of the protein (16,17). The art encoded protein is shorter in HIV-2 than it is in HIV-1 (100 versus 116 AA.), and most of its length is encoded by the last exon. Its most homologous part is located in a stretch of basic residues that has the potential to interact with nucleic acids.

Cross-Transactivation of HIV-1 and HIV-2.

The trans-activator gene (tat) has been shown to be indispensable for the replication and cytopathicity of HIV-1 (18) and it is important to investigate its existence in HIV-2. We constructed a plasmid, called pHIV2-CAT, containing the bacterial chloramphenicol acetyltransferase (CAT) gene under the control of the U3-R region of HIV-2 (150 bp of U3 and 250 bp of R). To test the trans-activation of HIV-2, cells were either infected with HIV-2 or mock infected, and five days later transfected with either pSVCAT (which contains the CAT gene under control of the SV40 early promoter) or pHIV2-CAT. At the time of transfection, the cells were not yet producing virus, but we observed a substantial increase in the amount of CAT expression in extracts of HIV2-infected versus mock-infected cells that had been transfected with pHIV2-CAT). The expression of the SV40 early promoter was not affected by HIV-2 infection.

To determine whether or not the tat gene of HIV-1 could transactivate the LTR of HIV-2 and vice-versa, we cotransfected SW480 cells, a cell-line derived from a colon carcinoma (19), with subgenomic fragments of HIV-1 or HIV-2 and pHIV2-CAT or a plasmid called pHIV1-CAT, which contains U3-R of HIV-1 (the entire U3 and 70 bp of R) directing transcription of the CAT gene. The plasmid pLET (given by Dr. S. Wain-Hobson) contains the region of the HIV-1 shown by others to encode the HIV-1 tat gene (16,17). The plasmid pME214, on the other hand, contains the HIV-2 open reading frame that shares homology with the tat gene of HIV-1. In both of these plasmids transcription is driven by the LTR of the respective virus, and the first AUG of the transcript is the first AUG of the putative tat gene. It should be noted that both of these plasmids also contain the coding potential for the art gene.

While the SV40 early promoter was not affected by either the HIV-1 tat nor the HIV-2 tat, both HIV-1 and HIV-2 LTRs were substantially activated by the HIV-1 tat gene. This is perhaps surprising in view of the difference in size of the R region of HIV-1 (where the transactivator responsive region, TAR, resides) and HIV-2. However , 35 of the 58 bases present in the first stem and loop secondary structure of the TAR region of HIV-1 are conserved, and an analogous stem and loop structure with the first 77 bases of R can be drawn for HIV-2 (15).

The HIV-2 LTR is trans-activated over 100-fold by pME214, but on the other hand, the HIV-1 LTR is not as well transactivated by this plasmid (about 5-10 fold). Similar results were obtained after transfection of Hela and HUT 78 cells and these experiments indicate that pME214 encodes a functional tat gene and that the template specificity of the HIV-2 tat is somewhat different from that of the HIV-1 tat. It will be important to determine whether or not this observation is isolate-specific.

DISCUSSION.

Origin of the Human Immune Deficiency Viruses.

HIV-1 and HIV-2 share a similar genomic organization, indicating a common evolutionary origin, but differ significantly in terms of nucleotide and amino-acid sequence : the more conserved gag and pol genes respectively display only 56 and 60 % nucleotide sequence homology and both less than 60 % of amino-acid identity. The calculation of the nucleotide sequence homology for the other genes gives even lower values making HIV-1 and 2 overall 42 % homologous. This confirms that these two viruses are distinct elements of the HIV family.

It was previously established that HIV-2 is more related to the simian immunodeficiency viruses (SIV) than it is to HIV-1. All of the SIV and HIV-2 proteins are antigenically cross-reactive, whereas their cross-reactivity to HIV-1 is restricted to gag and pol antigens. The N-terminal amino-acid sequence of the major core protein (corresponding to the $p25^{gag}$ of HIV-1 and $p26^{gag}$ of HIV-2) has been determined in one isolate of SIV obtained from Macaques with an AIDS-like disease (MnIV, 8). Out of the 23 AA determined, 21 match with the N-terminus of $p26^{gag}$ of HIV-2, whereas 13 (with one deletion) match to the p25 of HIV-1. Furthermore, while HIV-2 can infect, at least transiently, primate species which are evolutionarily more distantly related to humans (at least baboons and macaques), HIV-1 infects only humans and chimpanzees (R. Desrosiers, NERPRC, and P. Fultz, CDC, personal communication). In fact, it is not possible from current data to know whether SIV can be classified distinctly from HIV-2 or if they only differ as independent isolates of the same virus.

The almost simultaneous emergence of two foci of AIDS in distinct areas of the African continent is unlikely to be due to the recent emergence of two novel human pathogens, for example by simultaneous trans-species infection by animal retroviruses, or by the mutation of preexisting non pathogenic human retroviruses. Indeed, HIV-1 and HIV-2 are obviously retroviruses with a common origin, but highly divergent, and it is more likely that their time of divergence is anterior to the beginning of the current epidemics. Therefore a common ancestor, with similar properties and pathogenic potential, probably existed a long time ago in a human population, and the emergence of the AIDS epidemics is more likely due to simultaneous modifications of epidemiological parameters in West and Central Africa, such as uncontrolled urbanisation, leading to the infection of larger populations.

A question to be addressed is why the HIV were only recently detected if they existed for a long period. This may be due to the fact that the pathogenicity of an HIV-type retrovirus cannot be revealed until it has spread to a significant portion of the population. First, in undermedicalized areas of Africa, where other infections, such as malaria, represent primary causes of morbidity, isolated cases of AIDS could have been an undetectable clinical event. Then, the incubation time can vary considerably, and it cannot still be ruled out that a large fraction of individuals infected by a HIV will remain healthy carriers.

A retrovirus designated HTLV-4, but undiscernable from HIV-2 and SIV by the antigenicity of its proteins was identified in apparently healthy individuals in West Africa (20), an area were we have observed several typical AIDS cases caused by HIV-2. It is possible that the apparent non pathogenicity of HTLV-4 is due to a recent epidemic diffusion of the HIV-2/HTLV-4 in the West Africa, where AIDS cases still represent a minor fraction of the infected and seropositive individuals, whereas HIV-1 has diffused in major cities of the Central Africa or the USA some time before.

Implications for Vaccines and Diagnostics

The risk that HIV-2 infected blood samples may not be detected by standard screens, currently based upon the detection of anti-HIV-1 antibodies, urges the need of diagnostic means for HIV-2 infection. As the envelope, and especially its transmembrane part represents the primary target of the host antibody response, to the HIV infection, antigens from the envelope of HIV-2 will significantly improve the spectrum of the screening tests, allowing the detection of samples infected by HIV-2, and perhaps by other yet uncharacterized members of the HIV family.

As it shares most of the structural characteristics and biological properties of HIV-1, but displays a significative genetic divergence, HIV-2 represents a powerful tool to study the molecular biology of this group of retroviruses. We must take advantage of the precise delineation of the conserved structures to understand their molecular biology and develop new therapeutic tools, especially means for immunoprophylaxy that could be efficient in the eradication of these pathogens.

HIV-1 and probably HIV-2 recognize the T4 surface molecule as a receptor on helper/inducer T lymphocytes and perhaps on other cells expressing the T4 protein (21,22). In HIV-1, this interaction is mediated by the external envelope glycoprotein

(EGP, 23), and an important problem to address is the determination of the domain (s) of this protein that are involved in that interaction. Indeed, blocking this step of the virus life cycle, either by antibodies or drugs, could be an efficient means for preventing the infection or impeding its spread. As the receptor is made of a constant cellular protein, we can postulate that the binding domain of the envelope is conserved among the T4 tropic HIVs. The conserved domains of the EGP of HIV-1 and 2 are not numerous, and therefore it becomes possible to investigate their possible role in the virus-receptor interaction using a relatively limited set of site-directed mutations. Given the absence of antigenic cross-reactivity of the envelopes of the two HIVs, this T4-binding domain is probably not or poorly immunogenic --perhaps because of masking by glycosylation , poor exposure on the virion surface, or mimicking of "self" antigens. Nevertheless, its presentation to the immune system out of context of the virion, that is, as a peptide, might induce a neutralizing antibody response that is not attained, or with a low efficiency, with the complete native envelope from virions or expression systems (24-26).

AKNOWLEDGEMENTS

We thank Drs F. Brun-Vézinet, R. Desrosiers, P.Fultz, and M. Muesing for exchange of scientific information ; Drs. S. Wain-Hobson and M.L. Michel for providing plasmids ; M.E. is a fellow from the Leukemia Society of America, Inc. This work was in part accomplished in the Laboratoire de Biologie Moléculaire et Immunologie des Rétrovirus, Institut Pasteur.

REFERENCES.

1. Weiss, R.A. (1984). Human T-cell retroviruses. In Molecular biology of the tumor viruses : RNA tumor viruses, vol II, supplement, R. Weiss, N. Teich, H. Varmus, J. Coffin, eds. (Cold Spring Harbor, New York: Cold Spring Harbor Laboratory), vol II : supplement, pp. 405-485.
2. Quinn, T.C., Mann, J.M., Curran, J.W., & Piot, P. (1986). AIDS in Africa : an epidemiologic paradigm. Science **234**, 955-963.
3. Clavel, F., Guetard, D., Brun-Vézinet, F., Chamaret, S., Rey, M.A., Santos-Ferreira, M.O.,Laurent, A.G., Dauguet, C., Katlama, C.,Rouzioux, C., Klatzmann, D., Champelinaud, J.L., & Montagnier, L.(1986). Isolation of a new human retrovirus from West-African patients with AIDS. Science **233**, 343-346.

4. Brun-Vézinet, F. Rey, M.A., Katlama, C., Girard, P.M., Roulot, D., Yeni, P., Lenoble, L., Clavel, F., Alizon, M., Gadelle, S., Madjar, J.J., & Harzic, M. (1987). HIV/LAV-2 in AIDS and ARC patients : clinical and virological studies. Lancet **i**, 128-132
5. Clavel, F., Mansinho, K., Guétard, D., Chamaret, S., Santos-ferreira, M.O., Champalimaud, J.L., & Montagnier, L. (1987). N. Engl.J. Med. in press.
6. Daniel,M.D. Letvin, N.L., King, M.W., Kannagi, M., Seghal, P.K., Hunt, R.D., Kanki, P.J., Essex, M., & Desrosiers, R.C. (1985) Isolation of T-cell tropic HTLV-III-like retrovirus from macaques. Science **228** , 1199-1204.
7. Kanki, P.J., Alroy, J. & Essex, M. (1985). Isolation of T-lymphotropic retroviruses from wild-caught African Green Monkeys. Science **230**, 951-954.
8. Benveniste, R.E. et al. J.Virol. **60** , 483-490 (1986).
9. Murphey-Corb, M. et al. Nature **321**, 435-437 (1986).
10. Clavel, F., Guyader, M., Guétard, D., Sallé, M., Montagnier, L., & Alizon, M. Molecular cloning of the human immune deficiency virus type 2 (HIV-2) associated with AIDS in West Africa (1986). Nature **324**, 691-695.
11. Sonigo, P., Alizon, M., Staskus, K., Klatzmann, D., Cole, S., Danos, O., Retzel, E., Tiollais, P., Haase, A. & Wain-Hobson, S. (1985). Nucleotide sequence of the visna lentivirus : Relationship to the AIDS virus. Cell **42**, 369-382.
12. Montagnier L., & Alizon M. Human immune deficiency virus (HIV) : an update. (1987) Ann.Inst. Pasteur (Virol.) **138**, 3-11.
13. Chen, I.S.Y. (1986). Regulation of AIDS virus expression. Cell **47**, 1-2.
14. Alizon, M., Wain-Hobson, S., Montagnier, L., & Sonigo, P. (1986). Genetic variability of the AIDS virus : Nucleotide sequence analysis of two isolates from African patients. Cell **46**, 63-74.
15. Muesing, M.A., Smith, D.H., & Capon, D.J. (1987). Regulation of mRNA accumulation by a human immune deficiency virus trans-activator protein. Cell **48**, 691-701.
16. Dayton, A.I., Sodroski, J.G. Rosen, C.A., Goh, W.C. & Haseltine, W.A. (1986). Trans-activator gene of the human T-cell lymphotropic virus type III is required for replication. Cell **44**, 941-947.
17. Adachi, A. et al. J.Virol. **59**, 284-291 (1986).
18. Arya, S.K., Guo, C., Josephs, S.F., & Wong-Staal, F. (1985). Trans-activator gene of human T-lymphotropic virus type III (HTLV-III). Science **229**, 69-73.

19. Sodroski, J., Patarca, R., Rosen C., Wong-Staal, F. & Haseltine, W. (1985). Location of the trans-activating region on the genome of human T-cell lymphotropic virus type III. Science **229**, 74-77.
20. Kanki, P.J., Barin, F., M'Boup, S., Allan, J.S., Romet-Lemonne, J.L., Markink, R., McLane, M.F., Lee, T.H., Arbeille, B., Denis, F. & Essex, M. (1986). New human T-lymphotropic retrovirus related to simian T-lymphotropic virus type III (STLV-III_{AGM}). Science, **232**, 238-243.
21. Dalgleish, A.G., Beverley, P.C., Clapham, P.R., Crawford, D.H., Greaves, M.F. & Weiss, R.A. (1984). The CD4 (T4) antigen is an essential component of the receptor for the AIDS retrovirus. Nature **312**, 763-767.
22. Klatzmann, D., Champagne, E., Chamaret, S., Gruest, J., Guetard, D., Hercend, T., Gluckman, J.C. & Montagnier, L. (1984). T-lymphocyte T4 molecule behaves as the receptor for human retrovirus LAV. Nature **312**, 767-768.
23. MacDougal, J.S., Kennedy, M.S., Sligh, J.M., Cort, S.P., Mawle, A. & Nicholson, J.K.A. (1986). Binding of HTLV-III/LAV to $T4^+$ cells by a complex of the 110 k viral protein and the T4 molecule. Science **231**, 382-385.
24. Weiss, R.A., Clapham, P.R., Cheinsong-Popov, R., Dalgleish, A.G., Carne, C.A., Weller, I.A.D. & Tedder, R.C. (1985). Neutralization of human T-lymphotropic virus type III by sera of AIDS and AIDS-risk patients. Nature, **316**, 69-72.
25. Clavel, F., Klatzmann, D., & Montagnier, L. (1985). Deficient neutralizing capacity of sera from patients with AIDS or related syndromes. Lancet **I**, 879-880.

26. Lasky, L.A., Groopman, J.E., Fennie, C.W., Benz, P.W., Capon, D.J., Dowbenko, D.J., Nakamura, G.R., Nunes, W.M., & Berman, P.W. (1986). Neutralization of the AIDS retrovirus by antibodies to a recombinant envelope glycoprotein. Science **238**, 209-212.

Human Retroviruses, Cancer, and AIDS: Approaches to Prevention and Therapy, pages 43–56

LIKE HIV (HTLV-III), HTLV-IV, LAV-2 (HIV-2), SBLV-6669 AND STLV-III POSSESS FUNCTIONAL TRANSACTIVATOR GENE

Suresh K. Arya
Laboratory of Tumor Cell Biology, National Cancer Institute
National Institutes of Health
Bethesda, Maryland 20892, U.S.A.

INTRODUCTION

The human T-lymphotropic retroviruses (HTLVs) share many properties, including preferred tropism for OKT4+ T-lymphocytes, similar mode of transmission and likely African origin. They also differ from each other in significant ways forming two distinct groups. HTLV-I, a transforming virus, is the prototype of the first group. It causes adult T-cell leukemia (ATL) and appears to be involved in B-cell malignancies and in central nervous system disease (see references 1 and 2 for reviews). This group also includes HTLV-II[3] and variants of HTLV-I[4] which are associated with T-cell malignancies different from ATL. Human immune deficiency virus (HIV), also known as HTLV-III or lymphadenopathy virus (LAV), a non-transforming virus, is the prototype of the second group. It causes acquired immune deficiency syndrome (AIDS) and nervous system disorders. A remarkable spectrum of variants of HIV have been identified[5-8], differing from one another to varying degrees in their nucleotide sequence [9-11]. Because they share structural and immunobiological properties they have been considered as one virus type. Recently, new members of this group of non-transforming human retroviruses were isolated from individuals from different countries of West Africa[13-15]. These isolates show major antigenic characteristics that distinguish them from HIV, although they retain many features in common[12-15]. These new isolates have been termed HTLV-IV, LAV-2 and SBLV-6669. Current epidemiological studies suggest that some of these virus isolates cause immune deficiency whereas others may not or may be considerably less efficient at inducing immune deficiency. Remarkably, counterparts of both groups of human retroviruses also exist in old world subhuman primates. They have been termed simian T-lymphotropic virus-I and -III

(STLV-I and -III). STLV-III, related to HIV and even more closely to HTLV-IV/LAV-2/SBLV-6669[13-16] does not appear to cause AIDS in its natural host, the African green monkeys and related species. A novel feature of HTLV-I, -II and -III (HIV) is the possession of a gene, termed tat, which trans-activates the expression of genes linked to the viral long terminal repeat (LTR)[17-23]. These respective genes of HTLV-I and HTLV-III (HIV) are implicated in their pathobiology[17-25], even though they cause different diseases in humans. We report here that like HTLV-I, -II, and -III (HIV) the new West African human retroviruses, as well as STLV-III, possess the putative tat gene, irrespective of their pathogenic potential *in vivo*.

RESULTS AND DISCUSSION

The first isolate of the new subgroup of West African retroviruses, HTLV-IV (P190), was isolated from lymphocytes of a healthy female prostitute[13]. Another isolate, LAV-2 (FG), was obtained from the same patient with AIDS from which LAV-2[14] was previously isolated. A third isolate, SBLV-6669, was isolated from lymphocytes of an individual afflicted with early phase of lymphadenopathy[15]. All three isolates are antigenically related to HIV but more so to STLV-III than to HIV[12-15]. Thus far, HTLV-IV(P190) has not been linked to any disease in the natural host and appears not to be as cytopathic for human T-lymphocytes *in vitro* as HIV. Similarly, an isolate of $STLV\text{-}III_{AGM}$ (K1) has not been associated with disease in the natural simian host[13,16].

To test if the new non-transforming human retrovirus contained a transactivating gene, we cloned HTLV-IV and LAV-2 LTRs by way of cDNA cloning. Several independent clones containing 3'-LTR and sequences extending upstream were characterized. DNA sequence of some of these clones of HTLV-IV (V17b, V17 and V8) and LAV-2 (LV2 and LV2P), containing different lengths of sequences upstream from the putative transcriptional initiation (cap) site are shown in Figure 1. Several consensus and/or putative regulatory elements are noticeable (see Fig. 1). We also obtained and sequenced clones containing STLV-III 3'-LTR and additional 5'-sequence. The sequence of the STLV-III clone is more than 95% homologous to the sequence of HTLV-IV shown in Figure 1. LTR in this report refers to U3 and R and does not include U5. Additional longer clones of HTLV-IV, LAV-2 and STLV-III contain an open

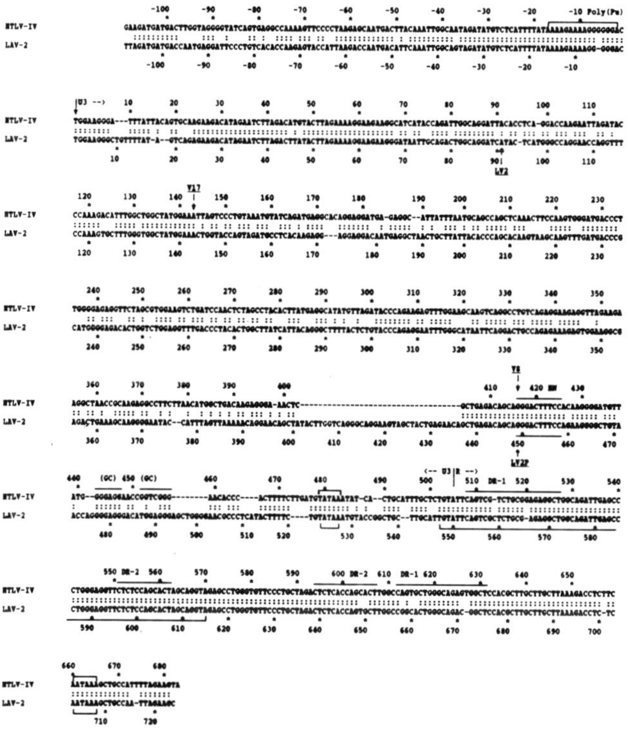

Figure 1: Nucleotide sequence of HTLV-IV LTR cDNA clones (V17b, V17 and V8) and LAV-2 LTR cDNA clones (LV2 and LV2P). The boundaries of the U3 region have not yet been experimentally determined but are based on the analogy with HTLV-III$_B$. The polypurine stretch [p(Pu)] of HTLV-IV and LAV-2 is identical to that of HTLV-III$_B$. TATA box and poly(A) signal sequence are boxed. A decanucleotide sequence, GGGACTTTCC, which is a putative enhancer in HTLV-III$_B$[29,30], is present at approximately the same distance upstream of the TATA box in HTLV-IV and LAV-2 as in HTLV-III. However, this sequence is repeated in HTLV-III$_B$ LTR, and HTLV-IV and LAV-2 contain only an imperfect repeat of this sequence. The potential "GC" box or SPI binding sites[29,30] are discernable. Two imperfect direct repeats (DR-1 and DR-2) are also indicated.

reading frame similar to and about 30% homologous with the 3'*orf* gene of HTLV-III$_B$ strain of HIV (data not shown).

The cloned HTLV-IV (V17, V17b and V8) and LAV-2 (LV2 and LV2P) DNAs were placed upstream of the bacterial chloramphenicol acetyltransferase (CAT) gene carried on a vector lacking promotor-enhancer sequences (pSVOCat)[27] and the resulting plasmids were termed pV17bCat, pV17Cat and pV8Cat for HTLV-IV LTR-Cat constructs and LV2Cat and LV2PCat for LAV-2 LTR-Cat constructs. These DNAs were placed in both 5'-3' and 3'-5' orientations in front of the CAT gene and were termed correct (c) and non-correct (nc) orientations, respectively. Two additional plasmids, pSV2Cat[27] and pC15Cat[22] respectively contained SV40 promoter-enhancer and HTLV-III$_B$ 3'-LTR linked to the CAT gene in correct orientation. The plasmid DNAs were transfected into virus infected and uninfected human HUT 78 cells by the DEAE-dextran protocol. The transactivation of the LTR-linked CAT gene was measured by conversion of chloramphenicol to its acetylated forms catalyzed by the enzyme in cellular extracts 44-48 hr after transfection as described[22]. Representative results are shown in Figure 2 and the more extensive data are summarized in Table 1.

The HTLV-IV and LAV-2 LTRs contain promoter-enhancer sequence elements, as expected. The CAT gene activity in uninfected HUT78 cells transfected with plasmid DNA with HTLV-IV or LAV-2 LTR linked in correct orientation to the CAT gene (e.g., pV17bCat or LV2Cat) was higher than that for the incorrect orientation (e.g., pV17bCat-nc or LV2 Cat-nc) or for the control plasmid lacking promoter-enhancer (pSVOCat) (Fig. 2.). The CAT gene activity under the control of HTLV-IV and LAV-2 LTRs in HUT 78 cells infected with new virus isolates and with STLV-III and HTLV-III$_B$, was markedly elevated as compared with uninfected cells (Fig. 2, Table 1). This suggests that the virus-infected cells contain a factor(s) which acts *in trans* in amplifying the expression of the CAT gene linked to HTLV-IV and LAV-2 LTRs. This activation was specific for plasmid DNAs where LTR was linked to the CAT gene in the correct orientation. HTLV-IV and LAV-2 LTRs responded to the transactivating factor in cells infected with all three of the HTLV-IV related viruses as well as those infected with STLV-III and HTLV-III$_B$. These results suggest that (i) all new isolates (HTLV-IV, LAV-2 and SBLV-6669) as well as STLV-III contain a transactivating gene, (ii) their

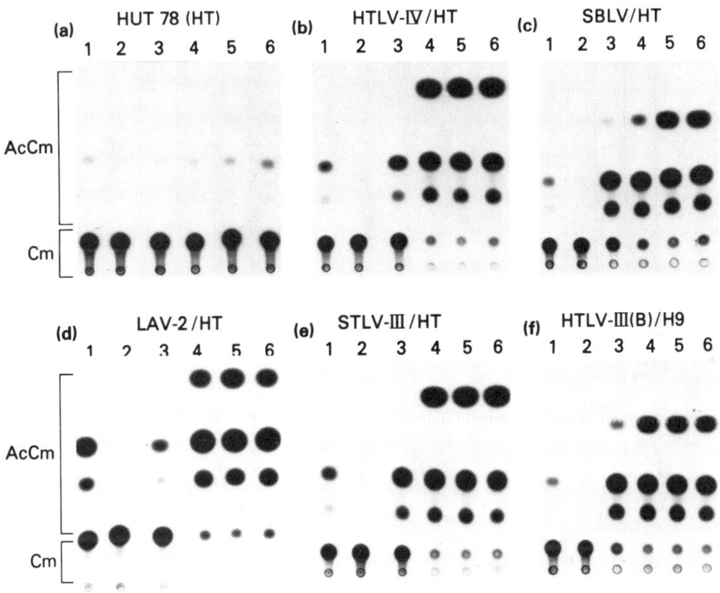

Figure 2: Activation of HTLV-IV, LAV-2 and HTLV-III$_B$ LTR-linked CAT gene in uninfected HUT78 cells (panel a), and cells infected with HTLV-IV (panel b), SBLV-6669 (panel c), LAV-2 (panel d), STLV-III (panel e), and HTLV-III$_B$ (panel f). Lanes 1-6 are for pSV2Cat(SV40), pSVOCat(none), pC15Cat(HTLV-III$_B$), pV17bCat(HTLV-IV), pV8Cat(HTLV-IV) and LV2Cat(LAV-2), respectively. About 10 x 10^6 cells were transfected with 10 μg of plasmid DNA by the DEAE-dextran protocol and assays were performed as described before (22). Cm, chloramphenicol; AcCm, acetylated chloramphenicol.

putative transactivating genes are structurally and/or functionally homologous, and (iii) their LTRs are also structurally and/or functionally related. The fact that HTLV-IV and LAV-2 LTRs are transactivated equally well in cells infected with HTLV-IV/LAV-2/SBLV-6669/STLV-III and HTLV-III$_B$ whereas

Table 1

TRANSACTIVATION OF HTLV-IV AND HTLV-III LTRs IN VIRUS-INFECTED CELLS

Plasmid	Regulatory Elements	% Conversion of Chloramphenicol to Acetylated Forms					
		HUT78[a]	HTLV-IV/HT[a]	SBLV-6669/HT[a]	LAV-2/HT[a]	STLV-III/HT[a]	HTLV-III$_B$/H9[a]
1. pSV2Cat	SV-40	2.4 ± 1.7	3.0 ± 0.35	0.7 ± 0.6	9.5 ± 1.0	4.5 ± 3.8	1.3 ± 0.3
2. pSV0Cat	None	0.12 ± 0.01	0.12 ± 0.01	0.14 ± 0.03	0.16 ± 0.18	0.15 ± 0.03	0.14 ± 0.01
3. pC15Cat	HTLV-III	0.43 ± 0.3	11.4 ± 1.9	21.5 ± 34.2	4.6	16.0 ± 9.1	96 ± 1.4
4. pV17bCat	HTLV-IV	1.4 ± 1.0	98.7 ± 0.9	62.9 ± 50.0	98.1 ± 0.2	96.2 ± 2.8	98 ± 0.3
5. pV8Cat	HTLV-IV	1.3 ± 0.8	98.7 ± 0.2	56.7 ± 39.0	98.3	98.0 ± 2.0	98 ± 0.8
6. pLV2Cat	LAV-2	---	99.1	---	96.9	---	99.2
7. pV17bCat(nc)	HTLV-IV	0.13 ± 0.8	0.2 ± 0.05	---	---	---	---

[a]Mean and standard deviation for 2 to 4 transfection experiments.

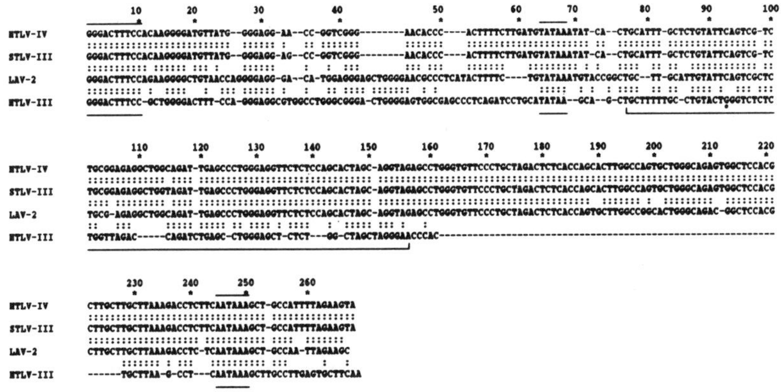

Figure 3: Comparison of the sequence of HTLV-IV, STLV-III, LAV-2 and HTLV-III$_B$ LTRs corresponding to the segments containing putative regulatory sequences and R region. The proposed HTLV-III$_B$ TAR sequence is underlined.

HTLV-III$_B$ LTR is highly transactivated only in cells infected with HTLV-III$_B$ suggests that HTLV-IV/LAV-2/SBLV-6669/STLV-III transactivating genes and LTRs may be more related among themselves than to HTLV-III$_B$ or HIV. Hybridization experiments with HTLV-IV-derived probes show that LAV-2 and SBLV-6669 as well as STLV-III contain homologous sequences. In fact, the sequences of the putative regulatory regions of HTLV-IV, LAV-2 and STLV-III LTRs can be aligned to display about 85-95% homology (Fig. 3.).

The fact that HTLV-IV LTR was also transactivated in HTLV-III$_B$ infected cells, and also when co-transfected with cloned

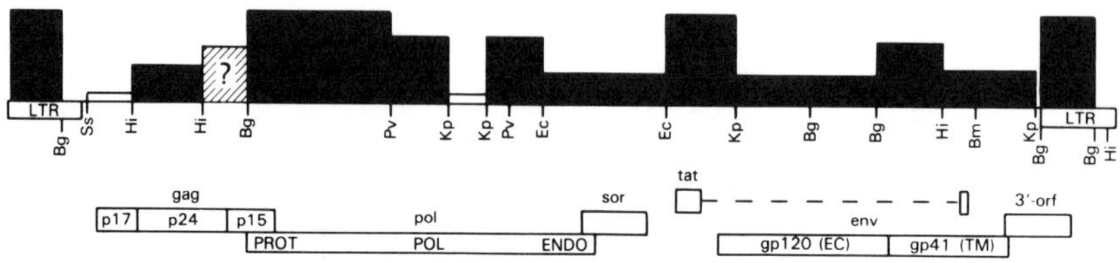

Figure 4: A qualitative description of the nucleotide homology between HTLV-IV and HTLV-III_B.

HTLV-III_B tat gene into uninfected cells (data not shown), suggests that the putative transactivating gene of HTLV-IV is related to the similar gene in HTLV-III_B. This was also indicated by the hybridization of HTLV-IV DNA to the cloned HTLV-III_B tat gene. In fact, HTLV-IV and HTLV-III_B show varying degrees of nucleotide homologies throughout their genomes. Fig. 4 depicts a qualitative description of homology between HTLV-IV and HTLV-III_B genomes. This map was constructed by hybridizing total HTLV-IV cDNA with genomic and subgenomic HTLV-III_B DNAs under varied stringencies of hybridization. A direct comparison of the DNA sequence of HTLV-IV compared with that of HTLV-III_B should provide a more quantitative evaluation of homology.

A specific sequence (TAR) in HTLV-III_B LTR responsible for optimal transactivation has been identified and localized between 6 bp and 76 bp downstream of the TATA box[27-29]. If such a specific sequence also exists in HTLV-IV and STLV-III LTRs, it must lie within 62 bp upstream and 202 bp downstream of the TATA box. This is the only sequence contained in the fully active clone V8. Furthermore, the LTR sequences of HTLV-IV/STLV-III/LAV-2 and HTLV-III_B can be aligned such that they are about 65% homologous downstream of the TATA box in the proposed TAR region of HTLV-III_B (Fig. 3).

Interestingly, HTLV-IV/LAV-2 LTR is equally well transactivated in HTLV-IV/LAV-2 and HTLV-III_B infected cells, while HTLV-III_B LTR is more transactivated in cells infected with HTLV-III_B than with HTLV-IV/LAV-2 (Figs. 5 and 6, and Table 1). It is possible that HTLV-IV/LAV-2 promoter-enhancer elements may be stronger than such elements in HTLV-III_B, thus

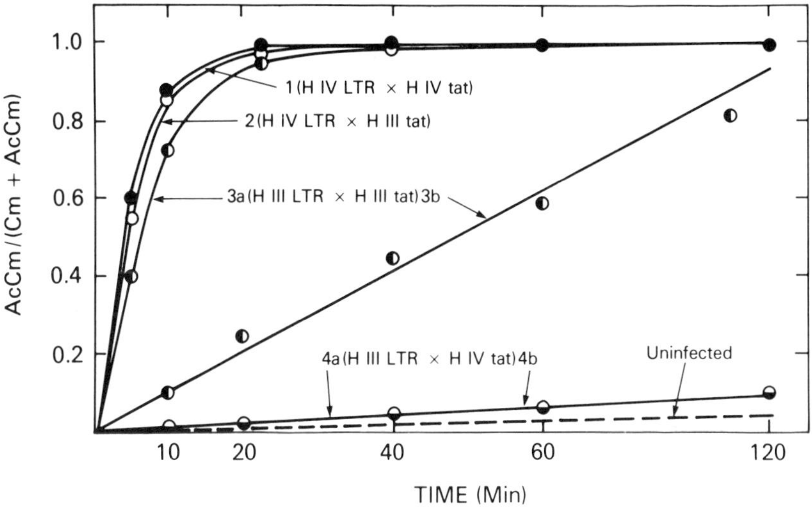

Figure 5: Kinetics of CAT activity induced in virus-infected cells transfected with viral LTR-Cat DNAs. About 10 x 10^6 cells were transfected with 10 µg of plasmid DNA and cells were processed 44 hr post-transfection to obtain 100 µl of cytoplasmic extract. Each time point in the assay corresponds to 10 µl of the cytoplasmic extract. Lines 3a and 3b are for two different HTLV-III_B LTR-Cat plasmids differing in sequence content upstream of the enhancer elements. Two different HTLV-III_B LTR clones differing in the content of upstream sequences were used.

achieving optimal transactivation even with heterologous HTLV-III_B transactivator. Additionally, it may be that the HTLV-IV/LAV-2 LTR transactivator interaction has a broader specificity than HTLV-III_B transactivator interaction. The possible broader specificity of HTLV-IV/LAV-2 LTR may make it more amenable to activation by other viral and cellular transactivating factors. The sequence of HTLV-IV/LAV-2 as well as HTLV-III_B LTR downstream of the putative transcriptional initiation site contains imperfect direct and indirect repeats. These sequences can be arranged to generate characteristic and analogous stem-loop structures for the 5'-end

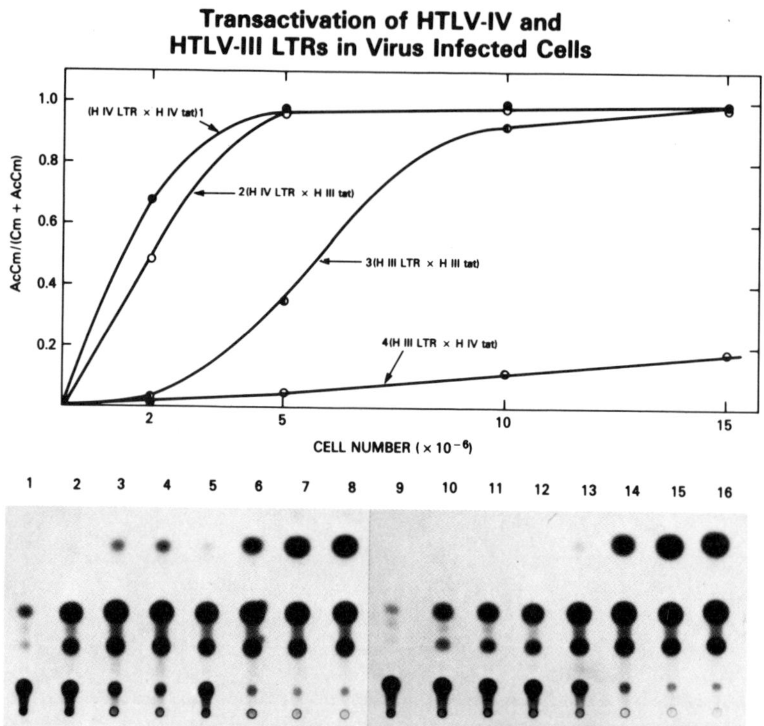

Figure 6: Activation of HTLV-IV and HTLV-III$_B$ LTR in HTLV-IV and HTLV-III$_B$ infected cells. Specified number of cells were transfected with 10 µg of LTR-CAT DNA and equal amounts of cytoplasmic extracts were assayed for CAT activity.

of the transcripts of HTLV-IV/LAV-2 and HTLV-III$_B$ (Fig. 7). These structures may provide overlapping sites for transactivator interactions.

The cells infected with all four virus isolates of the West African subgroup (HTLV-IV, LAV-2, SBLV-6669, and STLV-III) contain a factor that activates their LTRs in *trans*, thus suggesting that these viruses possess a functional transactivating gene. The transactivating gene of HIV has been implicated in its pathobiology. Since HTLV-IV and SLTV-III

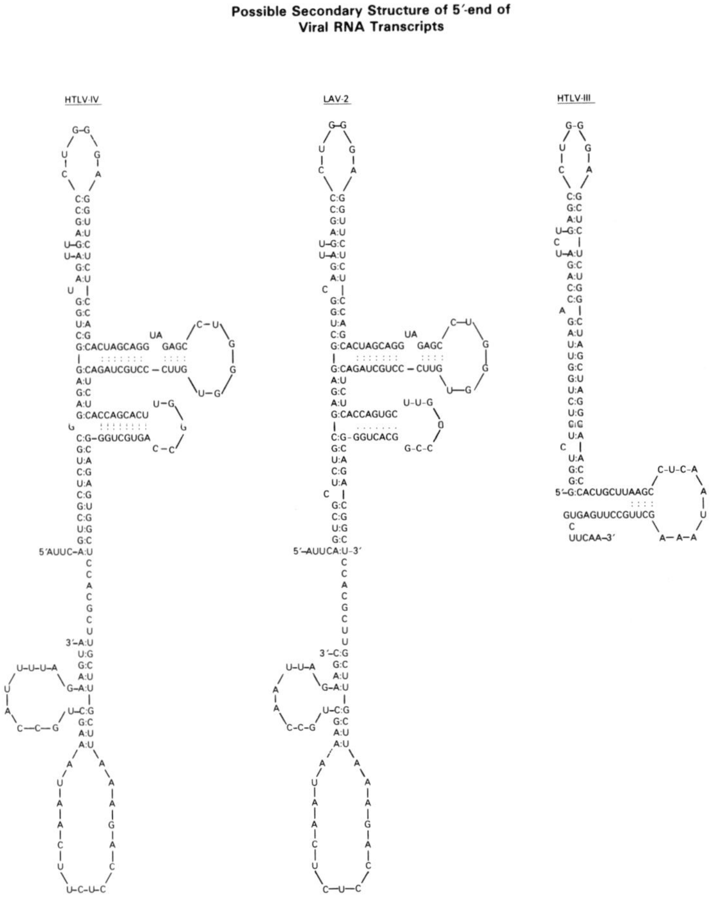

Figure 7: Predicted secondary structures of the 5′-end of the transcripts of HTLV-IV, LAV-2 and HTLV-III$_B$.

are not known to be pathogenic in their natural host, either their transactivating genes do not function in vivo, an unlikely possibility,or this gene function is not sufficient for pathogenicity. Host factors or other viral factors directly or indirectly may modulate the potential pathogenic role of the transactivating genes of these viruses.

ACKNOWLEDGMENTS

I thank B. Beaver and Dr. B. Ensoli for their assistance and contributions and Dr. L. Jagodzinski and co-workers for major part of the DNA sequencing. I am grateful to the following individuals who provided viruses and/or virus-infected cells which were propagated in the Laboratory of Tumor Cell Biology: Drs. M. Essex and P. Kanki for HTLV-IV and STLV-III; Dr. D. Zagury and collaborators for LAV-2; Drs. E. Norby, G. Biberfeld, J. Albert, and E. Fenyo for SBLV-6669. Finally, I thank Drs. F. Wong-Staal and R. C. Gallo for their support and encouragement.

REFERENCES

1. Wong-Staal F, Gallo RC (1985). Human T-lymphotropic retroviruses. Nature 317:395.
2. Gallo RC (1982). Human Retroviruses and the Diseases They Cause. In Smith LH, Wyngaarden JB (eds): "Cecil's Textbook of Medicine (18th Edition)," Philadelphia: Saunders Publication, in press.
3. Kalyanaraman VS, Sarngadharan MG, Robert-Guroff M, Miyoshi I, Blayney D, Golde D, Gallo RC (1982). A new subtype of human T-cell leukemia virus (HTLV-II) associated with a T-cell variant of hairy cell leukemia. Science 218:571.
4. Hahn BH, Shaw GM, Popovic M, Hoxie J, Gallo RC, Wong-Staal F (1985). Genomic diversity of the AIDS virus HTLV-III: different viruses exhibit greatest divergence in their envelope genes. Int J Cancer 34:613.
5. Barre-Sinoussi F, Cherman JC, Rey R, Nugeryte MT, Chamaret S, Gruest J, Dauget C, Axier-Blin C, Vezinet-Brun F, Rouzioux C, Rosenbaum W, Montagnier L (1983). Isolation of a T-lymphotropic retrovirus from a patient at risk for acquired immune deficiency syndrome (AIDS). Science 220:868.
6. Popovic M, Sarngadharan MG, Read E, Gallo RC (1984). Detection, isolation, and continued production of cytopathic retroviruses (HTLV-III) from patients with AIDS and pre-AIDS. Science 224:497.
7. Levy JA, Hoffman AD, Dramer SM, Kramer SM, Lamois JA, Shimabukuro JM, Oskiro LS (1984). Isolation of lymphocytopathic retroviruses from San Francisco patients with AIDS. Science 225:840.
8. Salahuddin SZ, Markham M, Popovic M, Sarngadharan MG, Orndorff S, Flandagar A, Patel A, Gold J, Gallo RC (1985). Isolation of infectious human T-cell leukemia/-

lymphotropic virus type-III (HTLV-III) from patients with acquired immunodeficiency syndrome (AIDS) or AIDS-related complex (ARC) and from healthy carriers: A study of risk groups and tissue sources. Proc Natl Acad Sci USA 82:5530.
9. Ratner L, Gallo RC, Wong-Staal F (1985). HTLV-III, LAV, and ARV are variants of the same AIDS virus. Nature 313:636.
10. Starcich BR, Hahn BH, Shaw GM, McNeely PD, Modrow S, Wolf H, Parks ES, Parks WP, Josephs SJ, Gallo RC, Wong-Staal F (1986). Identification and characterization of conserved and variable regions in the envelope gene of HTLV-III/LAV, the retrovirus of AIDS. Cell 45:637.
11. Hahn BH, Shaw GM, Taylor ME, Redfield RR, Markham PD, Salahuddin SZ, Wong-Staal F, Gallo RC, Parks ES, Parks WP (1986). Genetic variation in HTLV-III/LAV overtime in patients with AIDS or at risk for AIDS. Science 232:1548.
12. Barin F, M'Boup S, Denis F, Kanki P, Allan JS, Lee TH, Essex M (1985). Serological evidence for a virus related to Simian T-lymphotropic retrovirus-III in residents of West Africa. Lancet 2:1387.
13. Kanki PJ, Barin F, M'Boup S, Allan JS, Romet-Lemonne JL, Marlink R, McLane MF, Lee TH, Arbeille B, Denis F, Essex M (1986). New human T-lymphotropic retrovirus related to Simian T-lymphotropic virus type-III (STLV-III_{AGM}). Science 232:238.
14. Clowel F, Guetard D, Brun-Vezinet F, Chamaret S, Rey M, Santos-Ferreira MO, Laurent AG, Dauguet C, Katlama C, Rouzioux C, Klatzmann D, Champalimaud JL, Montagnier L (1986). Isolation of a new human retrovirus from West African patients with AIDS. Science 233:343.
15. Albert J, Bredberg K, Chiodi F, Bottiger B, Fenyo EM, Norrby E, Biberfeld G. A new pathogenic human retrovirus of West African origin (SBLV-6669) and its relationship to HTLV-IV, LAV-2, and HTLV-III_B. J Aids Res Human Retroviruses, in press.
16. Kanki PJ, Alroy J, Essex M (1985). Isolation of T-lymphotropic retrovirus related to HTLV-III/LAV from wild-caught African green monkeys. Science 230:951.
17. Sodroski JA, Rosen C, Haseltine WA (1984). Trans-acting transcriptional activation of the long terminal repeat of human T-lymphotropic viruses infected cells. Science 225:381.
18. Arya SK, Gallo RC, Hahn BH, Shaw GM, Popovic M, Salahuddin SZ, Wong-Staal F (1984). Homology of genomes of

AIDS-associated virus with genomes of human T-cell leukemia viruses. Science 225:927.

19. Felber BK, Paskalis H, Kleinman-Ewing C, Wong-Staal F, Pavlakis G (1985). The pX protein of human T-cell leukemia virus-I is a transcriptional activator of its long terminal repeats. Science 229:675.
20. Cann AJ, Rosenblatt JD, Wachsman W, Shah NP, Chen, ISY (1985). Identification of the gene responsible for human T cell leukemia virus transcriptional regulation. Nature 318: 517.
21. Sodroski JG, Rosen CA, Wong-Staal F, Salahuddin SZ, Popovic M, Arya SK, Gallo RC, Haseltine WA (1985). Trans-acting transcriptional regulation of human T-cell leukemia virus type III long terminal repeat. Science 227:171.
22. Arya SK, Guo C, Josephs SF, Wong-Staal F (1985). Trans-activator gene of human T-lymphotropic virus type III (HTLV-III). Science 229:69.
23. Arya SK, Gallo RC (1986). Three novel genes of human T-lymphotropic retrovirus-III (HTLV-III): immune reactivity of their products with sera from AIDS patients. Proc Natl Acad Sci USA 83:2209.
24. Sodroski JG, Patarca R, Rosen C, Haseltine WA (1985). Location of the trans-acting region on the genome of human T-cell lymphotropic virus type-III. Science 229:74.
25. Dayton AI, Sodroski JG, Rosen CA, Goh WC, Haseltine WA (1986). The trans-activator gene of the human T-cell lymphotropic virus type III is required for replication. Cell 44:941.
26. Fisher AG, Feinberg MB, Josephs SJ, Harper ME, Marselle LM, Reyes G, Gonda MA, Aldovini A, Debouk C, Gallo RC, Wong-Staal F (1986). The trans-activator gene of HTLV-III is essential for virus replication. Nature 320:367.
27. Gorman CM, Moffat LF, Howard BH (1982). Recombinant genomes which express chloramphenicol acetyltransferase in mammalian cells. Mol Cell Biol 2:1044.
28. Rosen CA, Sodroski JG, Haseltine WA (1985). Location of cis-acting regulatory sequences in the human T cell lymphotropic virus type III (HTLV-III/LAV) long terminal repeat. Cell 41:813.
29. Jones KA, Kadonaga JT, Luciw PA, Tjian R (1986). Activation of the AIDS retrovirus promoter by the cellular transcription factor, SP1. Science 232:755.
30. Muesing MA, Smith DH, Capon DJ (1987). Regulation of mRNA accumulation by a human immunodeficiency virus trans-activator protein. Cell 48:691.

Human Retroviruses, Cancer, and AIDS: Approaches to Prevention and Therapy, pages 57–74

MOLECULAR CLONING AND NUCLEOTIDE SEQUENCE ANALYSIS OF HTLV-4: COMPARISON TO OTHER HUMAN AND SIMIAN IMMUNODEFICIENCY-ASSOCIATED VIRUSES*

Beatrice H. Hahn,[1] Prasanna Kumar,[1] Marie E. Taylor,[1] Suresh K. Arya,[2] and George M. Shaw[1]

[1]Division of Hematology-Oncology, University of Alabama at Birmingham, Birmingham, Alabama 35294

[2]Laboratory of Tumor Cell Biology, National Institutes of Health, Bethesda, MD 20895

ABSTRACT Three independent isolates of HTLV-4 were analyzed by restriction endonuclease mapping, molecular cloning, and/or partial nucleotide sequencing. Restriction patterns of all isolates were indistinguishable from each other and from three independent isolates of STLV-3/AGM. Nucleotide sequences of LTR, env, 3' orf, and central viral regions were 99% identical, indicating that the HTLV-4 and STLV-3 isolates reported to date are all members of a single viral species. Comparison of STLV-3/HTLV-4 to HIV-2 (LAV-2) and HIV-1 demonstrated a similar genomic organization in all these viruses. STLV-3/HTLV-4 differed from

*This work was supported in part by National Institutes of Health grants AI 23616 and AI 23854 and by the U.S. Army Medical Research Acquisition Activity, Contract No. DAMD17-87-C-7038 and by a grant from Life and Health Insurance Medical Research Fund. B.H.H. is a Special Fellow of the Leukemia Society of America and G.M.S. is a Pew Scholar in the Biomedical Sciences.

HIV-2 in 25% of its nucleotide sequence, while both STLV-3/HTLV-4 and HIV-2 differed from HIV-1 in approximately 50% to 60% of their nucleotide sequence. Sequence alignment revealed that STLV-3/HTLV-4 and HIV-2 contain a novel, highly conserved potential coding region, termed X, that is not present in HIV-1. These data show that STLV-3/HTLV-4 and HIV-2 are equally distant from HIV-1 and suggest that STLV-3/HTLV-4 represents a third, phylogenetically-distinct subgroup of African immunodeficiency viruses.

INTRODUCTION

Human Immunodeficiency Virus Type 1 (HIV-1), formerly termed HTLV-3 or LAV, is the etiological agent of AIDS in central Africa, Europe, the United States, and most other countries worldwide. A second major group of human and primate T-lymphotropic, immunodeficiency-associated retroviruses related to but distinct from HIV-1 was discovered by Essex, Kanki, and co-workers in Africa in 1985 (1,2). Reasoning that HIV-1 could have evolved from a related primate retrovirus, these investigators screened sera from human and monkey populations for reactivity to HIV-1 and a related simian C-type retrovirus, STLV-3/MAC, discovered earlier in captive rhesus monkeys with AIDS-like illness (3,4). Healthy wild-caught African green monkeys and healthy Senegalese people at increased risk for sexually-transmitted disease showed strong serologic reactivity to a virus more closely related to STLV-3 than to HIV-1 (1,2). Subsequently, Kanki, et. al., reported the isolation of STLV-3/AGM from six African green monkeys (1) and HTLV-4 from three Senegalese prostitutes (2). At the same time French investigators reported the isolation of a West African retrovirus HIV-2 (LAV-2) which, like HTLV-4, was structurally and antigenetically more related to STLV-3 than to HIV-1 (5). However, unlike HTLV-4, this virus was isolated from patients with full-blown AIDS who had repeatedly been shown not to be infected with HIV-1. Thus, while HIV-1 infection in populations worldwide has been associated with immune suppression and AIDS, infection with the other STLV-3-related group of viruses has not uniformly been associated with disease.

In order to define more precisely the genetic relatedness of the STLV-3-like viruses to each other and to HIV-1 and to elucidate the genetic basis for their respective biological properties, considerable attention is now focusing on their nucleotide sequence and genetic structure. Recently, Mullins and co-workers published a detailed restriction enzyme analysis of six independent STLV-3 isolates from African green monkeys and three independent HTLV-4 isolates from healthy Senegalese prostitutes, finding all nine viral isolates plus three other STLV-3/MAC isolates virtually identical by careful restriction enzyme mapping (6). These remarkable similarities contrast with considerable differences in restriction enzyme cleavage patterns reported for isolates of HIV-1 (7), HIV-2 (19) and an STLV-3 isolate from a sooty mangabey (8) and, in turn, have raised questions as to the authenticity of these HTLV-4 and STLV-3 isolates (6,8). To determine on a nucleotide sequence level exactly how and to what extent HTLV-4 relates to STLV-3, HIV-2, and HIV-1 we have utilized a combination of restriction enzyme mapping, molecular cloning and nucleotide sequencing to analyze and compare different isolates of HTLV-4 with molecularly cloned and sequenced isolates of STLV-3, HIV-2 (LAV-2) and HIV-1.

RESULTS

Three HTLV-4 isolates (HTLV-4/PK82, HTLV-4/PK289, HTLV-4/PK190; ref. 2) and two STLV-3 isolates (STLV-3/AGM-K1, STLV-3/AGM-Mm6324; ref. 1) were obtained from Drs. Phyllis Kanki and Myron Essex. A virus-specific, partial cDNA clone was prepared from the RNA of isolate HTLV-4/PK190 and STLV-3/AGM-K1 (17). A virus-specific insert from one of these cDNA clones was then used to probe recombinant lambda phage libraries prepared from HTLV-4/PK82 and HTLV-4/PK289 infected DNA. Full-length proviral DNA clones including flanking cellular sequences were obtained for both HTLV-4 viruses. Southern blot analysis of STLV-3/AGM-K1, STLV-3/AGM-Mm6324, HTLV-4/PK82, and HTLV-4/PK289 infected cellular DNA as well as Southern blot analysis of the full-length lambda phage clones derived from the two HTLV-4 isolates demonstrated that all viral genomes were identical to each other in 19 out of 19 restriction enzyme sites mapped (9).

Proviral or cDNA clones of HTLV-4/PK82, HTLV-4/PK190

TABLE 1

NUCLEOTIDE SEQUENCE HOMOLOGY BETWEEN HTLV4/PK82 AND OTHER HUMAN AND SIMIAN IMMUNODEFICIENCY-ASSOCIATED RETROVIRUSES

viruses	basepairs compared	basepairs matched	basepairs unmatched (ins/del)	genomic regions compared	**% homology**
HTLV4/PK82 / HIV2/ROD	5391 / 5397	4138	175	central region, env 3'orf, LTR, gag	**77**
HTLV4/PK82 / HIV1/BH10	5391 / 5312	2928	519	"	**55**
HTLV4/PK82 / HIV1/LAVEli	5391 / 5311	2919	494	"	**55**
HIV2/ROD / HIV/BH10	5397 / 5312	2568	276	"	**48**
HIV2/ROD / HIV1/LAVEli	5397 / 5311	2872	521	"	**54**
HIV1/BH10 / HIV1/LAVEli	5312 / 5311	4702	49	"	**88**

Table 1 Continued

viruses	basepairs compared	basepairs matched	basepairs unmatched (ins/del)	genomic regions compared	**% homology**
HTLV4/PK82 / HTLV4/PK190	850 / 850	844	0	3'orf/LTR	**99**
HTLV4/PK82 / STLV3/K1	1178 / 1169	1163	9	3'orf/LTR	**99**
HTLV4/PK82 / STLV3/K2	4178 / 4175	4121	5	central region, env	**99**
HTLV4/PK82 / STLV3/K6	2670 / 2670	2654	0	env	**99**

HTLV-4/PK190 is represented by cDNA clone pV2, and STLV-3/K1 by cDNA clone pPBS3 (17). The nucleotide sequences of STLV-3/K2, HIV-2/ROD, HIV-1/BH-10 and HIV-1/LAVEli have been published (14,12,10,11) and the sequence of STLV-3/K6 was kindly provided by Drs. M. Reitz and G. Franchini prior to publication. All sequences were optimally aligned using the computer programs NUCALN and MICROGENIE. Homology is expressed as a percentage of the number of matching nucleotides divided by the total number of nucleotides compared (insertions and deletion are excluded).

and STLV-3/AGM-K1 were then subjected to DNA sequence analysis. For the proviral clone representing HTLV-4/PK82, the region sequenced included the entire LTR, gag p16 equivalent, central viral region, env, and 3' open reading frame (3' orf or F). For the cDNA clones representing HTLV-4/PK190 and STLV-3/AGM-K1, the sequence included R and U3 LTR regions and portions of 3' orf. Table 1 compares the nucleotide sequences of these clones with those of two other independent isolates of STLV-3, as well as with isolates of HIV-1 and HIV-2. The analysis shows that all five HTLV-4 and STLV-3 genomes are conserved to 99% in nucleotide sequence including various genomic regions like the central viral region, the envelope, 3'orf, LTR and gag. HIV-2 differs in 25% nucleotide sequence from STLV-3/HTLV-4 in these same regions. Comparison of STLV-3/HTLV-4 and HIV-2 to BH-10, an American prototype AIDS virus (10), and to LAVEli, an AIDS virus isolate from Zaire (11), demonstrates considerably less genome homology (40% to 50%), but also shows that HIV-1 is equally distant from both STLV-3/HTLV-4 and HIV-2.

The genomic regions of HTLV-4/PK82 selected for sequence analysis in this study were chosen because they correspond to regions in HIV-1 that are known to vary maximally (env, 3' orf) and because they include regions known to be unique to this group of immunodeficiency-associated viruses (tat, art/trs, sor, R, 3' orf). Figure 1 shows 5,391 basepairs of HTLV-4/PK82 sequence aligned with 5,397 basepairs of HIV-2 (LAV-2) sequence (12).

The sequence begins with the 3' terminus of a reading frame corresponding to the sor (or Q) of HIV-1 and HIV-2. The function of the sor protein in HIV-1 is unknown, although it has been observed that sor defective mutant viruses are morphologically normal in appearance but are poorly infectious (13).

The first major open reading frame in HTLV-4 and HIV-2 3' of sor is designated X. This region overlaps with the 3' terminus of sor and potentially encodes a protein of 112 amino acids in length. As shown in Figure 1, the X regions of HTLV-4 and HIV-2 are highly conserved having identical 94 out of 112 deduced amino acids. There is a methionine at amino acid position 2 of the X orf, and the deduced polypeptide sequence contains the unusual feature of seven contiguous proline residues at its carboxyterminus.

The reading frame following X in HTLV-4 and HIV-2 is

designated R. Its potential coding area is also highly conserved between HTLV-4 and HIV-2 and corresponds to an analogous region in HIV-1. The R region in HTLV-4 potentially encodes a polypeptide 97 amino acids in length compared to 105 amino acids in HIV-2. Although a biologic function for the R protein has not yet been determined, it is apparently made since HIV-1 infected individuals make antibodies to it (13).

Overlapping with R is a fourth open reading frame which is present both in HTLV-4 and HIV-2 and possesses considerable amino acid homology with the tat region of HIV-1. Although a transcriptional map of HTLV-4 is not available, by analogy with HIV-1 and HIV-2 the HTLV-4 tat gene is most likely comprised of three exons including a 5' leader sequence, a first coding exon in the central region, and a second coding region within the envelope region. Splice donor and acceptor sites likely to be utilized in HTLV-4 are shown in Figure 1 in comparison to analogous sites proposed for HIV-2 (12). Most of the homology in the deduced amino acid sequences of the HTLV-4 and HIV-2 tat genes is located in the 3' two-thirds of the first coding exon. It is this region that is believed to be important for the biological activity of the respective tat proteins.

The last open reading frame present in the central region of HTLV-4 and LAV-2 is designated art. This region most likely corresponds to the first coding exon of art/trs in HIV-1. In contrast to HIV-2, an open reading frame potentially encoding a protein of 125 amino acids is present in the sequence of HTLV-4. The same region in HIV-2 (and HIV-1) is abbreviated by a series of inframe stop codons. Whether or not this longer open reading frame in HTLV-4 has any biological significance is presently unknown. The second exon of art/trs can be better aligned and encodes a polypeptide of 84 amino acids in HTLV-4 which is 62% homologous to HIV-2 and 30% homologous to HIV-1. As for tat the region of highest amino acid conservation in art/trs highlights an area of basic, hydrophylic amino acid residues which most likely comprises a nucleic acid binding region.

The HTLV-4 and HIV-2 envelope open reading frames follow 3' to the central viral region. The first methionine codon of HTLV-4 corresponds in location to the first methionine codon of HIV-2. The length of the signal peptide of the HTLV-4 and HIV-2 envelope precursor has not yet been determined but is approximately 30 amino acids

```
                                                X M S D P R E R I P P G N S G E E T I G E
sor A H R Y Q V P S L Q Y L A L K V V S           D V R S Q G E N P T W K Q W R R D N R R
GAGCTCATAGGTACCAGGTACCAAGCCTACAGTACTTAGCACTAAAAGTAGTAAGC---GATGTCAGATCCCAGGGAGAGAATCCCACCTGGAAACAGTGGAGAAGAGACAATAGGAGAG  117  HTLV4/PK
GAGCTCATAGAGCCCAGGTACCGTCACTTCAATTTCTGGCCTTAGTGGTAGTGCAACAAAATGACAGACCCCAGAGAGACAGTACCACCAGGAAACAGCGGCGAAGAGACTATCGGAGAG  120  HIV2/LAV2
sor A H R A Q V P S L Q F L A L V V V Q Q N D R P Q R D S T T R K Q R R R D Y R R
                                                X M T D P R E T V P P G N S G E E T I G E

 A F E W L N R T V E E I N R E A V N H L P R E L I F Q V W Q R S W E Y W H D E Q
G L R M A K Q N S R G D K Q R G S K P P T K G A D F P G L A K V L G I L A *
GCCTTCGAATGGCTAAACAGAACAGTAGAGGAGATAAACAGAGAGGCAGTAAACCACCTACCAAGGGAGCTGATTTTCCAGGTTTGGCAAAGGTCTTGGGAATACTGGCATGATGAACAA  237  HTLV4/PK
GCCTTCGCCTGGCTAAACAGGACAGTAGAAGCCATAAACAGAGAAGCAGTGAATCACCTACCCCGAGAACTTATTTTCCAGGTGTGGCAGAGGTCCTGGAGATACTGGCATGATGAACAA  240  HIV2/LAV2
G L R L A K Q D S R S H K Q R S S E S P T P R T Y F P G V A E V L E I L A *
 A F A W L N R T V E A I N R E A V N H L P R E L I F Q V W Q R S W R Y W H D E Q

 G M S Q S Y V K Y R Y L C L M Q K A L F M H C K K G C R C L G E G H G A G G W R
GGGATGTCACAAAGCTATGTAAAATACAGATACTTGTGTTTAATGCAAAAGGCTTTATTTATGCATTGCAAGAAAGGCTGTAGATGTCTAGGGGAAGGACACGGGGCAGGGGGATGGAGA  357  HTLV4/PK
GGGATGTCAGAAAGTTACACAAAGTATAGATATTTGTGCATAATACAGAAAGCAGTGTACATGCATGTTAGGAAAGGGTGTACTTGCCTGGGGAGGGGACATGGGCCAGGAGGGTGGAGA  360  HIV2/LAV2
 G M S E S Y T K Y R Y L C I I Q K A V Y M H V R K G C T C L G R G H G P G G W R

 P G P P P P P P P P G L A *R M E E R P P E             N E G P Q R E P W D E W V V E V
CCAGGACCTCCTCCTCCTCCCCCTCCAGGACTAGCATAAATGGAAGAAAGACCTCCAGAA------------AATGAAGGCCCACAAAGGGAACCATGGGATGAATGGGTAGTGGAGGTT  465  HTLV4/PK
CCAGGGCCTCCTCCTCCTCCCCCTCCAGGTCTGGTCTA-ATGGCTGAAGCACCAACAGAGCTCCCCCCGGTGGATGGGACCCCACTGAGGGAGCCAGGGGATGAGTGGATAATAGAAATC  479  HIV2/LAV2
 P G P P P P P P P P G L V *R M A E A P T E L P P V D G T P L R E P G D E W I I E I

                                                               tat M E T P L R E Q E N S L E
 L E E L K E E A L K H F D P R L L T T L G N H I Y N R H G D T L E G A G E L I R
CTGGAAGAATTGAAAGAAGAAGCTTTAAAACATTTTGATCCTCGCTTGCTAACTACACTTGGTAATCATATCTATAATAGACATGGAGACACCCTTGAGGGAGCAGGAGAACTCATTAGA  585  HTLV4/PK
TTGAGAGAAATAAAAGAAGAAGCTTTAAAGCATTTTGACCCTCGCTTGCTAATTGCTCTTGGCAAATATATCTATACTAGACATGGAGACACCCTTGAAGGCGCCAGAGAGCTCATTAAA  599  HIV2/LAV2
 L R E I K E E A L K H F D P R L L I A L G K Y I Y T R H G D T L E G A R E L I K
                                                               tat M E T P L K A P E S S L K

                        art ? M Q P L Q N R P T W G R K S S L N Y T A L L R R A I T
 S S N E R S S C I L E A D A T T P E S A N L G E E I L S Q L Y R P L E A C Y N T
 I L Q R A L F M H F R G G C N H S R I G Q P G G G N P L S T I P P S *
ATCCTCCAACGAGCGCTCTTCATGCATTTTAGAGGCGGATGCAACCACTCCAGAATCGGCCAACCTGGGGGAGGAAATCCTCTCTCAACTATACCGCCCTCTTGAGGCGTGCTATAACAC  705  HTLV4/PK
GTCCTGCAACGAGCCCTTTTCACGCACTTCAGAGCAGGATGTGGCCACTCAAGAATTGGCCAGACAAGGGGAGGAAATCCTCTCTCAGCTATACCGACCCCTAGAAACATGCAATAACTC  719  HIV2/LAV2
 V L Q R A L F T H F R A G C G H S R I G Q T R G G N P L S A I P T P R N M Q *
 S C N E P F S R T S E Q D V A T Q E L A R Q G E E I L S Q L Y R P L E T C N N S

H A I V K S V A T I A S F V F L K R D W G Y V M S S H E R E E E L R K R L R L I
 C Y C K K C C Y H C Q F C F L K K G L G I C Y E Q S R K R R R T P K K A K A N T
ATGCTATTGTAAAAAGTGTTGCTACCATTGCCAGTTTTGTTTTCTTAAAAAGGGATTGGGGATATGTTATGAGCAGTCACGAAAGAGAAGAAGAACTCCGAAAAAGGCTAAGGCTAATAC  825  HTLV4/PK
ATGCTATTGTAAGCGATGCTGCTACCATTGTCAGATGTGTTTTCTAAACAAGGGGCTCGGGATATGTTATGAACGAAAGGGCAGACGAAGAAGGACTCCAAAGAAAACTAAGACTCATCC  839  HIV2/LAV2
 C Y C K R C C Y H C Q M C F L N K G L G I C Y E R K G R R R R R T P K K T K T H P
                                                          art M N E R A D E E G L Q R K L R L I

H L L H Q T S K Y G M S W E S A A Y R H L A F K C L W D L L Y S I C H S L L W C
 S S A S N K *
               env M G C L G N Q L L I A I L L L S V Y G I Y C T Q Y V T V F Y G V
ATCTTCTGCATCAAACAAGTAAGTATGGGATGTCTTGGGAATCAGCTGCTTATCGCCATCTTGCTTTTAAGTGTCTATGGGATCTATTGTACTCAATATGTCACAGTCTTTTATGGTGTA  945  HTLV4/PK
GTCTCCTACACCAGACAAGTGAGTATG---------ATGAATCAGCTGCTTATTGCCATTTTATTAGCTAGTGCTTGCTTAGTATATTGCACCCAATATGTAACTGTTTTCTATGGCGTA  950  HIV2/LAV2
               env M             M N Q L L I A I L L A S A C L V Y C T Q Y V T V F Y G V
 S P T P D K *
P L L H Q T S E Y           D E S A A Y C H F I S *

T S L E E C D N S P L L C N Q E *
 P A W R N A T I P L F C A T K N R D T W G T T Q C L P D N G D Y S E L A L N V T
CCAGCTTGGAGGAATGCGACAATTCCCCTCTTCTGTGCAACCAAGAATAGGGATACTTGGGGAACAACTCAGTGCCTACCAGATAATGGTGATTATTCAGAATTGGCCCTTAATGTTACA  1065  HTLV4/PK
CCCACGTGGAAAAATGCAACCATTCCCCTCTTTTGTGCAACCAGAAATAGGGATACTTGGGGAACCATACAGTGCTTGCCTGACAATGATGATTATCAGGAAATAACTTTGAATGTAACA  1070  HIV2/LAV2
 P T W K N A T I P L F C A T R N R D T W G T I Q C L P D N D D Y Q E I T L N V T
```

Figure 1, part 1

```
E  S  F  D  A  W  E  N  T  V  T  E  Q  A  I  E  D  V  W  Q  L  F  E  T  S  I  K  P  C  V  K  L  S  P  L  C  I  T  M  R
GAAAGCTTTGATGCTTGGGAGAATACAGTCACAGAACAGGCAATAGAGGACGTATGGCAACTCTTTGAGACCTCAATAAAGCCTTGTGTAAAATTATCCCCATTATGCATTACTATGAGA  1185  HTLV4/PK
GAGGCTTTTGATGCATGCAATAATACAGTAACAGAACAAGCAATAGAAGATGTCTGGCATCTATTCGAGACATCAATAAAACCATGTGTCAAACTAACACCTTTATGTGTAGCAATGAAA  1190  HIV2/LAV2
E  A  F  D  A  C  N  N  T  V  T  E  Q  A  I  E  D  V  W  H  L  F  E  T  S  I  K  P  C  V  K  L  T  P  L  C  V  A  M  K

C  N  K  S  E  T  D  R  W  G  L  T  K  S  S  T  T  I  T  T  A  A  P  T  S  A  P  V  S  E  K  I  D  M  V  N  E  T  S  S
TGCAATAAAAGTGAGACAGATAGATGGGGATTGACAAAATCATCAACAACAATAACAACAGCAGCACCAACATCAGCACCAGTATCAGAAAAAATAGACATGGTCAATGAGACTAGTTCT  1305  HTLV4/PK
TGCAGCAGCACAGAGAGCAGCACAGGGAACAACACAACCTCAAAGAGCACAAGCACAACCACAACCACACCCACAGACCAGGAGCAAGAGATAAGT------------GAGGATACTCCA  1298  HIV2/LAV2
C  S  S  T  E  S  S  T  G  N  N  T  T  S  K  S  T  S  T  T  T  T  T  P  T  D  Q  E  Q  E  I  S              E  D  T  P

C  I  A  Q  N  N  C  T  G  L  E  Q  E  Q  M  I  S  C  K  F  T  M  T  G  L  K  R  D  K  T  K  E  Y  N  E  T  W  Y  S  T
TGTATAGCTCAGAATAATTGCACAGGCTTGGAACAAGAGCAAATGATAAGCTGTAAATTCACCATGACAGGGTTAAAAAGAGACAAGACAAAGGAGTACAATGAAACTTGGTACTCTACA  1425  HTLV4/PK
TCGCCACGCGCAGACAACTGCTCAGGATTGGGAGAGGAAGAAACGATCAATTGCCAGTTCAATATGACAGGATTAGAAAGAGATAAGAAAAAACAGTATAATGAAACATGGTACTCAAAA  1418  HIV2/LAV2
S  P  R  A  D  N  C  S  G  L  G  E  E  E  T  I  N  C  Q  F  N  M  T  G  L  E  R  D  K  K  K  Q  Y  N  E  T  W  Y  S  K

D  L  V  C  E  Q  G  N  S  T  D  N  E  S  R  C  Y  I  N  H  C  N  T  S  V  I  Q  E  S  C  D  K  H  Y  W  D  T  I  R  F
GATTTGGTTTGTGAACAAGGGAATAGCACTGATAATGAAAGCAGATGCTACATAAATCACTGTAACACTTCTGTTATCCAAGAGTCTTGTGACAAACATTATTGGGATACTATTAGATTT  1545  HTLV4/PK
GATGTGGTTTGTGAGACAAATAATAGCACA---AATCAGACCCAGTGTTACATGAACCATTGCAACACATCAGTCATCACAGAATCATGTGACAAGCACTATTGGGATGCTATAAGGTTT  1535  HIV2/LAV2
D  V  V  C  E  T  N  N  S  T     N  Q  T  Q  C  Y  M  N  H  C  N  T  S  V  I  T  E  S  C  D  K  H  Y  W  D  A  I  R  F

R  Y  C  A  P  P  G  Y  A  L  L  R  C  N  D  T  N  Y  S  G  F  M  P  K  C  S  K  V  V  V  S  S  C  T  R  M  M  E  T  Q
AGGTATTGTGCACCTCCAGGTTATGCTTTGCTTAGATGTAATGACACAAATTATTCAGGCTTTATGCCTAAATGTTCTAAGGTGGTGGTCTCTTCATGCACAAGGATGATGGAGACACAG  1665  HTLV4/PK
AGATACTGTGCACCACCGGGTTATGCCCTATTAAGATGTAATGATACCAATTATTCAGGCTTTGCACCCAACTGTTCTAAAGTAGTAGCTTCTACATGCACCAGGATGATGGAAACGCAA  1655  HIV2/LAV2
R  Y  C  A  P  P  G  Y  A  L  L  R  C  N  D  T  N  Y  S  G  F  A  P  N  C  S  K  V  V  A  S  T  C  T  R  M  M  E  T  Q

T  S  T  W  F  G  F  N  G  T  R  A  E  N  R  T  Y  I  Y  W  H  G  R  D  N  R  T  I  I  S  L  N  K  Y  Y  N  L  T  M  K
ACTTCTACTTGGTTTGGCTTTAATGGAACTAGAGCAGAAAATAGAACTTATATTTACTGGCATGGTAGGGATAATAGGACTATAATTAGTTTAAATAAGTATTATAATCTAACAATGAAA  1785  HTLV4/PK
ACTTCCACATGGTTTGGCTTTAATGGCACTAGAGCAGAGAATAGAACATATATCTATTGGCATGGCAGAGATAATAGAACTATCATCAGCTTAAACAAATATTATAATCTCAGTTTGCAT  1775  HIV2/LAV2
T  S  T  W  F  G  F  N  G  T  R  A  E  N  R  T  Y  I  Y  W  H  G  R  D  N  R  T  I  I  S  L  N  K  Y  Y  N  L  S  L  H

C  R  R  P  G  N  K  T  V  L  P  V  T  I  M  S  G  L  V  F  H  S  Q  P        I  N  D  R  P  K  Q  A  W  C  W  F  G  G
TGTAGAAGACCAGGAAATAAGACAGTTTTACCAGTCACCATTATGTCTGGATTGGTTTTCCACTCACAACCA------ATCAATGATAGGCCAAAGCAGGCATGGTGTTGGTTTGGAGGA  1899  HTLV4/PK
TGTAAGAGGCCAGGGAATAAGACAGTGAAACAAATAATGCTTATGTCAGGACATGTGTTTCACTCCCACTACCAGCCGATCAATAAAAGACCCAGACAAGCATGGTGCTGGTTCAAAGGC  1895  HIV2/LAV2
C  K  R  P  G  N  K  T  V  K  Q  I  M  L  M  S  G  H  V  F  H  S  H  Y  Q  P  I  N  K  R  P  R  Q  A  W  C  W  F  K  G

K  W  K  D  A  I  K  E  V  K  Q  T  I  V  K  H  P  R  Y  T  G  T     N  N  T  D  K  I  N  L  T  A  P  G  G  G  D  P  E
AAATGGAAGGATGCAATAAAAGAGGTGAAACAGACCATTGTCAAACATCCCAGGTATACTGGAACTA---ACAATACTGATAAAATCAATTTAACGGCTCCTGGAGGAGGAGATCCAGAA  2016  HTLV4/PK
AAATGGAAAGACGCCATGCAGGAGGTGAAGGAAACCCTTGCAAAACATCCCAGGTATAGAGGAACCAATGACACAAGGAATATTAGCTTTGCAGCGCCAGGAAAAGGCTCAGACCCAGAA  2015  HIV2/LAV2
K  W  K  D  A  M  Q  E  V  K  E  T  L  A  K  H  P  R  Y  R  G  T  N  D  T  R  N  I  S  F  A  A  P  G  K  G  S  D  P  E

V  T  F  M  W  T  N  C  R  G  E  F  L  Y  C  K  M  N  W  F  L  N  W  V  E  D  R  D  V  T  T  Q  R  P  K  E  R  H  R  R
GTTACCTTCATGTGGACAAATTGCAGAGGAGAGTTCCTCTACTGTAAAATGAATTGGTTTCTAAATTGGGTAGAGGATAGGGATGTAACTACCCAGAGGCCAAAGGAACGGCATAGAAGG  2136  HTLV4/PK
GTAGCATACATGTGGACTAACTGCAGAGGAGAGTTTCTCTACTGCAACATGACTTGGTTCCTCAATTGGATAGAGAATAAGACACACCGC------------------------------  2105  HIV2/LAV2
V  A  Y  M  W  T  N  C  R  G  E  F  L  Y  C  N  M  T  W  F  L  N  W  I  E  N  K  T  H  R

N  Y  V  P  C  H  I  R  Q  V  I  N  T  W  H  K  V  G  K  N  V  Y  L  P  P  R  E  G  D  L  T  C  N  S  T  V  T  S  L  I
AATTACGTGCCGTGTCATATTAGACAAGTAATCAACACTTGGCATAAAGTAGGCAAAAATGTTTATTTGCCTCCAAGAGAGGGAGACCTCACGTGTAACTCCACAGTGACCAGTCTCATA  2256  HTLV4/PK
AATTATGCACCGTGCCATATAAAGCAAATAATTAACACATGGCATAAGGTAGGGAGAAATGTATATTTGCCTCCCAGGGAAGGGGAGCTGTCCTGCAACTCAACAGTAACCAGCATAATT  2225  HIV2/LAV2
N  Y  A  P  C  H  I  K  Q  I  I  N  T  W  H  K  V  G  R  N  V  Y  L  P  P  R  E  G  E  L  S  C  N  S  T  V  T  S  I  I

A  N  I  D  W  T  D  G  N  Q  T  N  I  T  M  S  A  E  V  A  E  L  Y  R  L  E  L  G  D  Y  K  L  V  E  I  T  P  I  G  L
GCAAACATAGATTGGACTGATGGAAACCAAACTAATATCACCATGAGTGCAGAGGTGGCAGAACTGTATCGATTGGAGTTGGGAGATTATAAATTAGTAGAGATCACTCCGATCGGCTTG  2376  HTLV4/PK
GCTAACATTGACTGGCAAAACAATAATCAGACAAACATTACCTTTAGTGCAGAGGTGGCAGAACTATACAGATTGGAGTTGGGAGATTATAAATTGGTAGAAATAACACCAATTGGCTTC  2345  HIV2/LAV2
A  N  I  D  W  Q  N  N  N  Q  T  N  I  T  F  S  A  E  V  A  E  L  Y  R  L  E  L  G  D  Y  K  L  V  E  I  T  P  I  G  F

A  P  T  D  V  K  R  Y  T  T  G  G  T  S  R  N  K  R  G  V  F  V  L  G  F  L  G  F  L  A  T  A  G  S  A  M  G  A  A  S
GCCCCCACAGATGTGAAGAGGTACACTACTGGTGGCACCTCAAGAAATAAAAGAGGGGTCTTTGTGCTAGGGTTCTTGGGTTTTCTCGCAACGGCAGGTTCTGCAATGGGCGCGGCGTCG  2496  HTLV4/PK
GCACCTACAAAAGAAAAAAGATACTCCTCTGCTCACGGG---AGACATACAAGAGGTGTGTTCGTGCTAGGGTTCTTGGGTTTTCTCGCAACAGCAGGTTCTGCAATGGGCGCGGCGTCC  2462  HIV2/LAV2
A  P  T  K  E  K  R  Y  S  S  A  H  G     R  H  T  R  G  V  F  V  L  G  F  L  G  F  L  A  T  A  G  S  A  M  G  A  A  S
```

Figure 1, part 2

```
L T L T A Q S R T L L A G I V Q Q Q Q Q L L D V V K R Q Q E L L R L T V W G T K
TTGACGCTGACCGCTCAGTCCCGGACTTTATTGGCTGGGATAGTGCAGCAACAGCAACAGCTGTTGGACGTGGTCAAGAGACAACAAGAATTGTTGCGACTGACCGTCTGGGGAACAAAG  2616  HTLV4/PK
CTGACCGTGTCGGCTCAGTCCCGGACTTTACTGGCCGGGATAGTGCAGCAACAGCAACAGCTGTTGGACGTGGTCAAGAGACAACAAGAACTGTTGCGACTGACCGTCTGGGGAACGAAA  2682  HIV2/LAV2
L T V S A Q S R T L L A G I V Q Q Q Q Q L L D V V K R Q Q E L L R L T V W G T K

N L Q T R V T A I E K Y L K D Q A Q L N T W G C A F R Q V C H T T V P W P N A S
AACCTCCAGACTAGGGTCACTGCCATCGAGAAGTACTTAAAGGACCAGGCGCAGCTGAATACTTGGGGATGTGCGTTTAGACAAGTCTGCCACACTACTGTACCATGGCCAAATGCAAGT  2736  HTLV4/PK
AACCTCCAGGCAAGAGTCACTGCTATAGAGAAGTACCTACAGGACCAGGCGCGGCTAAATTCATGGGGATGTGCGTTTAGACAAGTCTGCCACACTACTGTACCATGGGTTAATGATTCC  2702  HIV2/LAV2
N L Q A R V T A I E K Y L Q D Q A R L N S W G C A F R Q V C H T T V P W V N D S

L T P D W N N D T W Q E W E R K V D F L E E N I T A L L E E A Q I Q Q E K N M Y
CTAACACCAGACTGGAACAATGATACTTGGCAAGAGTGGGAGCGAAAGGTTGACTTCTTGGAGGAAAATATAACAGCCCTCCTAGAAGAGGCACAAATTCAACAAGAGAAGAACATGTAT  2856  HTLV4/PK
TTAGCACCTGACTGGGACAATATGACGTGGCAGGAATGGGAAAAACAAGTCCGCTACCTGGAGGCAAATATCAGTAAAAGTTTAGAACAGGCACAAATTCAGCAAGAGAAAAATATGTAT  2822  HIV2/LAV2
L A P D W D N M T W Q E W E K Q V R Y L E A N I S K S L E Q A Q I Q Q E K N M Y

E L Q K L N S W D V F G N W F D L A S W I K Y I Q Y G I Y V V V G V I L L R I V
GAATTACAAAAGTTAAATAGCTGGGATGTGTTTGGCAATTGGTTTGACCTTGCTTCTTGGATAAAGTATATACAATATGGAATTTATGTAGTTGTAGGAGTAATACTGTTAAGAATAGTG  2976  HTLV4/PK
GAACTACAAAAATTAAATAGCTGGGATATTTTTGGCAATTGGTTTGACTTAACCTCCTGGGTCAAGTATATTCAATATGGAGTGCTTATAATAGTAGCAGTAATAGCTTTAAGAATAGTG  2942  HIV2/LAV2
E L Q K L N S W D I F G N W F D L T S W V K Y I Q Y G V L I I V A V I A L R I V

                       art A S V L F P T L L F P V D S Y P T G P G T A N Q R
              tat G R G I G Q C S L P H P L I S S R L I P N R T R H C Q P E K
I Y I V Q M L A K L R Q G Y R P V F S S P P S Y F Q * T H T Q Q D P A L P T R E
ATCTATATAGTACAAATGCTAGCTAAGTTAAGGCAGGGGTATAGGCCAGTGTTCTCTTCCCCACCCTCTTATTTCCAGTAGACTCATACCCAACAGGACCCGGCACTGCCAACCAGAGAA  3096  HTLV4/PK
ATATATGTAGTACAAATGTTAAGTAGGCTTAGAAAGGGCTATAGGCCTGTTTTCTCTTCCCCCCCCGGTTATATCCAACAGATCCATATCCACAAGGACCGGGGACAGCCAGCCAACGAA  3062  HIV2/LAV2
I Y V V Q M L S R L R K G Y R P V F S S P P G Y I Q Q I H I H K D R G Q P A N E
          tat V G L E R A I G L F S L P P P V I S N R S I S T R T G D S Q P T K
                       art A C F L F P P R L Y P T D P Y P Q G P G T A S Q R

R Q R R R R W R R R W Q Q L L A L A D R I Y S F P D P P T D T P L D L A I Q Q L
 A K K E T V E K A V A T A P G L G R *
 G K E G D G G E G G G N S S W P W Q I E Y I H F L I R Q L I R L L T W L F S N C
GGCAAAGAAGGAGACGGTGGAGAAGGCGGTGGCAACAGCTCCTGGCCTTGGCAGATAGAATATATTCATTTCCTGATCCGCCAACTGATACGCCTCTTGACTTGGCTATTCAGCAACTGC  3216  HTLV4/PK
GAAACAGAAGAAGACGGTGGAAGCAACGGTGGAGACAGATACTGGCCCTGGCCGATAGCATATATACATTTCCTGATCCGCCAGCTGATTCGCCTCTTGACCAGACTATACAGCATCTGC  3182  HIV2/LAV2
 E T E E D G G S N G G D R Y W P W P I A Y I H F L I R Q L I R L L T R L Y S I C
 K Q K K T V E A T V E T D T G P G R *
R N R R R R W K Q R W R Q I L A L A D S I Y T F P D P P A D S P L D Q T I Q H L

                                                                     3'orf M G G
Q N L A I E S I P D P P T N T P E A L C D P T K D S R S P Q D *
 R T L L S R A Y Q I L Q P I L Q R L S A T L R R I R E V L R T E L T Y L Q Y G W
AGAACCTTGCTATCGAGAGCATACCAGATCCTCCAACCAATACTCCAGAGGCTCTCTGCGACCCTACGAAGGATTCGAGAAGTCCTCAGGACTGAACTGACCTACCTACAATATGGGTGG  3336  HTLV4/PK
AGGGACTTACTATCCAGGAGCTTCCTGACCCTCCAACTCATCTACCAGAATCTC---------------------AGAGACTGGCTGAGACTTAGAACAGCCTTCTTGCAATATGGGTGC  3281  HIV2/LAV2
 R D L L S R S F L T L Q L I Y Q N L                           R D W L R L R T A F L Q Y G C
Q G L T I Q E L P D P P T H L P E S                           Q R L A E T *
                                                                     3'orf M G A

 A I S M R R S K P A G D L R Q K L L R A R G E T Y G R L L G E V E D G S S Q S L
 S Y F H E A V Q A G W R S A T E T L A G A W G D L W E T L R R G G R W I L A I P
AGCTATTTCCATGAGGCGGTCCAAGCCGGCTGGAGATCTGCGACAGAAACTCTTGCGGGCGCGTGGGGAGACTTATGGGAGACTCTTAGGAGAGGTGGAAGATGGATCCTCGCAATCCCT  3456  HTLV4/PK
GAGTGGATCCAAGAAGCATTCCAGGCCGCCGCGAGGGCTACAAGAGAGACTCTTGCGGGCGCGTGCAGGGGCTTGTGGAGGGTATTGGAACGAATCGGGAGGGGAATACTCGCGGTTCCA  3401  HIV2/LAV2
 E W I Q E A F Q A A A R A T R E T L A G A C R G L W R V L E R I G R G I L A V P
 S G S K K H S R P P R G L Q E R L L R A R A G A C G G Y W N E S G G E Y S R F Q

R R I R Q G L E L T L L *
 G G L G K G L S S R S C E G Q K Y N Q G Q Y M N T P W R N P A E E K E K L A Y R
AGGAGGATTAGGCAAGGGCTTGAGCTCACGCTCTTGTGAGGGACAGAAATACAATCAGGGGCAGTATATGAATACTCCATGGAGAAACCCAGCTGAAGAAAAGGAAAAATTAGCATACAG  3576  HTLV4/PK
AGAAGGATCAGACAGGGAGCAGAAATCGCCCTCCTGTGAGGGACGGCAGTATCAGCAGGGAGACTTTATGAATACTCCATGGAAGGACCCAGCAGCAGAAAGGGAGAAAAATTTGTACAG  3521  HIV2/LAV2
 E G S D R E Q K S P S C E G R Q Y Q Q G D F M N T P W K D P A A E R E K N L Y R
R R I R Q G A E I A L L *
```

Figure 1, part 3

```
 K  Q  N  M  D  D  I  D  E  E  D  D  D  L  V  G  V  S  V  R  P  K  V  P  L  R  A  M  T  Y  K  L  A  I  D  M  S  H  F  I
AAAACAAAATATGGATGATATAGATGAGGAAGATGATGACTTGGTAGGGGTATCAGTGAGGCCAAAAGTTCCCCTAAGAGCAATGACTTACAAATTGGCAATAGATATGTCTCATTTTAT  3696  HTLV4/PK
GCAACAAAATATGGATGATGTAGATTCAGATGATGATGACCAAGTAAGAGTTTCTGTCACACCAAAAGTACCACTAAGACCAATGACACATAGATTGGCAATAGATATGTCACATTTAAT  3641  HIV2/LAV2
 Q  Q  N  M  D  D  V  D  S  D  D  D  D  Q  V  R  V  S  V  T  P  K  V  P  L  R  P  M  T  H  R  L  A  I  D  M  S  H  L  I

polypurine tract |--->LTR
 K  E  K  G  G  L  E  G  I  Y  Y  S  A  R  R  R  R  I  L  D  M  Y  L  E  K  E  E  G  I  I  P  D  W  Q  D  Y  T  S  G  P
AAAAGAAAAGGGGGACTGGAAGGGATTTATTACAGTGCAAGAAGACGTAGAATCTTAGACATGTACTTAGAAAAGGAAGAAGGCATCATACCAGATTGGCAGGATTACACCTCAGGACC  3816  HTLV4/PK
AAAAACAAGGGGGGGACTGGAAGGGATGTTTTACAGTGAAAGAAGACATAAAATCTTAAATATATACTTAGAAAAGGAAGAAGGGATAATTGCAGATTGGCAGAACTACACTCATGGGCC  3761  HIV2/LAV
 K  T  R  G  G  L  E  G  M  F  Y  S  E  R  R  H  K  I  L  N  I  Y  L  E  K  E  E  G  I  I  A  D  W  Q  N  Y  T  H  G  P
polypurine tract |--->LTR

 G  I  R  Y  P  K  T  F  G  W  L  W  K  L  V  P  V  N  V  S  D  E  A  Q  E  D  E  R  H  Y  L  M  Q  P  A  Q  T  S  K  W
AGGAATTAGATACCCAAAGACATTTGGCTGGCTATGGAAATTAGTCCCTGTAAATGTATCAGATGAGGCACAGGAGGATGAGAGGCATTATTTAATGCAGCCAGCTCAAACTTCCAAGTG  3936  HTLV4/PK
AGGAGTAAGATACCCAATGTTCTTTGGGTGGCTATGGAAGCTAGTACCAGTAGATGTCCCACAAGAAGGGGAGGACACTGAGACTCACTGCTTAGTACATCCAGCACAAACAAGCAAGTT  3881  HIV2/LAV2
 G  V  R  Y  P  M  F  F  G  W  L  W  K  L  V  P  V  D  V  P  Q  E  G  E  D  T  E  T  H  C  L  V  H  P  A  Q  T  S  K  F

 D  D  P  W  G  E  V  L  A  W  K  S  D  P  T  L  A  Y  T  Y  E  A  Y  V  R  Y  P  E  E  F  G  S  K  S  G  L  S  E  E  E
GGATGACCCTTGGGGAGAGGTTCTAGCGTGGAAGTCTGATCCAACTCTAGCCTACACTTATGAGGCATATGTTAGATACCCAGAAGAGTTTGGAAGCAAGTCAGGCCTGTCAGAGGAAGA  4052  HTLV4/PK
TGATGACCCGCATGGGGAGACACTAGTCTGGGAGTTTGATCCCTTGCTGGCTTATAGTTACGAGGCTTTTATTCGGTACCCAGAGGAATTTGGGCACAAGTCAGGCCTGCCAGAGGAAGA  4001  HIV2/LAV2
 D  D  P  H  G  E  T  L  V  W  E  F  D  P  L  L  A  Y  S  Y  E  A  F  I  R  Y  P  E  E  F  G  H  K  S  G  L  P  E  E  E

                                                                                                        core enhancer
 V  R  R  R  L  T  A  R  G  L  L  N  M  A  D  K  R  E  T                                            R  *
GGTTAGAAGAAGGCTAACCGCAAGAGGCCTTCTTAACATGGCTGACAAGAGGGAAACTC---------------------------------------GCTGAGACGGCAGGGACTTTCCA  4138  HTLV4/PK
GTGGAAGGCGAGACTGAAAGCAAGAGGAATAC----CATTTAGTTAAAGACAGGAACAGCTATACTTGGTCAGGGCAGGAAGTAACTAACAGAAACAGCTGAGACTGCAGGGACTTTCCA  4117  HIV2/LAV2
 W  K  A  R  L  K  A  R  G  I     P  F  S  *
                                                                                                        core enhancer

     SP1                      SP1       SP1                     tata box
CAAGGGGATGTTAT-------------GGGGAGGAGCCGGTCGGGAACACCCACTTTCTTGATGTATAAATATCACTGCATTTCGCTCTGTA--TTCAGTCGCTCTGCGGAGAGGCTGGT  4243  HTLV4/PK
GAAGGGGCTGTAACCAAGGGAGGGACATGGGAGGAGCTGGTGGGGAACGCCCTCATATTCTCTGTATAAATATACCCGCTAGCTTGCATTGTACTTCGGTCGCTCTGCGGAGAGGCTGGC  4237  HIV2/LAV2
     SP1                SP1       SP1       SP1                 tata box

AGATTGAGCCCTGGGAGGTTCTCTCCAGCACTAGCAGGTAGAGCCTGGGTGTTCCCTGCTAGACTCTCACCAGCACTTGGCCAGTGCTGGGCAGAGTGGCTCCACGCTTGCTTGCTTAAA  4363  HTLV4/PK
AGATTGAGCCCTGGGAGGTTCTCTCCAGCAGTAGCAGGTAGAGCCTGGGTGTTCCCTGCTAGACTCTCACCAGCACTTGGCCGGTGCTGGGCAGAC-GGCCCCACGCTTGCTTGCTTAAA  4356  HIV2/LAV2

      polyA signal
GACCTCTTCAATAAAGCTGCCATTTTAGAAGTAAGCCAGTGTGTGTTCCCATCTCTCCTAGTCGCCGCCTGGTCAACTCGGTACTCGGTAATAAGGGGACCCCTGGTCTGTTAGGACCCT  4483  HTLV4/PK
AACCTCCTTAATAAAGCTGCCAGTTAGAAGCAAGTTAAGTGTGTGCTCCCATCTCTCCTAGTCGCCGCCTGGTCATTCGGTGTTCACCTGAGTAACAAGACCCTGGTCTGTTAGGACCCT  4476  HIV2/LAV2
      polyA signal

                                LTR<---|  primer binding site
TTCTGCTTTGGGAAACCGAGGCAGGAAGATCCCTAGCAGGTTGGCGCCCGAACAGGGACTTGAAGGAGAGTGAGAGACTCCTGAGTACGGCTGAGTGAAGGCGGTAAGGGCGGCAGGAAC  4603  HTLV4/PK
TCTTGCTTTGGGAAACCGAGGCAGGAAAATCCCTAGCAGGTTGGCGCCTGAACAGGGACTTGAAGAAGACTGAGAAGTCTTGGAACACGGCTGAGTGAAGGCAGTAAGGGCGGCAGGAAC  4596  HIV2/LAV2
                                LTR<---|  primer binding site

CAACCACG-CGGAGTGCTCCTATAAAGGCGCGGGTCGGTACCAGACG----GCGTGAGGAGCGGGAGAGGAGGAGGCCTCCG-GTGCAGGTAAGTGCAACACAAAAAAGAAATAGCTGT-  4716  HTLV4/PK
AAACCACGACGGAGTGCTCCTAGAAAGGCGCGGGCCGAGGTACCAAAGGCAGCGTGTGGAGCGGGAGGAGAAGAGGCCTCCGGGTGAAGGTAAGTACCTACACCAAAAACTGTAGCCGAA  4716  HIV2/LAV2

                                      gag M  G  A  R  N  S  V  L  S  G  K  K  A  D  K  L  E  K  I  R  L  R  P  G  G
----CTTGTTATCCAAGAAGGGATAATAAGATAGA--GTGGGAGATGGGCGCGAGAAACTCCGTCTTGTCAGGGAAGAAAGCAGATAAATTAGAAAAAATTAGGCTACGACCCGGCGGAA  4830  HTLV4/PK
AGGGCTTGCTATCCTACCTTTAGACAGGTAGAAGATTGTGGGAGATGGGCGCGAGAAACTCCGTCTTGAGAGGGAAAAAAGCAGATGAATTAGAAAGAATCAGGTTACGGCCCGGCGGAA  4836  HIV2/LAV2
                                      gag M  G  A  R  N  S  V  L  R  G  K  K  A  D  E  L  E  R  I  R  L  R  P  G  G

K  K  K  Y  M  L  K  H  V  V  W  A  A  N  E  L  D  R  F  G  L  A  E  S  L  L  E  N  K  E  G  C  Q  K  I  L  S  V  L  A
AGAAAAAGTACATGTTGAAGCATGTAGTATGGGCAGCAAATGAATTAGATAGATTTGGATTAGCAGAAAGCCTGTTGGAGAACAAAGAAGGATGTCAAAAAATACTTTCGGTCTTAGCTC  4950  HTLV4/PK
AGAAAAAGTACAGGCTAAAACATATTGTGTGGGCAGCGAATAAATTGGACAGATTCGGATTAGCAGAGAGCCTGTTGGAGTCAAAAGAGGGTTGTCAAAAAATTCTTACAGTTTTAGATC  4956  HIV2/LAV2
K  K  K  Y  R  L  K  H  I  V  W  A  A  N  K  L  D  R  F  G  L  A  E  S  L  L  E  S  K  E  G  C  Q  K  I  L  T  V  L  D
```

Figure 1, part 4

```
P  L  V  P  T  G  S  E  N  L  K  S  L  Y  N  T  V  C  V  I  W  C  I  H  A  E  E  K  V  K  H  T  E  E  A  K  Q  I  V  Q
CATTAGTGCCAACAGGCTCAGAAAATTTAAAAAGCCTTTATAATACTGTCTGCGTCATCTGGTGCATTCACGCAGAAGAGAAAGTGAAACACACTGAGGAAGCAAAACAGATAGTGCAGA  5070  HTLV4/PK
:: : :: :: ::::: :::::::::::::::: :::: :::::::::::::::::: :::::::: :::::::::::::::::::: : ::::: : ::::::::: ::::::: ::
CAATGGTACCGACAGGTTCAGAAAATTTAAAAAGTCTTTTTAATACTGTCTGCGTCATTTGGTGCATACACGCAGAAGAGAAAGTGAAAGATACTGAAGGAGCAAAACAAATAGTGCGGA  5076  HIV2/LAV2
P  M  V  P  T  G  S  E  N  L  K  S  L  F  N  T  V  C  V  I  W  C  I  H  A  E  E  K  V  K  D  T  E  G  A  K  Q  I  V  R

R  H  L  N  V  E  T  G  T  A  E  T  M  L  K  T  S  R  P  T  A  P  S  S  G  R  E  G  N  Y  P  V  Q  Q  I  G  G  N  Y  V
GACACCTAATGGTGGAAACAGGAACAGCAGAAACTATGCTAAAAACAAGTAGACCAACAGCACCATCTAGCGGCAGAGAAGGAAATTACCCAGTACAACAAATAGGTGGTAACTATGTCC  5190  HTLV4/PK
:::: ::: :::  ::::::::::: : :  :::: ::  ::::::::::::::::::::::::::::::  :  : ::::::::::::::: :::::   :::: :: :::::   ::
GACATCTAGTGGCAGAAACAGGAACTGCAGAGAAAATGCCAAGCACAAGTAGACCAACAGCACCATCTAGCGAGAAGGGAGGAAATTACCCAGTGCAACATGTAGGCGGCAACTACACCC  5196  HIV2/LAV2
R  H  L  V  A  E  T  G  T  A  E  K  M  P  S  T  S  R  P  T  A  P  S  S  E  K  G  G  N  Y  P  V  Q  H  V  G  G  N  Y  T

H  L  P  L  S  P  R  T  L  N  A  W  V  K  L  I  E  E  K  K  F  G  A  E  V  V  P  G  F  Q  A  L  S  E  G  C  T  P  Y  D
ACCTGCCATTAAGCCCGAGAACATTAAATGCCTGGGTAAAATTGATAGAGGAAAAGAAATTTGGAGCAGAAGTAGTGCCAGGATTTCAGGCACTGTCAGAAGGCTGCACCCCCTATGACA  5310  HTLV4/PK
:  : ::  : :: ::  ::::  ::::::::::::::::::::  :::::::::: :: :: :: :::::::::::::::::::::::::::::: :::::::::::::: :::::::: :
ATATACCGCTGAGTCCCCGAACCCTAAATGCCTGGGTAAAATTAGTAGAGGAAAAAAAGTTCGGGGCAGAAGTAGTGCCAGGATTTCAGGCACTCTCAGAAGGCTGCACGCCCTATGATA  5316  HIV2/LAV2
H  I  P  L  S  P  R  T  L  N  A  W  V  K  L  V  E  E  K  K  F  G  A  E  V  V  P  G  F  Q  A  L  S  E  G  C  T  P  Y  D

I  N  Q  M  L  N  C  V  G  D  H  Q  A  A  M  Q  I  I  R  D  I  I  N  E  E  A  A  ...
TTAATCAGATGTTAAATTGTGTGGGAGACCATCAAGCGGCTATGCAGATTATCAGAGATATTATAAATGAGGAGGCTGCAG  5391                                          HTLV4/PK
: :: :: ::: : :::::::::::: :::::::::: :: :::::::: ::::: :: : :::: ::::::::: :: :::
TCAACCAAATGCTTAATTGTGTGGGCGACCATCAAGCAGCCATGCAGATAATCAGGGAGATTATCAATGAGGAAGCAGCAG  5397                                          HIV2/LAV2
I  N  Q  M  L  N  C  V  G  D  H  Q  A  A  M  Q  I  I  R  E  I  I  N  E  E  A  A  ...
```

Figure 1: Nucleotide sequence comparison between HTLV-4 and HIV-2. 5391 bp of HTLV-4/PK82 sequence and 5397 bp of HIV-2 sequence (12) are shown along with the deduced amino acid sequences of corresponding putative viral proteins. Sequences were aligned using the computer program NUCALN (18). The putative viral genes are translated starting with the first methionine. A splice donor site at position 843 and a splice acceptor site at position 3054 (underlined) most likely correspond to the splice sites utilized to express the art and tat genes of HTLV-4. They are shown in comparison to analogous sites in HIV-2. The reading frames R, tat, art, env, 3' orf, and gag have been designated in accordance with analogous genomic regions in HIV-1 (10). An additional reading frame, X, is designated in accordance with HIV-2 (12). The envelope reading frame in HTLV-4 contains a premature, inframe stop codon at position 3055 which is not present in HIV-2. The polypurine tracts and the primer binding sites of HTLV-4 and HIV-2 are underlined, and core enhancer sequences, SP1 binding sites, tata box and poly A signal are overscored by a dotted line.

long. A hydrophobic region, RNKR, most likely represents the cleavage site between the exterior envelope glycoprotein and the membrane-bound domain in HTLV-4. The corresponding sequence in HIV-2 is RHTR. A third hydrophobic region in the middle of the membrane-associated envelope domain probably represents the actual membrane spanning region. The envelope reading frame in HTLV-4/PK82 is interrupted by an inframe stop codon at position 3,055 (compare Figure 1). This stop codon, which is not present in HIV-2, is located 209 amino acids 3' to the putative cleavage site of the membrane-associated envelope protein and could explain the smaller size of this protein in HTLV-4 (32 kd) compared to HIV-2 (40 kd) and HIV-1 (41 kd). Interestingly, a stop codon in identical location was recently detected in three other independent STLV-3 clones as well as in a biologically-active molecular clone of HTLV-4 (14, M. Reitz and G. Franchim personal communication), indicating that the truncation of the transmembrane protein is a characteristic feature of STLV-3/HTLV-4 and does not prevent the production of infectious virus.

The last open reading frame 3' of the env is designated 3' orf, or F (see Figure 1). This region overlaps both env and LTR and a similarly located reading frame is present both in HIV-2 and HIV-1. The 3' orf is among the least well conserved genes between HTLV-4 and HIV-2 and between these viruses and HIV-1 (data not shown). Yet, there are two regions within 3' orf that are highly conserved. These correspond to amino acids 97-131 and 145 to 181 (HTLV-4 sequence). It is likely that these correspond to biologically-important domains.

The LTR region of HTLV-4 is 808 basepairs in length, compared to 854 basepairs for HIV-2 (12). The boundaries of both HTLV-4 and HIV-2 LTRs are demarcated by short inverted repeats (5' CTG-CAG 3') adjacent to the polypurine tract at the 3' LTR and the primer binding site at the 5' LTR. Interestingly, the polypurine tract for HTLV-4 is identical to that of HIV-1, but differs from HIV-2 at 3 of 16 nucleotides (compare Figure 1). Similarly, the primer binding site of HTLV-4 is identical to the primer binding site of HIV-1 but differs in one basepair to the primer binding site of HIV-2. HTLV-4, like HIV-1, contains three potential SP1 transcription factor binding sequences, whereas HIV-2 contains four such regions (6). With gaps introduced to optimize alignment, the overall LTR sequence of HTLV-4 is 76% homologous to HIV-2. The

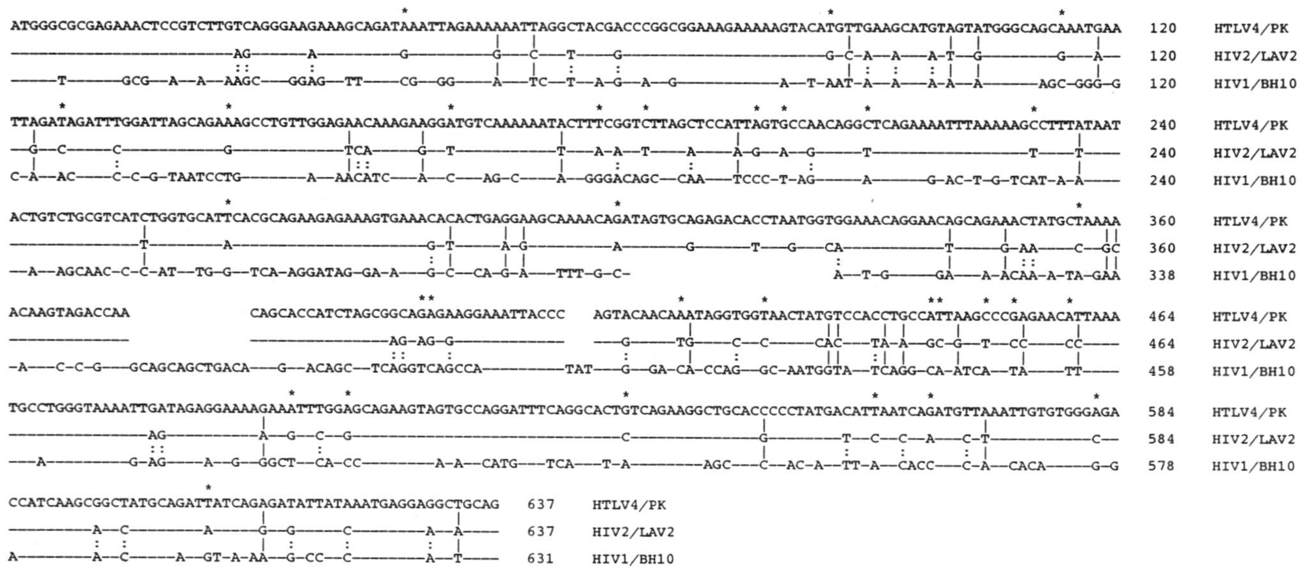

Figure 2: Nucleotide sequence alignment of a portion of the gag open reading frame of HTLV-4/PK82, HIV-2 and HIV-1/BH-10. 637 bp of HTLV-4/PK82 and HIV-2 gag sequence (12) are compared to each other and to 631 bp of HIV-1/BH-10 gag sequence (10). The sequences start with the initiation codon and encompas the gag p16 equivalent and parts of p25 equivalent. Dashes indicate nucleotide sequence identity between HTLV-4/PK82 and HIV-2 as well as between these viruses and HIV-1/BH-10. Vertical lines indicate sequence identity between HTLV-4/PK82 and HIV-1/BH-10, while two dots indicate sequence identity between HIV-2 and HIV-1/BH-10, only. Asterisks mark basepair changes that differ in all three viruses.

most remarkable differences are two large insertions in the U3 region of the HIV-2 LTR which do not seem to result from a mere duplication of adjacent LTR sequences.

One of the most conserved genomic regions among retroviruses is the gag gene. We have sequenced and compared 636 basepairs of gag (compare Figure 1) and found 84% nucleotide sequence homology and 87% amino acid sequence homology between HTLV-4 and HIV-2. Similarly, this region is also highly conserved between HIV-1, HTLV-4, and HIV-2, respectively. We found 59% nucleotide sequence homology between HTLV-4 and a prototype HIV-1 virus BH10 (56% amino acid sequence homology) and 58% nucleotide sequence homology between HIV-2 and BH-10 (54% amino acid sequence homology). The apparent equidistance of HTLV-4 and HIV-2 to HIV-1 prompted us to align the nucleotide sequence of all three viruses in this region. Figure 2 shows such an alignment and depicts 99 nucleotide sequence differences between HTLV-4 and HIV-2 (excluding insertions and deletions). Thirty-one of these point mutations differ among all three viruses. In 33 of these changes HTLV-4 is identical to HIV-1 and in 35 of these changes HIV-2 is identical to HIV-1. Thus, HIV-2 is not closer to HIV-1 than is STLV-3/HTLV-4 which suggests that these virus evolved from a common ancestral virus long before the onset of the current AIDS epidemic.

DISCUSSION

The results of this study and others (6,14) indicate that at a nucleotide sequence level 6 STLV-3/AGM, 3 STLV-3/MAC, and 3 HTLV-4 viruses previously isolated in two separate laboratories are virtually identical. This degree of similarity among proportedly independent virus isolates must have one of two extreme explanations: Either the various HTLV-4 and STLV-3 isolates understudy have resulted from laboratory contamination and thus do not represent independent viral isolates from different subjects, or this newly discovered family of retroviruses possesses a remarkably stable genome under conditions of chronic infection in three different species. Although there are precedents in other retroviral systems for strong conservation in genomic sequence upon repeated _in vitro_ or _in vivo_ passage (15, 16), the finding of 99% sequence homology in independent human and simian retrovirus isolates is extraordinary. Given the biological, clinical, and public health implications of this data, reisolation and characterization of additional HTLV-4 viruses from West African populations is imperative.

Regardless of the origin of the HTLV-4/PK82, 190, and 289 cell cultures, the STLV-3/HTLV-4 virus group represents an important species whose natural host is presumably the African green monkey. Because of its integral relation to HIV-2 and HIV-1, molecular analaysis of STLV-3/HTLV-4 can provide important clues as to the evolutionary origins of these viruses. STLV-3/HTLV-4 and HIV-2 are clearly more related to each other than to HIV-1, and all three are more related to each other than to other known retroviruses. These genomic similarities are consistent with the observed antigenic cross-reactivity amongst these viruses and imply a common evolutionary origin for them as a group. However, STLV-3/HTLV-4 is actually quite dissimilar from HIV-2 in overall nucleotide sequence and deduced amino acid sequences. In particular, the LTR of STLV-3/HTLV-4 differs from HIV-2 in overall size (808 basepairs versus 854 basepairs), number of potential SP1 binding regions, and in the sequence of the adjacent polypuring tract and primer binding site. In comparison, the LTRs of 5 widely divergent isolates of HIV-1 vary in size by only one basepair, and contain identical potential SP1 binding regions, polypurine tracts and primer binding sites. These data suggest that STLV-3/HTLV-4 may represent a viral subgroup distinct from HIV-2. Furthermore, since STLV-3/HTLV-4 and HIV-2 are both equally distinct from HIV-1 (Figure 2, Table 1), it is unlikely that STLV-3/HTLV-4 or HIV-2 represent an immediate or recent predecessor to HIV-1. Instead all three viruses appear to share a common ancestral virus and most likely have evolved independently over a long period of time.

In addition to providing important phylogenetic information, the availability of detailed sequence information for STLV-3/HTLV-4, HIV-2, and HIV-1 will provide a powerful tool for investigating molecular structure function relationships for these viruses. Highly conserved genomic regions in these otherwise rather distinct viruses are likely to correspond to biologically critical domains in their respective proteins. Furthermore, identification of genes and gene products that are present in all virus groups, or in some but not others, will assist in the rational development of preventative, therapeutic, and diagnostic reagents specific for this family of immunodeficiency-associated viruses.

ACKNOWLEDGEMENTS

We thank Drs. Phyllis Kanki and Myron Essex for HTLV-4 and STLV-3 infected cell lines, Drs. Marvin Reitz and Genoveffa Franchini for exchanging envelope sequence information of STLV-3/AGM-K6 prior to publication, and Ms. Sheila Chastain for careful preparation of the manuscript.

REFERENCES

1. Kanki PJ, Alroy J, and Essex M (1985). Isolation of T-lymphotropic retrovirus related to HTLV-III/LAV from wild-caught African green monkeys. Science 230:951.
2. Kanki PJ, Barin F, M'Boup S, Allan JS, Romet-Lemonne JL, Marlink R, McLane MF, Lee TH, Arbeille B, Denis F, and Essex M (1986). New human T-lymphotropic retrovirus related to simian T-lymphotropic virus type III (STLV-IIIAGM). Science 232:238.
3. Daniel MD, Letvin NL, King NW, Kannagi M, Sehgal PK, Hunt RD, Kanki PJ, Essex M, and Desrosiers RC (1985). Isolation of T-cell tropic HTLV-III-like retrovirus from macaques. Science 228:1201.
4. Kanki PJ, McLane MF, King NW Jr, Letvin NL, Hunt RD, Sehgal P, Daniel MD, Desrosiers RC, and Essex M (1985). Serologic identification and characterization of a macaque T-lymphotropic retrovirus closely related to HTLV-III. Science 228:1199.
5. Clavel F, Guetard D, Brun-Vezinet F, Chamaret S, Rey MA, Santos-Ferreira MO, Laurent AG, Dauguet C, Katlama C, Rouzious C, Klatzmann D, Champalimaud JL, and Montagnier L (1986). Isolation of a new human retrovirus from West African patients with AIDS. Science 233:343.
6. Kornfeld H, Riedel N, Viglianti G, Hirsch V, and Mullins JI (1987). Molecular cloning and biological activity of human T-lymphotropic virus type 4 and its relation to sub-human primate viruses and human immunodeficiency viruses. Nature 326:610.
7. Hahn BH, Shaw GM, Taylor ME, Redfield RR, Markham PD, Salahuddin SZ, Wong-Staal F, Gallo RC, Parks ES, and

Parks WP (1986). Genetic variation in HTLV-III/LAV over time in patiens with AIDS or at risk for AIDS. Science 232:1548.
8. Desrosiers RC, Daniel MD, Letvin NL, King NW, and Hunt RD (1987). Origins of HTLV-4. Nature 327:107.
9. Hahn BH, Kumar P, Taylor ME, Arya SK, and Shaw GM. Molecular characterization of HTLV-4, manuscript submitted.
10. Ratner L, Haseltine W, Patarca R, Livak KJ, Starcich B, Josephs SF, Doran ER, Rafaiski JA, Withehorn EA, Baumeister K, Ivanoff L, Petteway SR Jr, Pearson ML, Lautenberger JA, Papas TS, Ghrayeb J, Chang NT, Gallo R, and Wong-Staal F (1985). Complete nucleotide sequence of the AIDS virus, HTLV-III. Nature 313:277.
11. Alizon M, Wain-Hobson S, Montagnier L, and Sonigo P (1986). Genetic variability of the AIDS virus: nucleotide sequence analysis of two isolates from African patients. Cell 46:63.
12. Guyader M, Emerman M, Sonigo P, Clavel F, Montagnier L, and Alizon M (1987). Genome organization and transactivation of the human immunodeficiency virus type 2. Nature 326:662.
13. Wong-Staal F, paper presented at the UCLA Symposium on Human Retroviruses, Cancer, and AIDS, April 1-6, 1987, Keystone, Colorado.
14. Hirsch V, Riedel N, and Mullins JI (1987). The genome organization of STLV-3 is similar to that of the AIDS virus except for a truncated transmembrane protein. Cell 49:307.
15. Bryant ML, Gardner MB, Marx PA, Maul DH, Lerche NW, Osborn KG, Lowenstine LJ, Bodgen A, Arthur LO, and Hunter E (1986). Immunodeficiency in Rhesus monkeys associated with the original Mason-Pfizer monkey virus JNCI 77:957.
16. Desrosiers RC, Daniel MD, Butler CV, Schmidt DK, Letvin NL, Hunt RD, King NW, Barber CS, and Hunter E (1985). Retrovirus D/New England and its relation to Mason-Pfize monkey virus. J Virol 54:552.
17. Arya SK, et. al. Submitted.
18. Wilbur WJ, and Lipman DJ (1983). Rapid similarity searches of nucleic acid and protein data banks. Proc Natl Acad Sci USA 80:726.
19. Clavel F, Guyader M, Guetard D, Salle M, Montagnier L, and Alizon M (1986). Molecular cloning and polymorphism of the human immune deficiency virus type 2. Nature 324:691.

Human Retroviruses, Cancer, and AIDS:
Approaches to Prevention and Therapy, pages 75–88

CHARACTERIZATION OF THE ENV GENE AND OF TWO NOVEL CODING REGIONS OF THE HUMAN SPUMARETROVIRUS

B. Maurer, H. Bannert, A. Rethwilm,
G. Darai*, and R.M. Flügel

Institute of Virus Research, German Cancer Research Center,
P.O. Box 101949, 6900 Heidelberg, FRG, and
*Institute of Medical Virology, University of Heidelberg,
Im Neuenheimer Feld 324, 6900 Heidelberg, FRG

ABSTRACT Recombinant clones harboring retroviral DNA were established. The nucleotide sequence of the central and 3' region of the genome of the human spumaretrovirus was determined. The 5' end of the deduced protein sequence was homologous to the endonuclease domain of retroviral reverse transcriptases. A small intergenic region is followed by a long open reading frame of 985 amino acid residues that according to its genomic location and structural features is a typical retroviral env gene. Surprisingly, the post-env region contains two open reading frames that encodes two novel retroviral genes, termed bel-1 and bel-2. The 3' LTR is 963 nucleotides long and contains the signal sequences characteristic for transcriptional regulation of retrovirus genomes.

INTRODUCTION

Spumaretroviruses, also called foamy viruses which constitute the third subfamily of the retrovirus family have been isolated from a number of mammalian species, including primates (1).

[1]This work was supported by the Deutsche Forschunggemeinschaft (Re 627/7).

They seem to induce persistent infections in their natural hosts without a recognizable pathological disease. They induce, however, charcteristic cytopathic effects that lead to the degeneration of the infected cells. In contrast to the onco-, and lentiviruses, which have been characterized in detail, spumaretroviruses have been neglected. There are a number of different reasons why research on this subfamily has been neglected. The reasons are the poor growth properties of the virus in cell culture and in vivo and the apparent absence of pathological disease. In addition, there have been attempts to molecularly clone the virus by different groups without much success. It turns out that the genome of the foamy virus has structural features that makes the molecular cloning difficult when standard cloning procedures are used, e.g. parts of the long terminal repeat sequences (U3) have been found to be relatively unstable during this establishment in bacterial plasmid vectors.

Furthermore, while molecular cloning the foamy virus genome, we happened to isolate a clone that contained part of a human retrotransposon (2). Another unusual feature of the foamy viral genome is its large size. To date, the genome of the human spumaretrovirus (HSRV) that was isolated in 1971 by Achong and Epstein (3) from a nasopharynx carcinoma patient and that we work with exceeds even the lentiviral genomes in size. In order to study the biological role of foamy viruses and to ascertain whether or not it really has no pathological role in vivo, we decided to characterize the viral genome of HSRV in more detail.

RESULTS

The stragey used for the molecular cloning of HSRV DNA relies on two independent sources of viral DNA. As a source for proviral and viral DNAs, HSRV-infected human embryonic lung (HEL) cells were used to prepare DNA fragments that hybridized to ^{32}P-labeled DNA complimentary to HSRV DNA (cDNA). As a second source, cDNA was separately synthesized from purified HSRV virions in larger amounts by using reverse transcriptase. Subsequently, and separately, recombinant lambda clones were constructed that harbored inserts of either viral or cDNA (4). Those phage clones that hybridized to separately synthesized cDNA were subcloned into bacterial plasmid vectors, e.g. pAT153 and pSP65. In this way, a number of recombinant plasmid clones were established two of which (C55 and B52) were characterized in more detail and will be described here. The molecular cloning of the HSRV genome is the subject of a manuscript in preparation.

1. Nucleotide Sequence Analysis

Recombinant clone C55 was characterized by restriction mapping. It contained a 5.4 kbp insert of HSRV DNA that had originally been cloned from cDNA, and subcloned into the Hind III sites of the bacterial plasmid pAT153. The detailed analysis revealed that C55 DNA overlaps part of B52 DNA, a recombinant clone that was established from viral DNA. Fig. 1 shows the restriction mapping of both recombinant clones that resulted in a unique and unambiguous physical map. The determination of the nucleotide sequence of C55 DNA allowed us to correlate its physical map to its genetic map by analogy to other retroviral genomes (Fig. 1).

In the following, the DNA sequence shown in fig. 2 will be described starting from the 5' end.

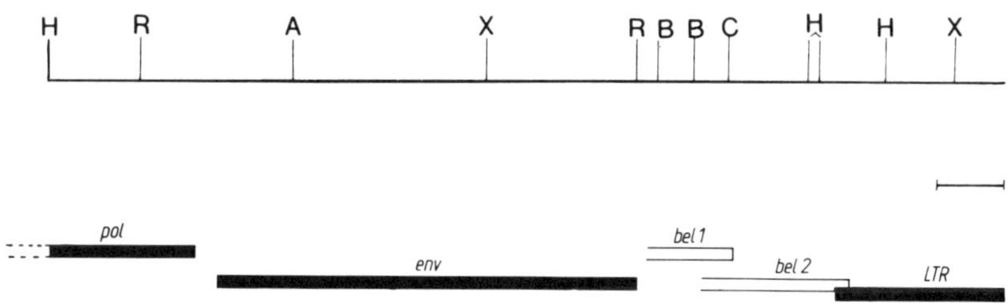

FIGURE 1. Restriction mapping of some enzymes (upper part) and proposed genetic map of the central and 3' region of the HSRV genome (lower part). H = Hind III, R = Eco RI, A = Hpa I, X = Xba I, B = Bam HI, and C = Cla I. The scale marks 500 bp.

a) The 3' pol and pol/env intergenic region. The nucleotide sequence shown in fig. 2 starts with the Hind III site of C55 DNA. The first 1032 nucleotides are homologous to the endonuclease (integrase) domain of the pol genes of most retroviruses (4). The deduced amino acid sequences show a relatively high degree of homology of 21-31% to the corresponding protein sequences of the retroviral reverse transcriptases (data not shown) (4).

```
             10         20         30         40         50         60         70         80         90        100
   1 AAGCTTGCCA CCCAAGGAAG TTATGTGGTT AATTGTAATA CCAAAAAACC AAACCTGGAT GCAGAGTTGG ATCAATTATT ACAGGGTCAT TATATAAAAG
 101 GATATCCCAA ACAATATACA TATTTTTTAG AAGATGGCAA AGTAAAAGTT TCCAGACCTG AAGGGGTTAA AATTATTCCC CCTCAGTCAG ACAGACAAAA
 201 AATTGTGCTT CAAGCCCACA ATTTGGCTCA CACCGGACGT GAAGCCACTC TTTTAAAAAT TGCCAACCTT TATTGGTGGC CAAATATGAG AAAGGATGTG
 301 GTTAAACAAC TAGGACGCTG TCAACAGTGT TTAATCACAA ATGCTTCCAA CAAAGCCTCT GGTCCTATTC TAAGACCAGA TAGGCCTCAA AAACCTTTTG
 401 ATAAATTCTT TATTGACTAT ATTGGACCTT TGCCACCTTC ACAGGGATAC CTATATGTAT TAGTAGTTGT TGATGGAATG ACAGGATTCA CTTGGTTATA
 501 CCCCACTAAG GCTCCTTCTA CTAGCGCAAC TGTTAAATCT CTCAATGTAC TCACTAGTAT TGCAATTCCA AAGGTGATTC ACTCTGATCA AGGTGCAGCA  pol
 601 TTCACTTCTT CAACCTTTGC TGAATGGGCA AAGGAAAGAG GTATACATTT GGAATTCAGT ACTCCTTATC ACCCCCAAAG TGGTAGTAAG GTGGAAAGGA
 701 AAAATAGTGA TATAAAACGA CTTTTAACTA AACTGCTAGT AGGAAGACCC ACAAAGTGGT ATGACCTATT GCCTGTTGTA CAACTTGCTT TAAACAACAC
 801 CTATAGCCCT GTATTAAAAT ATACTCCACA TCAACTCTTA TTTGGTATAG ATTCAAATAC TCCATTTGCA AATCAAGATA CACTTGACTT GACCAGAGAA
 901 GAAGAACTTT CTCTTTTACA GGAAATTCGT ACTTCTTTAT ACCATCCATC CACCCCTCCA GCCTCCTCTC GTTCCTGGTC TCCTGTTGTT GGCCAATTGG
1001 TCAGGAGAGG GTGGCTAGGC CTGCTTCTTT GAGACCTCGT TGGCATAAAC CGTCTACTGT ACTTAAGGTG TTGAATCCAA GGACTGTTGT TATTTTGGAC
1101 CATCTTGGCA ACAACAGAAC TGTAAGTATA GATAATTTAA AACCTACTTC TCATCAGAAT GGCACCACCA ATGACACTGC AACAATGGAT CATTTGGAAA
1201 AAAATGAATA AAGCGCATGA GGCACTTCAA AATACAACAA CTGTGACTGA ACAGCAGAAG GAACAAATTA TACTGGACAT TCAAAATGAA GAAGTACAAC
1301 CAACTAGGAG AGATAAATTT AGATATCTGC TTTATACTTG TTGTGCTACT AGCTCAAGAG TATTGGCCTG GATGTTTTTA GTTTGTATAT TGTTAATCAT
1401 TGTTTTGGTT TCATGCTTTG TGACTATATC CAGAATACAA TGGAATAAGG ATATTCAGGT ATTAGGACCT GTAATAGACT GGAATGTTAC TCAAAGAGCT
1501 GTTTATCAAC CCTTACAGAC TAGAAGGATT GCACGTTCCC TTAGAATGCA GCATCCTGTT CCAAAATATG TGGAGGTAAA TATGACTAGT ATTCCACAAG
1601 GTGTATACTA TGAACCCCAT CCGGAACCCA TAGTGGTGAA GGAGAGGGTC CTAGGTCTTT CTCAAATTCT GATGATTAAT TCAGAAAACA TTGCTAATAA
1701 TGCTAATTTG ACACAAGAAG TAAAGAAGTT GTTAACTGAA ATGGTTAATG AAGAAATGCA AAGTTTGTCA GATGTAATGA TTGACTTTGA AATTCCTTTA
1801 GGAGACCCTC GTGATCAAGA ACAATATATA CATAGAAAAT GCTATCAAGA ATTTGCAAAT TGTTATTTAG TAAAATATAA AGAACCCAAA CCGTGGCCTA
1901 AGGAGGGCCT TATAGCTGAT CAATGCCCAT TACCAGGTTA CCATGCTGGA TTAACCTATA ATAGACAGTC TATTTGGGAT TACTATATTA AAGTGGAGAG
2001 TATTAGACCT GCAAATTGGA CAACAAAGAG TAAATATGGA CAAGCTAGAC TAGGAAGTTT TTATATTCCT AGCAGCCTGA GACAAATCAA TGTTAGTCAT
2101 GTACTATTCT GTAGTGATCA ATTATATTCT AAATGGTATA ATATAGAAAA TACCATAGAA CAAAACGAGC GGTTTCTGCT TAATAAACTA AATAACCTTA
2201 CATCTGGAAC CTCAGTATTG AAGAAAAGAG CTCTTCCGAA GGATTGGAGT TCTCAAGGTA AAAATGCTCT GTTTAGAGAA ATCAATGTGT TAGATATCTG
2301 CAGTAAACCT GAATCTGTAA TACTATTGAA TACTTCATAC TATTCCTTCT CTTTATGGGA AGGAGATTGT AATTTTACTA AAGATATGAT TTCTCAGTTG
2401 GTTCCAGAAT GTGATGGATT TTATAACAAT TCTAAGTGGA TGCATATGCA TCCATATGCT TGTAGATTCT GGAGAAGTAA GAAGAATGAA AAAGAAGAAA
2501 CTAAATGTAG AGATGGGGAA ACTAAGAGAT GTCTGTATTA TCCTTTATGG GACAGTCCCG AATCTACATA TGATTTTGGT TATTTAGCAT ACCAAAAGAA
2601 TTTTCCTTCC CCTATCTGTA TAGAACAACA GAAAATTAGA GATCAAGATT ATGAAGTCTA TTCTTTGTAT CAAGAACGCA AAATAGCTTC TAAAGCATAT  env
2701 GGAATTGATA CAGTTTTATT CTCTCTAAAG AATTTTCTTA ATTATACAGG AACTCCTGTA AATGAAATGC CTAATGCAAG AGCTTTTGTA GGCCTAATAG
2801 ATCCCAAGTT TCCTCCTTCC TATCCCAATG TTACTAGGGA ACATTATACT TCCTGTAATA ATAGGAAAAG AAGAAGTGTT GATAATAACT ATGCTAAGTT
2901 AAGGTCTATG GGGTATGCAC TTACAGGAGC AGTGCAAACC TTATCTCAAA TATCAGATAT TAATGATGAA AACTTACAGC AAGGAATATA TTTATTAAGG
3001 GATCATGTAA TAACCTTAAT GGAAGCTACA TTGCATGATA TATCTGTTAT GGAAGGAATG TTTGCTGTAC AACATTTGCA TACACATTTG AATCATTTGA
3101 AGACAATGCT TCTAGAAAGA AGAATAGACT GGACCTATAT GTCTAGTACT TGGCTACAAC AACAATTACA GAAATCTGAT GATGAGATGA AAGTAATAAA
3201 GAGAATTGCT AGAAGTTTGG TATATTATGT TAAACAAACC CATAGTTCTC CCACAGCTAC AGCCTGGGAG ATTGGATTAT ATTATGAATT GGTTATACCT
3301 AAACATATTT ACTTGAATAA TTGGAATGTT GTCAATATAG GTCACTTAGT TAAATCAGCT GGACAATTGA CTCATGTAAC TATAGCTCAT CCTTATGAAA
3401 TAATCAATAA GGAATGTGTA GAGACTATAT ATCTGCATCT TGAGGACTGC ACAAGACAAG ATTATGTCAT ATGTGATGTG GTAAAGATAG TGCAGCCTTG
3501 TGGCAATAGC TCAGACACGA GTGATTGTCC TGTCTGGGCT GAAGCTGTAA AAGAACCATT TGTGCAAGTC AATCCTCTGA AAAACGGAAG TTATCTGGTT
3601 TTGGCAAGTT CCACAGACTG TCAGATCCCA CCATATGTTC CTAGCATCGT GACTGTTAAT GAAACAACGT CATGCTTTGG ACTGGACTTT AAAAGGCCAC
3701 TGGTTGCGGA AGAAAGATTG AGCTTTGAGC CACGACTGCC AAATCTACAA CTAAGATTAC CACATTTGGT TGGAATTATT GCAAAAATCA AAGGGATAAA
3801 AATAGAAGTC ACATCCTCTG GAGAAAGTAT AAAAGAGCAG ATTGAAAGAG CAAAAGCTGA GCTCCTTCGA CTGGACATTC ACGAGGGAGA TACTCCTGCC
3901 TGGATACAAC AGCTAGCTGC AGCAACAAAG GACGTCTGGC CAGCAGCAGC TTCTGCTCTA CAAGGAATTG GTAACTTTTT ATCTGGGACT GCCCAAGGAA
4001 TATTTGGAAC TGCCTTTAGT CTCTTGGGAT ACTTAAAGCC TATCCTAATA GGAGTAGGGG TCATTCTCTT GGTTATTCTT ATATTTAAGA TTGTATCATG
4101 GATTCCTACG AAAAAGAAGA ATCAGTAGCC TCCACCTCTG GAATTCAGGA CCTGCAGACT CTGAGTGAGC TTGTTGGCCC TGAAAATGCC GGAGAGGGAG
4201 AGCTGACTAT TGCTGAGGAA CCTGAAAGAA AATCCTCGAC GCCCCAGACG ATATACCAAA AGAGAAGTCA AATGTGTGTC TTATCATGCA TATAAAGAAA
4301 TTGAGGACAA ACATCCTCAA CATATTAAAC TGCAGGATTG GATCCCCACA CCAGAGGAAA TGAGTAAGTC ACTCTGTAAA AGACTTATTT TATGTGGATT
4401 GTATAGTGCA GAAAAGGCCT CAGAGATTTT AAGGATGCCT TTTACAGTTT CTTGGGAACA ATCAGATACT GACCCTGACT GTTTTATTGT AAGCTATACA
4501 TGTATATTTT GTGATGCTGT AATACATGAT CCCATGCCCA TAAGATGGGA TCCTGAAGTT GGAATTTGGG TAAAATATAA ACCCCTCAGA GGAATTGTTG  bel-1
4601 GATCTGCTGT GTTTATTATG CATAAACATC AAAGAAACTG TTCTCTTGTT AAACCTTCTA CCAGTTGCTC AGAAGGTCCA AAACCAAGAC CTAGGCACGA
4701 TCCTGTCCTT CGCTGTGACA TGTTTGAAAA GCATCACAAG CCTCGGCAGA AACGACCCAG GAGACGATCC ATCGATAATG AGTCATGTGC TTCCAGTAGT
4801 GACACCATGG TCAATGAGCC ATGATCACTA TGCACCAACC CTCTTTGGAA TCCTTGACCG CTACTATCAG GGCTACTTGA AGAGTCCAGC AACCTACCAA
4901 ACTTGGAAGT TCACATGTCA GGTGGACCCT TCTGGGAAGA GGTTTATGGA GACTCAATTT TGGGTCCCCC CTCTGGGTCA GGTGAACATT CAGTTTTATA
5001 AGAATTATCA GATTCTAACT TGCTGTCAGG CTGTAGACCC ATTTGCTAAT ATTTTTCATG GTACTGATGA AGAAATGTTT GACATTGATT CAGGTCCTGA
5101 TGTTTGGTGT TCTCCCTCTT TGTGTTTCAA GGTAATTTAT GAAGGGGCAA TGGGCCAAAA GCAAGAACAA AAAACATGGC TGTGCAGACT AGGACATGGT  bel-2
5201 CATCGTATGG GAGCATGCGA TTACCGTAAA GTAGATCTGT ATGCAATGAG ACAAGGAAAA GAAAACCCTT ATGGAGATAG GGGTGATGCA GCTTTGCAAT
5301 ATGCTTATCA GGTTAAAAGG GGCTGTAAAG CAGGGTGCTT GGCATCACCT GTACTTAACT ACAAAGCTTT GCAGTTTCAT AGAACCATTA TGGCAGACTT
```

Fig. 2

Fig. 2 (continued)

```
5401 CACCAATCCT AGGATTGGAG AAGGACATCT TGCTCATGGT TACCAAGCAG CTATGGAAGC TTATGGACCT CAGAGAGGAA GTAACGAGGA GAGGGTGTGG
5501 TGGAATGTCA CTAGAAACCA GGGAAAACAA GGAGGAGAGT ATTACAGGGA AGGAGGTGAA GAACCTCATT ACCCAAATAC TCCTGCTCCT CATAGACGTA
5601 CCTGGGATGA GAGACACAAG GTTCTTAAAT TGTCCTCATT CGCTACTCCC TCTGACATCC AACGCTGAAC TACTAAAGCA TTGCCTTATG GCTGGAAAGT
5701 GGTCACCGAA AGCGGAAATG ATTATACTAG CCGCAGAAAG ATCAGAACAT TGACAGAGAT GACTCAGGAT GAAATTAGAA AAAGGTGGGA AAGTGGATAT
5801 TGTGACCCCT TCATTGACTC AGGAAGTGAC TCAGATGGAC CCTTCTAAAA GCCACAGACA GTAAAAATGT GTTAGCACTT TATACAATAT TATATCTGCT
5901 TAAGCTATAG AAGCTTTCAC ATACTCAGTA\GCTGTTTCAC AATCAACAAA ACAATGATGA TGTAATCATA AGGAAGTAGT TTAAAATAGG TTAAGTAAGT
6001 TTACTGCAGT AGATAATCCC TGGGGAGGAT CTGGCTCTGT AAGCTGGAAC AGCAATGTTT TCAGTTCCAA TCCTCTCAAA GGAGAACCAG AGGGATGATG
6101 TGTTAGTTCA AATCCCATTA TCCTCATGGT TCCCTTTTCC ATAGTTTACT ATATTAATTT AAGGATAAGG TATAAGGATT AAGGTATGAG GTGTGTGGCT
6201 CAACACGTAG GGTGACAAGA AAATCTACTG TAATAGGACA CAACACCTCT AAAGTTGCCC GTGGGAAGGT GAAGTGAGAT CGAATCTTTC CTTAACGCAG  LTR
6301 ACAGCTTTTT ATCCACTAGG GATAATGTTT TAAGGAATAC TATAGTAATA GATTGATAGT TTTAACAATG ATAGAAATAG TATATAAGGA TAGTTTCTAG
6401 ATTGTACGGG AGGCTCTTCA CTACTCGCTG CGTCGAGAGT GTACGAGACT CTCCAGGTTT GGTAAGAAAT ATTTTATATT GTTATAATGT TACTATGATC
6501 CATTAACACT CTGCTTATAG ATTGTAAGGG TGATTGCAAT GCTTTCTGCA TAAAACTTTG GTTTTCTTGT TAATCAATAA ACCGACTTGA TTCGAGAACC
6601 AACTCCTATA TTATTGTCTC TTTTATACTT TATTAAGTAA AAGGATTTGT ATATTAGCCT TGCTAAGGGA GACATCTAGT GATATAAGTG TGAACTACAC
6701 TTATCTTAAA TGATGTAACT CCTTAGGATA ATCAATATAC AAAATTCCAT GACAA
```

FIGURE 2. Nucleotide sequence of the HSRV DNA. The sequence starts with the Hind III site at position 1 as the 5' terminus and extends to the end of the 3' LTR. Gene locations are given at the right margin. Stop codons are boxed, the putative env initiator is marked by horizontal arrow; potential splice acceptor sites for the bel genes are indicated by vertical arrowheads. The polypurine tract upstream of the 3' LTR is doubly underlined. The TATA-box and the polyA-addition signal is marked by a broken line. Cleavage sites for the restriction enzymes shown in fig. 1 are underlined.

The 3' pol region is followed by a relatively short intergenic sequence of 127 nucleotides. It is at this location that a long open reading frame (orf) coding for 995 amino acid residues is identified. This long orf lies in a frame different from that of the pol gene product and will be described below in detail. Overlapping the pol gene and the long orf in the third reading frame a short orf (S1) of only 87 amino acids was found. Since it is so short and not homologous to any of the other lentiviral genes that have been described to occur at a comparable genetic location including the S1 gene of equine infectious anemia virus (EIV) (5) we consider it unlikely that S1 of HSRV is expressed.

The env gene. There are three initiation codons in the first 70 nucleotides of the major long open reading frame that opens at position 1141 (Fig. 2). Only the second ATG and its neighboring sequences conform to those of a typical eukaryotic initiator (6). This initiator is located at position 1171, eleven tripletts inside the major orf that according to its size and to certain peculiar but typical structural features is the HSRV env precursor protein.

It extends for 985 codons to position 4126 where it stops (fig. 3). Its hydrophobicity profile was calculated according to Kyte and Doolittle (7) and is shown in fig. 4. There are two long hydrophobic domains and at least one that is less hydrophobic that deserve to be described. The first hydrophobic region corresponds to the signal peptide, since it is located close to the NH_2-terminus of the env precursor. It is of interest that the first 62 amino acids residues after the initiator at 1171 are clearly hydrophilic in character as is the case for the env precursors of visna virus (VIV) and mouse mammary tumour virus (MMTV) which are of similar lengths and hydrophilicity (8-11). The proper signal peptide comprises residues 74 to 87 (see fig. 3). There is a strongly basic

```
             10         20         30         40         50         60
  1 NLLLIRMAPP MTLQQWIIWK KMNKAHEALQ NTTTVTEQQK EQIILDIQNE EVQPTRRDKF
 61 RYLLYTCCAT SSRVLAWMFL VCILLIIVLV SCFVTISRIQ WNKDIQVLGP VIDWNVTQRA
121 VYQPLQTRRI ARSLRMQHPV PKYVEVNMTS IPQGVYYEPH PEPIVVKERV LGLSQILMIN
181 SENIANNANL TQEVKKLLTE MVNEEMQSLS DVMIDFEIPL GDPRDQEQYI HRKCYQEFAN
241 CYLVKYKEPK PWPKEGLIAD QCPLPGYHAG LTYNRQSIWD YYIKVESIRP ANWTTKSKYG
301 QARLGSFYIP SSLRQINVSH VLFCSDQLYS KWYNIENTIE QNERFLLNKL NNLTSGTSVL  OMP
361 KKRALPKDWS SQGKNALFRE INVLDICSKP ESVILLNTSY YSFSLWEGDC NFTKDMISQL
421 VPECDGFYNN SKWMHMHPYA CRFWRSKKNE KEETKCRDGE TKRCLYYPLW DSPESTYDFG
481 YLAYQKNFPS PICIEQQKIR DQDYEVYSLY QERKIASKAY GIDTVLFSLK NFLNYTGTPV
541 NEMPNARAFV GLIDPKFPPS YPNVTREHYT SCNNRKRRSV DNNYAKLRSM GYALTGAVQT
601 LSQISDINDE NLQQGIYLLR DHVITLMEAT LHDISVMEGM FAVQHLHTHL NHLKTMLLER
661 RIDWTYMSST WLQQQLQKSD DEMKVIKRIA RSLVYYVKQT HSSPTATAWE IGLYYELVIP
721 KHIYLNNWNV VNIGHLVKSA GQLTHVTIAH PYEIINKECV ETIYLHLEDC TRQDYVICDV  TMP
781 VKIVQPCGNS SDTSDCPVWA EAVKEPFVQV NPLKNGSYLV LASSTDCQIP PYVPSIVTVN
841 ETTSCFGLDF KRPLVAEERL SFEPRLPNLQ LRLPHLVGII AKIKGIKIEV TSSGESIKEQ
901 IERAKAELLR LDIHEGDTPA WIQQLAAATK DVWPAAASAL QGIGNFLSGT AQGIFGTAFS
961 LLGYLKPILI GVGVILLVIL IFKIVSWIPT KKKNQ*
```

FIGURE 3. Deduced amino acid sequence of the HSRV env gene. The methionine residue that initiates the env precursor is marked by a flag. Hydrophobic regions are underlined, sites for N-linked glycosylations are boxed. The proteolytic cleavage sites for generating the OMP and TMP is marked by a vertical arrow.

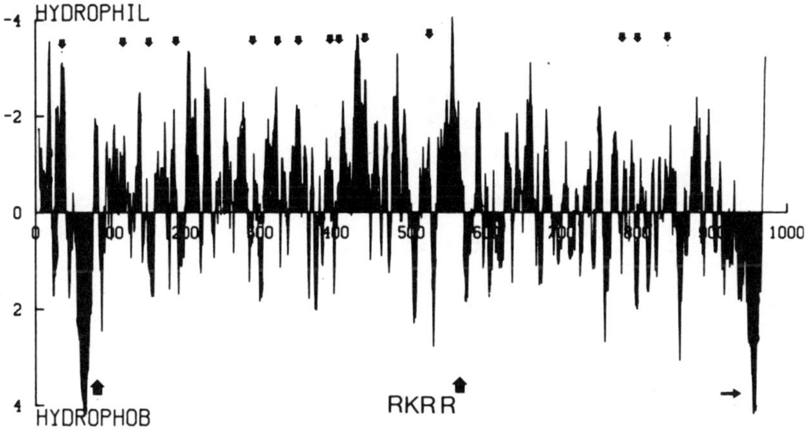

FIGURE 4. Hydropathic profile of the HSRV env precursor polypeptide. The hydrophilic (upper) and hydrophobic (lower) profile was calculated using a 5-amino acid-window size (7). Potential N-linked glycosylation sites are marked with arrows in the upper part. The two thick arrows in the lower part mark the potential processing sites of the env precursor into the mature OMP and TMP. The horizontal arrow indicates the transmembrane peptide.

sequence Arg-Lys-Arg-Arg (fig. 3 and 4) that represents the site for proteolytic processing of the HSRV env precursor into the outer membrane protein (OMP) and into the transmembrane protein (TMP). TMP is located at the carboxy terminus of the env polypeptide (12).

This proteolytic cleavage site is followed by a second less hydrophobic region that corresponds to the so-called fusion peptide region of other retroviral TMPs (13). The third, carboxyterminal, hydrophobic domain of the HSRV env protein is 37 residues long and shows a remarkable resemblance to the corresponding transmembrane domains of HIV-1 and VIV (14,8).

The molecular weight of the OMP of HSRV is predicted to be 53.7 kd, whereas that of a related simian foamy virus type 1 was found to be 70 kd (15). However, this comparison does not take into account the varying degree of glycosylation of these env proteins.

There are 14 potential glycoslyation signals of the type Asn-X-Ser/Thr in the env precursor protein sequence of HSRV (fig. 4). All but three are found in the OMP part of the env protein. The number and distribution of these signal sites resemble the pattern found in other retroviral env protein sequences, and particularly the lentiviruses, HIV, VIV, and EIV. As anticipated, there is little, if any homology at the level of amino acids, but it is worth mentioning that on the nucleotide level the degree of homology of the HSRV env gene to the VIV env gene is 52.1%.

The bel-1 and bel-2 sequences. The post-env region of HSRV is unusually long. It encompasses 1663 nucleotides (fig. 2), ranging from the end of the env gene to the start of the 3' LTR. Two open reading frames are identified in this region that are 205 (bel-1) and 364 (bel-2) amino acid residues long (fig. 5 and 6). It is interesting that both putative bel genes could be generated from spliced viral mRNAs or alternatively could start from initiators, resulting in slightly smaller versions of the predicted polypeptides. The presumed splice acceptor sites conform to those that are found in the HTLV-1 genome for mRNAs from which the px or tat proteins are derived and in which the corresponding initiator codon is located on a RNA leader sequence that is derived from the 5' end of the genome (16,17).

The deduced protein sequences are interesting for a number of different reasons. With respect to their genomic location they could correspond to either the x genes of HTLV-I and II or the 3'-orf of HIV. Alternatively, they can be compared to v-oncogenes of oncoviruses. It is noteworthy that bel-1 and bel-2 do not show any significant homology to any protein sequences of the NBFR protein data bank. On the other hand, they display some structural peculiarities (Fig. 5 and 6). Both are relatively rich in cysteine residues (there are 10 cysteine residues in bel-1 and 12 cys residues in bel-2), and have either one (bel-2) or two (bel-1) glycosylation signals, properties that are reminiscent of certain hormone sequences. The bel-2 has one Arg-Gly-Asp sequence, a versatile cell recognition signal that is crucial for interacting with its cell surface receptor (18). Furthermore, both bel sequences possess potential phosphorylation sites of the type Arg-Arg-Ser or -Thr. Finally, on the other hand, both putative genes show remarkably long stretches of strong basic residues that are reminiscent of similar regions in the tat proteins of HIV (16). It remains to be studied if the bel genes are expressed and what functions they possess.

```
                  bel-1
          10        20         30         40

  1 LLLRNLKENP RRPRRYTKRE VKCVSYHAYK EIEDKHPQHI
 41 KLQDWIPTPE EMSKSLCKRL ILCGLYSAEK ASEILRMPFT
 81 VSWEQSDTDP DCFIVSYTCI FCDAVIHDPM PIRWDPEVGI
121 WVKYKPLRGI VGSAVFIMHK HQRNCSLVKP STSCSEGPKP
161 RPRHDPVLRC DMFEKHHKPR QKRPRRRSID NESCASSSDT
201 MVNEP*
```

FIGURE 5. Amino acid sequence of the bel-1 coding region. The thick vertical arrow marks the position of the splice acceptor site corresponding to that shown in fig. 2. N-linked glycosylation sites are boxed; cysteine residues are underlined. The strongly basic amino acid stretches is doubly underlined.

The LTR Region

There are 107 nucleotides between the termination codon of the bel-2 open reading frame and the start of the 3' LTR. The LTR sequence is 963 nucleotides long and is located at the 3' end of the B52 DNA. It contains a number of key features of regulatory signals shown to be required for retroviral replication and transcription. There is a characteristic sequence, AGAA AAAGGTGGGAAAG, the polypurine tract (figure 3), that defines the 5' boundary of the HSRV LTR and is found in all retroviral genomes at this location and is the putative primer for plus strand DNA synthesis of retroviruses. Within the 3' presumed LTR there is one poly(A)-addition signal AATAAA (position 6576 to 6581) which perfectly matches the canonical consensus sequence. If the location of the poly(A)-signal is assumed to be nonvariant with respect to the polyadenylation-site of HSRV, one can draw an analogy to the LTRs of HIV and VIV (14,8), and place the polyadenylation site 24 bp downstream of the poly(A)-addition signal at CA (position 6600). Similar arguments indicate that the cap site starts with a G close to position 6412. A perfect and multiple TATATA-box precedes the presumptive RNA initiation

```
                10          20          30          40
  1  NINPSEELLD  LLCLLCINIK  ETVLLLNLLP  VAQKVQNQDL
 41  GTILSFAVTC  LKSITSLGRN  DPRDDSSIMS  HVLSVVTPWS
 81  MSHDHYAPTL  FGILDRYYQG  YLKSSATYQT  WKFTCTVDPS
121  GKRFMGTQFW  VPPLGQVNIQ  FYKNYQILTC  CQAVDPFANI
161  FHGTDEEMFD  IDSGPDVWCS  PSLCFKVIYE  GAMGQKQEQK
201  TWLCRLGHGH  RMGACDYRKV  DLYAMRQGKE  NPYGDRGDAA
241  LQYAYQVKRG  CKAGCLASPV  LNYKALQFHR  TIMADFTNPR
281  IGEGHLAHGY  QAAMEAYGPQ  RGSNEERVWW  NVTRNQGKQG
321  GEYYREGGEE  PHYPNTPAPH  RRTWDERHKV  LKLSSFATPS
361  DIQR*
```

bel-2

FIGURE 6. Amino acid sequence of the bel-2 gene. The thick arrow marks the position of the splice acceptor site as shown in fig. 2. The cell recognition Arg-Gly-Asp (RGD) (18) is doubly underlined. A putative N-linked glycosylation signal is boxed and cysteine residues are underlined.

site by 31 bp. Thus, the HSRV LTR can be subdivided into three regions. The R and U5 regions were calculated to be 193 and 154 bp, respectively. The U3 region was estimated to be 616 bp long. Restriction fine mapping of another recombinant clone that was derived from viral DNA and that contained sequences from the 5'-region of the HSRV genome resulted in DNA fragment sizes that were consistent with those obtained with the 3' LTR sequences from B52 DNA (R.M. Flügel, unpublished observation).

Although the HSRV LTR is unusually long, open reading frames for encoding proteins of more than 30 amino acid residues were not found. Furthermore, the HSRV LTR has little if any sequence homology to the LTRs of other retrovirus, in particular to those of HIV-I, HTLV-II, VIV, MMTV, and HIV-2 (14,17,18,10,19). In addition, no significant sequence homology was found to human endogenous retrovirus-like sequences including the 968 bp long LTR sequence of human endogenous retroviral HERV genes (20).

There are ten octamer sequences and six nonamers that form direct repeats within the LTR. The indirect repeats include a decamer at position 6646 and 6743 with a loop size of 78 bp and two octamers with a relatively small loop size of 34 and 5 bp, respectively. The significance of these repeats with respect to the regulation of transcription remains to be elucidated.

DISCUSSION

There are a number of common as well as distinguishing features when the HSRV genome is compared to the genomes of other retroviruses. In general, the characteristics typical for a retrovirus have been readily identified in foamy viruses in the past. It has an RNA genome composed of two subunits and a virion reverse transcriptase, concomitant with a RNAse H activity (1, and references cited therein). The fact that we succeeded in molecular cloning proviral DNA from HSRV-infected human cells and that we can sequence across the 5' LTR into the cellular flanking regions unambiguously proves that HSRV integrates into the host DNA. Furthermore, the protein sequences deduced from the DNA sequence of the HSRV pol gene and their comparison with the corresponding reverse transcriptase domains of other retroviruses clearly show that the HSRV pol gene product can be subdivided into a RNAse H and an endonuclease (integrase) domain.

Furthermore, the HSRV genome contains 3' to the pol gene an env gene, that is about as long as the env genes of lentiviruses. Although the primary structure of the HSRV env gene is unique, its overall structural organization and hydropathic profile is that of a typical retroviral env gene. It is rich in cysteine residues, contains many glycosylation sites, a signal peptide at its NH_2-terminus, and a proteolytic processing site of the same type as HIV-1 and VIV env gene products, that generates the mature env proteins that are essential for the budding process and necessary for the attachment of infectious virus to the surface receptors of the host cell.

On the other hand, spumaretroviruses seem to have properties that set them apart from the other subfamilies of retroviruses, namely from the onco- and lentiviruses, and from other members of the retrovirus family, e.g. the HTLV/BLV and the D- and B-type viruses. The large size of the HSRV genome can be accounted for in broad terms, since the different genes (gag, pol, env) and genomic regions (LTR and post-env) were found to be of a correspondingly greater size. The LTR is quite large, with a size of 963 bp as are the gag, pol, and env genes. Moreover, the bel coding regions that are located in the post-env part of the HSRV genome are unique with respect to size when compared to other retroviral genomes. Apparently, HSRV does not have a sor gene like HIV-1 and VIV do.

In conclusion, HSRV has a unique genomic structure that differs from those of other retroviruses in certain respects. A final and definitive phylogenetic placement will be possible when the 5' part of the HSRV DNA sequence will be determined which is currently underway. The fascinating aspect of the elucidating functions for the bel coding regions will allow to determine whether or not they can be correlated with the regulation of foamy virus expression. It will be of interest to study what regions of the HSRV genome are responsible for the cytopathic effects and to find out if foamy viruses cause a human disease.

ACKNOWLEDGEMENT

We thank Dr. Ronald C. Montelaro, Louisiana State University, for communicating his results to us. The expert editorial assistance of Ms. M. Kasamasch is gratefully acknowledged.

REFERENCES

1. Weiss R, Teich N, Coffin J (eds) (1985) Taxonomy of retroviruses. In "RNA Tumor Viruses", New York: Cold Spring Harbor Laboratory, 2nd edition, 2, p 25.
2. Flügel RM, Maurer B, Bannert H, Rethwilm A, Schnitzler P, Darai G (1987). Nucleotide sequence analysis of a cloned DNA fragment from human cells reveals homology to retrotransposons. Mol Cell Biol 7:231.
3. Achong BG, Mansell PW, Epstein MA, Clifford P (1971). An unusual virus in cultures from a human nasopharyngeal carcinoma. J Nat Cancer Inst 46:299.

4. Flügel RM, Rethwilm A, Maurer B, Darai G (1987). Nucleotide sequence analysis of the env gene and its flanking regions of the human spumaretrovirus reveals two novel genes. EMBO J
5. Rushlow K, Olsen K, Steigler G, Payne SL, Montelaro RC, Issel CJ (1986). Lentivirus genomic organization: the complete nucleotide sequence of the env gene region of equine infectious anemia virus. Virology 155:309.
6. Kozak M (1984). Compilation and analysis of the sequences upstream from the transcriptional start site in eukaryotic mRNAs. Nucleic Acids Res 12:857.
7. Kyte J, Doolittle RF (1982). A simple method for displaying the hydropathic character of a protein. J Mol Biol 157:105.
8. Sonigo P, Alizon M, Staskus K, Klatzmann C, Cole S, Danos O, Retzel E, Tiollais P, Haase A, Wain-Hobson S (1985). Nucleotide sequence of the visna lentivirus: relationship to the AIDS virus. Cell 42:369.
9. Fasel N, Pearson K, Buetti E, Diggelmann H (1982). The region of mouse mammary tumor virus DNA containing the long terminal repeat includes a long coding sequence and signals for hormonally regulated transcription. EMBO J 1:3.
10. Majors JE, Varmus HE (1983). Nucleotide sequencing of an apparent proviral copy of env mRNA defines determinants of expression of the mouse mammary tumor virus env gene. J Virol 47:495.
11. Redmond SMS, Dickson C (1983). Sequence and expression of the mouse mammary tumor virus env gene. EMBO J 2:125.
12. Coffin JM (1986). Genetic variation in AIDS viruses. Cell 46:1.
13. Bolognesi DP, Montelaro RC, Frank H, Schäfer W (1978). Assembly of type C oncornaviruses: a model. Science 199:183.
14. Ratner L, Haseltine W, Patarca R, Livak KJ, Starcich B, Josephs SF, Doran ER, Rafalski JA, Whitehorn EA, Baumeister K, Ivanoff L, Petteway SR jr, Pearson ML, Lautenberger JA, Papas TS, Ghrayeb J, Chang NT, Gallo RC, Wong-Staal F (1985). Complete nucleotide sequence of the AIDS virus, HTLV-III. Nature 313:277.
15. Benzair A-B, Rhodes-Feuillette A, Lasneret J, Emanoil-Ravier R, Périès J (1985). Purification and characterization of the major envelope glycoprotein of simian foamy virus type 1. J Gen Virol 66:1449.
16. Sodroski J, Rosen C, Wong-Staal F, Salahuddin SZ, Popovic M, Arya SK, Gallo RC, Haseltine WA (1985). Trans-acting

transcriptional regulation of human T-cell leukemia virus type III long terminal repeat. Science 227:171.
17. Shimotohno K, Wachsman W, Takahashi Y, Golde DW, Miwa M, Sugimura T, Chen ISY (1984). Nucleotide sequence of the 3' region of an infectious human T-cell leukemia virus type II genome.
18. Ruoshlat E, Pierschbacher MD (1986). Arg-Gly-Asp: a versatile cell recognition signal. Cell 44:517.
19. Clavel F, Guyader, M, Guétard D, Sallé M, Montagnier L, Alizon M (1986). Molecular cloning and polymorphism of the human immune deficiency virus type 2. Nature 324:691.
20. Ono M. (1986). Molecular cloning and long terminal repeat sequences of human endogenous retrovirus genes related to types A and B retrovirus genes. J Virol 58:937.

CORRECTION

The nucleotide sequence analysis of another recombinant clone of proviral DNA of HSRV revealed that the LTR region is longer by 298 bp. This results in a total length of 1216 bp for the LTR, with a U3 region of 814 bp. Correspondingly, the 3' LTR overlaps the bel-2 gene by 53 nucleotides, so that the polypurine tract at position 5472 to 5496 has to be postulated to be primer for plus strand DNA synthesis in analogy to all other retroviruses.

Accordingly, the 3'-LTR regions shown in fig. 1 and 2 should be redrawn to represent the overlap into the bel-2 part of the HSRV genome.

II. BIOLOGY AND GENETICS OF HIV

Human Retroviruses, Cancer, and AIDS:
Approaches to Prevention and Therapy, pages 91–100

BIOLOGIC, SEROLOGIC AND MOLECULAR DIFFERENCES AMONG HUMAN IMMUNODEFICIENCY VIRUSES (HIV)[1]

Jay A. Levy, Louise A. Evans, Masatoshi Tateno, Christopher Walker, Jacques Homsy, and Cecilia Cheng-Mayer

Department of Medicine and Cancer Research Institute, University of California, School of Medicine, San Francisco, California, 94143

ABSTRACT Studies on a wide variety of HIV isolated from different body tissues and fluids, as well as from individuals from different parts of the world, indicate an extensive heterogeneity. HIV isolates can be distinguished by biologic features which include cell tropism, replicating properties, and production of cytopathology in infected cells. In addition, some can induce a latent state which may be related to their production of the orf-B protein. Serotypes of HIV can be identified using selective sera. These serologic differences are probably the results of genomic variations in the envelope gene as reflected by restriction enzyme sensitivity patterns. An understanding of this heterogeneity of HIV, that occurs at several different levels of viral infection, is important in the design of effective antiviral therapy and a vaccine.

INTRODUCTION

The acquired immune deficiency syndrome (AIDS) is caused by a human retrovirus (1-3) now termed the human immunodeficiency virus (HIV) (4). Our laboratory has isolated over 400 different HIV from peripheral mononuclear cells, autopsy tissues and a variety of body fluids, including urine, saliva, tears, semen, vaginal/cervical secretions, cerebrospinal fluid, and blood. These isolates

[1]This work was supported by a grant from the California State Universitywide Task Force on AIDS.

have been recovered from individuals living in different parts of the world, including Africa and the Caribbean. In evaluating distinct features of these HIV, differences in the biologic, serologic and molecular characteristics were noted. They are the subject of this report.

Biologic Heterogeneity of HIV.

Peripheral mononuclear cells (PMC) from seronegative individuals are the most susceptible to acute infection by HIV (1-3,5). In order to obtain long term cultures of the virus, however, established human hematopoietic cells have been extremely useful. We first demonstrated that the HUT-78 T cell line was very susceptible to both acute and chronic infection with HIV (3). In subsequent studies, we found that only about 50% of HIV isolates can productively infect HUT-78 cells (5). Moreover, in using other established T cell lines (CEM, Jurkat, MOLT-4), differences in the replicating ability of individual HIV could be noted. Some isolates productively infected all the established T cell lines, while others could only replicate in one or two (5,6). Furthermore, when monocyte and EBV-transformed lymphoblastoid B cell lines were used, differences in the infection and replication of various HIV could be noted (5,6). Finally, in evaluation of PMC from 11 seronegative individuals coming from Oriental, Black and Caucasian backgrounds, differences in susceptibility and kinetics of replication by distinct HIV were observed (5). Thus, although PMC are the major target cells for HIV, they can also vary in their susceptibility to infection.

HIV isolated from brain tissues and cerebrospinal fluid, as well as from PMC, also differ in their ability to infect cultured human brain cells. In collaboration with Drs. Mark Rosenblum and James Rutka, we have demonstrated that early passaged fetal brain cells and established human cell lines from glioma tissue show differences in their sensitivity to infection by HIV. No distinct host range pattern was associated with viruses isolated from the brain as compared to those from PMC. Since cells bearing the glial fibrillary acid protein (GFAP), an astrocyte specific marker, were the most susceptible to HIV, these cells may be an important target for HIV in the brain (7).

Cytopathology.

Another heterogeneous characteristic of HIV is their relative ability to fuse and form multinucleated cells in tissue culture eventually leading to balloon or ghost cells (Figure 1).

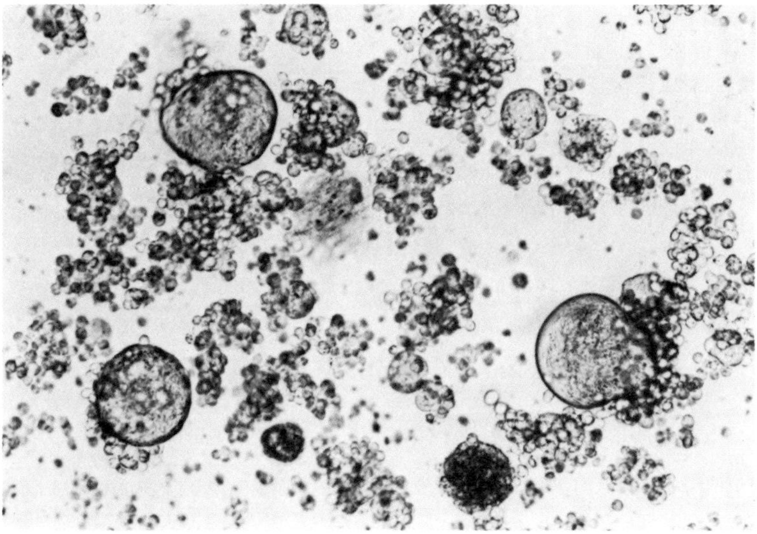

FIGURE 1. Human peripheral mononuclear cells infected with HIV_{SF2}. Note the large ballooning multinucleated cells. (x25).

One feature that seems to correlate with the extent of cytopathology is the induction of plaques in the established MT-4 T cell lines (6). This assay, first described by Harada, et al. (8) appears to reflect an enhanced ability of certain isolates to replicate rapidly and to form multinucleated cells. Some HIV can readily form plaques whereas others cannot (Table 1). Thus this procedure can be used for detecting differences among HIV as well as for neutralization assays.

TABLE 1
PLAQUE ASSAY OF DIFFERENT HIV ISOLATES

HIV_{SF} Isolates	Source	Plaque Forming	PFU/ml
4	PMC-SF	+	$3x10^4$
33	PMC-Phila.	+	$2x10^5$
128A	Brain-SF	-	
128B	LN-SF	-	
170	PMC-Africa	-	

PMC - peripheral mononuclear cells; SF - San Francisco; Phila. - Philadelphia, PFU - plaque forming units.

Latent Virus Infection.

We and others have noted that HIV can induce a latent virus infection in established human cells (9,10). Following a certain period of time post-infection, virus replication decreases and cells cease to release HIV. On addition of halogenated pyrimidines, such as iododeoxyuridine (IUDR), virus production is again resumed. We have noted differences among HIV in their ability to establish latency. Some take 20-30 days, whereas others enter this state in a much shorter period of time. One isolate (HIV_{SF247}), obtained from the PMC of an individual in the Dominican Republic, establishes latency in the human Jurkat T cell line within 6 days. In fact, virus replication after inoculation is not noted at all, and can only be revealed by induction with IUDR (10).

This difference in the ability of various HIV to establish latency is the subject of substantial research in our laboratory. Preliminary data suggest that the orf-B region of the viral genome may play a role in determining latency. In collaboration with Dr. Paul Luciw, we have noted, through mutational analysis of the HIV_{SF2} genome, that mutants in the orf-B region have enhanced replicating ability and progeny production (11). The orf-B region thus appears to down-regulate HIV replication. We are examining the possibility that enhanced production of the p27 orf-B protein affects the extent of HIV production and the establishment of a latent state. Isolates that easily enter latency may have very high levels of p27 protein production. Most importantly, this region might be manipulated to create a latent infection in individuals, and thus, delay the progression of disease. By blocking virus replication, this state would prevent HIV spread in the host.

Serologic Differences Among HIV.

Studies have been conducted to examine the extent of antigenic differences among HIV. Using selected sera from HIV-positive individuals, three HIV serotypes have been identified based on their susceptibility to serum neutralization. Some HIV are easily neutralized by most sera, others by only a few, and finally, one isolate (HIV_{SF170}) from Africa is not neutralized by most sera from HIV-infected individuals.

TABLE 2
NEUTRALIZATION OF HIV ISOLATES

HIV_{SF} (Source)	Location	Serum (End Titer) 1	2	3*
Serotype A				
2 (PMC)	San Francisco	1000	100	10
4 (PMC)	San Francisco	1000	100	100
33 (PMC)	San Francisco	1000	100	10
Serotype B				
128A (CNS)	San Francisco	100	-	-
247 (PMC)	Santo Domingo	100	-	-
Serotype C				
170 (PMC)	Kigali, Rwanda	-	-	-

* Serum from HIV_{SF2}-infected chimpanzee.

CNS - central nervous system; a negative indicates no neutralization at a 1:10 serum dilution.

It is noteworthy that HIV_{SF2} (formerly ARV-2) is extremely sensitive to neutralization by antisera. This isolate can be neutralized up to 1,000 times more efficiently than many other HIV. The reason for these observations is unknown, but suggests that unique epitopes are presented by different serotypes. These antigenic differences among HIV will be important in the eventual design of an effective vaccine.

Envelope Changes in HIV: Molecular Studies.

The identification of serotypes most likely reflects differences in the envelope portion of HIV. We have reported our assessment of changes in the envelope region of HIV using oligonucleotide probes to define variable regions of the envelope genome (12). These regions were recognized by comparing ARV-2 with LAV and HTLV-III. The latter viruses are very similar and thus their variable regions differed to the same extent from ARV-2. In collaboration with Drs. Dino Dina and Chuck Stabin, we produced labeled probes to these variable regions and evaluated a variety of HIV isolates in our laboratory. These analyses indicated that the variable region was different among some isolates, but in other HIV, this portion of the genome was conserved. This observation suggested that there may not be an unlimited number of changes in the variable region in HIV, and thus serotyping of HIV might be possible. Our results on neutralization noted above support this conclusion (Table 2).

Changes in HIV Over Time.

Recently, studies have been directed at evaluating possible biologic changes in HIV over time in the same host. In the patient from whom we recovered HIV_{SF2}, we were able to isolate a virus five months later. At that time, he had progressed from oral candidiasis to Kaposi's sarcoma and *Pneumocystis carinii* pneumonia. The virus isolated (HIV_{SF13}) had the same host range and serotype properties as HIV_{SF2}, but it now produced more cytopathology in PMC and could readily plaque in the MT-4 cell line (Tables 3, 4). Moreover, HIV_{SF13} had the same envelope variable region as HIV_{SF2}, as evaluated by the oligonucleotide probes (10,12).

TABLE 3
CHANGE IN HIV OVER TIME IN AN INFECTED INDIVIDUAL

	HIV_{SF2}	HIV_{SF13}
Clinical state	Oral candida	KS, PCP (5 mos.)
Host range	HUT-78, U-937	same
Cytopathology	+	++
Plaque formation	-	+
Neutralization	++	++

It is intriguing to speculate that the enhanced cytopathology of HIV_{SF13} may have been responsible for the increased pathology observed in this individual.

In a similar manner, we have isolated a virus (HIV_{SF2A}) from a chimpanzee that was inoculated one year previously with HIV_{SF2}. This HIV_{SF2A} isolate had the same host range in culture as HIV_{SF2}, but it was not longer susceptible to neutralization by the same sera that neutralize the parental virus (Table 4).

TABLE 4
SEROLOGIC PROPERTIES OF HIV RECOVERED OVER TIME

Serum	HIV_{SF2}	HIV_{SF13} (5 mos.)	HIV_{SF2A}* (1 year)
1	100	100	10
2	1000	1000	10
3	1000	100	-
4	1000	1000	-
5	100	100	10
6	1000	100	-

* chimpanzee isolate. Reciprocal of the end-dilution of serum showing greater than 66% reduction in reverse transcriptase activity is given. - less than 10.

Moreover, as noted for HIV_{SF13}, this isolate induced cytopathology readily in PMC and plaques in the MT-4 cell line. These two examples suggest that HIV can change biologically over time in an individual. Thus, the HIV from one person may show not only differences in restriction enzyme sensitivity (13), but also, most importantly, in certain biologic and serologic properties that can influence approaches at controlling HIV infection. In fact, when HIV_{SF2}, HIV_{SF13}, and HIV_{SF2A}, were evaluated by preliminary restriction enzyme analyses, a small difference was noted only with the Kpn-1 and Sac-1 enzymes. Alternatively, our results may indicate that one isolate in an individual infected with several HIV can emerge over time. In any case, these observations demonstrate that measurements of biologic features among different HIV isolated over time from the same individual may be a better indication of the important changes in HIV that could affect pathogenesis and therapy. They also pose important problems in the development of effective antiviral therapy.

CONCLUSIONS

These observations in our laboratory indicate the extensive heterogeneity among HIV as reflected in their biologic, serologic and molecular features. Individual HIV show different cell tropisms, and replicating properties. They vary in their kinetics of replication, production of cytopathology in cells, and ability to establish a latent state. Serotypes of HIV can be identified using selected sera from HIV-infected individuals. These serologic differences may be the result of variations in the *env* portion of the genome as reflected by the restriction enzyme sensitivity patterns and envelope variable regions. All these heterogeneous features can be observed in HIV when they infect different subjects. Moreover, changes may also emerge as the virus replicates within the same host. These observations suggest areas of research in which the biologic properties of the virus might be modified with antiviral therapy (e.g., *orf-B* protein), and underline the difficulties that may be encountered in developing effective therapies and a vaccine.

REFERENCES

1. Barre-Sinoussi F, Chermann JC, Rey R, Nugeyre MT, Chamaret S, Gruest J, Dauguet C, Axler-Blin C, Vezinet-Brun F, Rouzioux C, Rosenbaum W, Montagnier L (1983) Isolation of a T-lymphotropic retrovirus from a patient at risk for acquired immune deficiency syndrome (AIDS). Science 225:868.

2. Gallo RC, Salahuddin SZ, Popovic M, Shearer GM, Kaplan M, Haynes BF, Palker TJ, Redfiend R, Oleske J, Safai B, White G, Foster P, Markham PD (1984). Frequent detection and isolation of cytopathic retroviruses (HTLV-III) from patients with AIDS and at risk for AIDS. Science 224:500.

3. Levy JA, Hoffman AD, Kramer SM, Landis JA, Shimabukuro JM, Oshiro LS (1984) Isolation of lymphocytopathic retroviruses from San Francisco patients with AIDS. Science 235:840.

4. Coffin J, Haase A, Levy JA, Montagnier L, Oroszlan S, Teich N, Temin H, Toyoshima K, Varmus H, Vogt P, Weiss R (1986) Human immunodeficiency viruses. Science 235:697.

5. Evans LA, McHugh TM, Stites DP, Levy JA (1987) Differential ability of human immunodeficiency virus isolates to productively infect human cells. J Immunol (in press).

6. Levy JA, Evans LA, Pan L-Z, Tateno M, Reed MF, Walker C, Homsy J, Cheng-Mayer C (1987) The biologic heterogeneity of HIV and host immune response during HIV infection. In: Ginsburg H, Lerner R, Chanock R (eds): Vaccines 1987 (in press).

7. Cheng-Mayer C, Rutka JT, Rosenblum ML, McHugh T, Stites DP, Levy JA (1987) The human immunodeficiency virus (HIV) can productively infect cultured human glial cells. Proc Natl Acad Sci (USA) (in press).

8. Harada S, Koyanagi Y, Yamamoto N (1985) Infection of human T-lymphotropic virus type-1 (HTLV-I)-bearing MT-4 cells with HTLV-III (AIDS virus): Chronological studies of early events. Virology 146:272.

9. Folks T, Powell DM, Lightfoote MM, Benn S, Martin MA, Fauci AS (1986) Induction of HTLV-III/LAV from a non-virus-producing T cell line: Implications for Latency. Science:

231:600.

10. Levy JA, Evans LA, Cheng-Mayer C, Pan L-Z, Lane A, Staben C, Dina D, Wiley C, Nelson J (1987) The biologic and molecular properties of the AIDS-associated retrovirus that affect antiviral therapy. Ann Inst Pasteur 138:101.

11. Luciw PA, Cheng-Mayer C, Levy JA (1987) Mutational analysis of the human immunodeficiency virus (HIV): The orf-B region down-regulates virus replication. Proc Natl Acad Sci (USA) 84:1434.

12. Staben C, Shimabukuro J, Stephens JC, Barr PJ, Sabin B, Parkes D, Luciw PA, Steimer KS, Levy JA, Dina D (1986) The nature and significance of sequence variation among independent AIDS retrovirus isolates. In:Vaccine '86, Cold Spring Harbor Laboratory, p 345.

13. Hahn BH, Shaw GM, Taylor ME, Redfield RR, Markham PD, Salahuddin SZ, Wong-Staal F, Gallo RC, Parks ES, Parks WP (1986) Genetic variation in HTLV-III/LAV over time in patients with AIDS or at risk for AIDS. Science 232:1548.

**Human Retroviruses, Cancer, and AIDS:
Approaches to Prevention and Therapy, pages 101–114**

GENETIC VARIATION OF HUMAN IMMUNODEFICIENCY VIRUS TYPE 1 (HIV-1) *IN VITRO* AND *IN VIVO*[1]

Joseph Gibbons,[2] Michael S. Saag,[2] Elizabeth S. Parks,[3] Wade P. Parks,[3] Beatrice H. Hahn,[2] George M. Shaw,[2]

[2]Departments of Internal Medicine and Biochemistry
University of Alabama at Birmingham
Comprehensive Cancer Center, BHS 288
Birmingham, Alabama 35294

[3]Department of Pediatrics
University of Miami School of Medicine
Miami, Florida 33101

ABSTRACT Genetic variation of HIV-1 is a prominent viral property which may contribute importantly to viral persistence and disease pathogenesis. In this report, we present data indicating that the observed genetic diversity among independent HIV-1 isolates is the result of genetic changes that have occurred during natural infection *in vivo*, and are not the result of *in vitro* changes in the virus. The extent of HIV-1 diversity present in infected individuals at any one time is extensive, and is the result of rapid and progressive changes in the viral genome. Accordingly, "isolates" of HIV-1 from infected patients, unless biologically or molecularly cloned, are generally comprised of complex mixtures of genotypically-distinct, albeit related, viral forms. The implications of these findings in regard to AIDS pathogenesis and studies of HIV-1 biology are discussed.

[1]This work was supported in part by National Institutes of Health grants AI 23616 and AI 23854, by the U.S. Army Medical Research Acquisition Activity, Contract No. DAMD17-87-C-7038, and by a grant from the Life and Health Insurance Medical Research Fund. B.H.H. is a Special Fellow of the Leukemia Society of American and G.M.S. is a Pew Scholar in the Biomedical Sciences.

INTRODUCTION

The biology of HIV-1 infection and the pathogenesis of AIDS are known to be extraordinarily complex (1-3). Effective prophylaxis and treatment of retroviral infections in man and animals is unprecedented and is made especially difficult by the chronicity of viral infection, the propensity of virus to integrate as proviral DNA within the host's genome, the down-regulation of viral replication *in vivo*, the propensity for genetic variation over time, and the fact that HIV-1 not only establishes chronic infection but also infects and destroys a critical component of the immune system which otherwise would participate in the elimination of the infecting virus (4,5).

Genetic variation among independent isolates of HIV-1 was recognized early on as a prominent property of this virus (6,7). Subsequent studies by numerous investigators have shown that HIV-1 isolates from different parts of the United States, Europe, Haiti, and Africa vary by as much as 25% in the amino acid sequence of the outer envelope (8-11). With few exceptions, every reported isolate of HIV-1 has been readily distinguishable by restriction enzyme cleavage analysis.

Given the observed differences in restriction patterns and nucleotide sequences among different HIV-1 isolates, the question is raised whether these differences are the result of genetic changes that occurred in these viruses *in vivo* during persistent viral infection, or *in vitro* during viral cultivation and propagation prior to analysis. We summarize here a series of experiments whose results indicate that the observed genetic differences among independent HIV-1 isolates are the result of mutations in the viral genome that have occurred *in vivo*, not *in vitro*. That these genotypic changes occurred *in vivo* during persistent viral infection has important implications concerning the pathobiology of AIDS and HIV-1 infection.

RESULTS

An example of the extent of variation in restriction enzyme cleavage patterns that is evident among independent isolates of HIV-1 is shown in Figure 1.

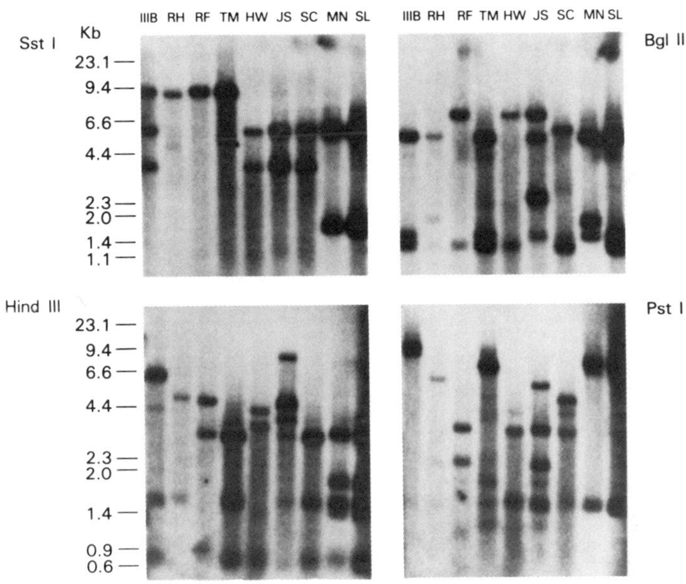

FIGURE 1. Heterogeneity of independent HIV-1 virus isolates based on restriction cleavage - Southern blot analysis (from Science 229:759, 1985). Virus was cultured from patient lymphocytes and propagated in normal donor lymphocytes or in immortalized T-cell lines.

Subsequent mapping studies (12-14) have confirmed that most HIV-1 isolates are quite readily distinguishable on the basis of restriction mapping as well as nucleotide sequencing.

In order to determine if such differences in restriction enzyme cleavage patterns of HIV-1 isolates could have resulted from *in vitro* mutations occurring during virus cultivation and propagation, the restriction pattern of a viral isolate cultivated from brain tissue was compared in its restriction pattern to that of proviral DNA in fresh, *uncultured* brain tissue from the same patient (Figure 2).

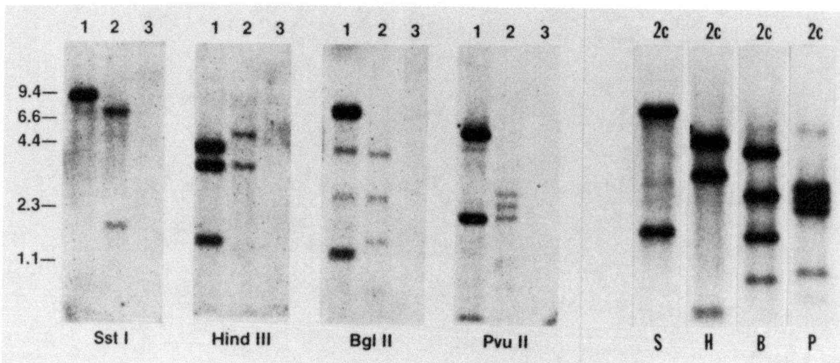

FIGURE 2. Southern blot comparison of the restriction enzyme cleavage pattern of HIV-1 (isolate BB) that was cultured from brain tissue and propagated in normal donor lymphocytes (lanes 2c) with provirus present in fresh, uncultured brain tissue (lanes 2). In this experiment, brain tissue from an infant with AIDS encephalopathy was

(continued)

obtained at necropsy; a portion of this brain specimen was co-cultured with normal donor lymphocytes and a second portion extracted directly for high molecular weight DNA. Lanes 1 and 3 represent unrelated positive and negative control DNAs. Note that the proviral restriction fragments for Sst I (S), Hind III (H), Bgl II (B), and Pvu II (P) are identical for cultured (2c) and uncultured (2) proviruses. This analysis demonstrated that the virus cultured from this patient was indistinguishable from the predominant viral form present in situ (in vivo), thus providing direct evidence that the genomic differences among independent HIV-1 isolates illustrated in Figure 1 are not due to changes that occurred during in vitro virus cultivation.

A second experimental approach taken to address the question of in vitro viral changes was to passage an HIV-1 isolate in vitro and to examine its genome before and after passage for genotypic changes. In this experiment, isolate HIV-1/WMJ-1 (13) was utilized. Cell-free virus was passed through a 0.45 micron filter, serially diluted from 10^{-1} through 10^{-6}, and then each 10-fold dilution was applied to uninfected H9 cells. The culture corresponding to the last dilution of supernatant which still gave rise to a positive culture after four weeks was taken as the end-point or terminal dilution. Supernatant from this culture was similarly passed through a 0.45 micron filter, diluted to 10^{-6}, and all dilutions again applied to uninfected H9 cells. This sequence was repeated five times. In this manner, cell-free virus was forced over a six month period to undergo a very large number of replicative cycles including the error-prone reverse transcriptase step. As Figure 3 illustrates, after six months of in vitro propagation, the genomic restriction pattern of the WMJ-1 virus (T.D.5) was indistinguishable from that observed before passage.

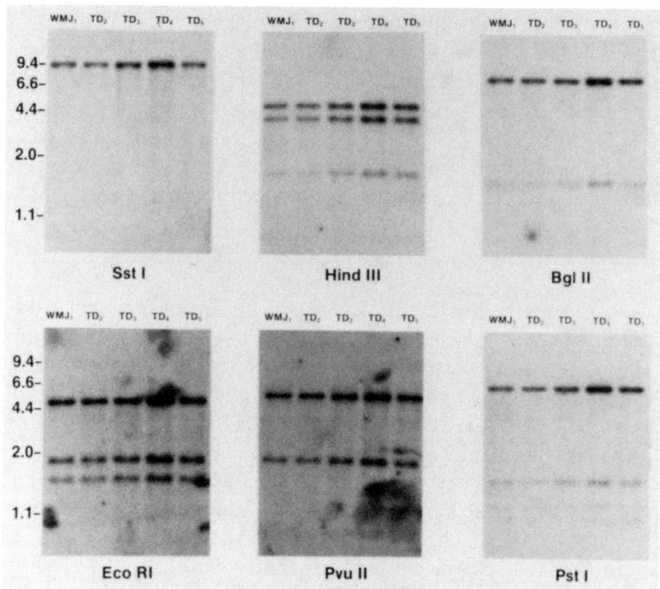

FIGURE 3. Restriction enzyme-Southern blot comparison of HIV-1 virus isolate WMJ-1 (13) before and after five sequential end-point dilutions and cell-free transmissions (see text for experimental details).

The third experimental approach taken to analyze the nature and significance of genomic heterogeneity in independent HIV-1 isolates was to compare the extent of restriction enzyme differences among virus isolates from different patients with differences in sequential virus isolates from individual patients. Figure 4 depicts the restriction fragment analysis of five sequential virus isolates of patient WMJ obtained over a period of one year

(13). All five isolates are identical in Sst I, EcoRI, and Pst I patterns and nearly identical in Bgl II and Pvu II. If restriction site changes had resulted from *in vitro* viral propagation, one would expect a spectrum of diversity in the sequential WMJ isolates (Figure 4) equal to that for isolates from different patients (Figure 1). This was not the case. Finally, we have also taken blood samples from HIV-1 infected individuals, divided the specimens, co-cultivated them with different normal donor lymphocytes, and found their restriction patterns to be identical (data not shown).

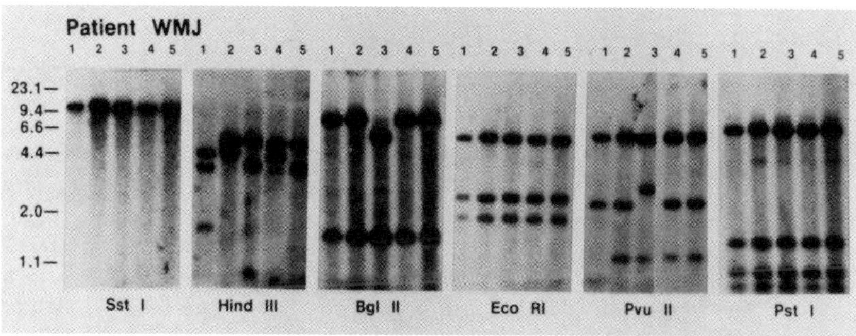

FIGURE 4. Restriction patterns of five sequential virus isolates obtained from patient WMJ over a one-year period.

The experimental data cited above thus argue strongly that genotypic differences among independent AIDS virus isolates are, in fact, the result of mutations that have occurred in vivo, and not in vitro during virus cultivation. We have previously analysed the extent and nature of genotypic variation occurring in sequential virus isolates that were obtained over a one- to two-year period from three patients (13). That study led to the conclusion that the rate of viral genetic change for HIV-1 is actually quite high, approximately 10^{-3} nucleotide substitutions per site per year, a rate equal to that of Influenza A (13). With that study and the experiments described in this paper in mind, we decided to determine the extent of HIV-1 genotypic diversity that might exist within an individual patient at any one point in time. That is, are individuals generally infected with a single genotype of virus at a time, or are they infected with a constellation of genotypically-distinct viruses? Our earlier studies (6,7,13) had suggested that individuals were infected with only one or a limited group of HIV-1 viruses but could not determine whether or not genotypic variants of these predominant viral forms were also present. To study this question, three virus isolates were obtained from the peripheral blood of two patients with AIDS-related complex (WMF-I; WMF-II; and RJS-IV). The Southern blot analyses of these isolates have been reported elsewhere (ref. 13; Figure 1), and were shown to contain two apparent predominant viral genotypes in each isolate. However, when recombinant DNA libraries were prepared from these "isolates," it was found that there were 14 distinct full-length genotypic forms of HIV-1 in isolate RJS-4, 9 distinct full-length HIV-1 genotypes in isolate WMF-1, and 5 different genotypes in WMF-3 (Table 1).

TABLE 1
GENOTYPIC DIVERSITY WITHIN HIV-1 "ISOLATES"[a]

HIV-1 Isolate	# of Full-length Clones Analysed	# of Genotypically-Distinct Clones
RJS-4	28	14
WMF-1	17	9
WMF-3	8	5
WMJ-1 (TD-5)	10	1

(continued)

[a]Recombinant DNA libraries were prepared from virally-infected cellular DNA of isolates RJS-4, WMF-1, and WMF-3 described in reference 13, and from isolate WMJ-1 (Terminal Dilution #5) described in this paper. Recombinant clones were mapped with six enzymes.

The predominant restriction patterns visualized by Southern analysis of virally-infected cellular DNA of each of these isolates corresponded to the recombinant proviral clones that were most abundant in the libraries. Yet, as shown in Table 1, there were a surprisingly large number of genotypically-distinct viral forms present in each "isolate" that were not apparent in the Southern blot analyses of the virally-infected cellular DNAs. These genotypically-distinct viral forms, although differing from each other in some restriction sites, were all closely related to each other, thus indicating that they had evolved from a common progenitor virus, most likely within that infected individual. In contrast, a recombinant DNA library prepared from cellular DNA of a biologically-cloned isolate (WMJ Terminal Dilution #5; Figure 3) did not contain this genotypic diversity, with nine of 10 clones being identical and one clone differing in only a single restriction site out of 20 mapped.

These data, along with prior studies of genetic diversity (6-13), thus indicate that a striking degree of genomic variation of HIV-1 develops *in vivo* during persistent infection of the host. A model for the generation of this diversity is presented in Figure 5.

GENERATION OF VARIANT HIV VIRUSES WITHIN AN INFECTED INDIVIDUAL

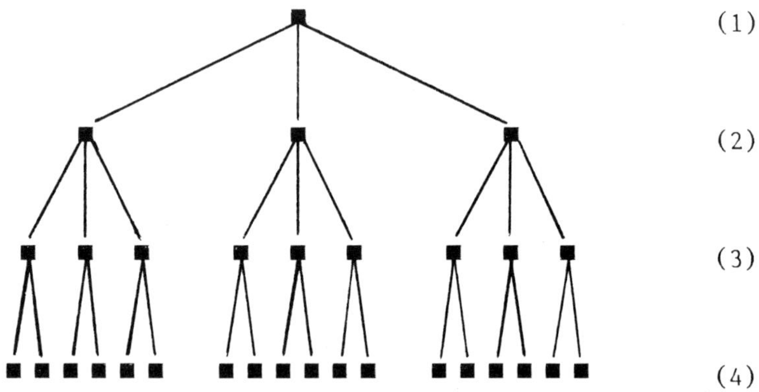

FIGURE 5. The experimental observation that individuals are persistently infected by a group of highly related, yet distinguishable and changing viral genotypes (7,13), suggests that individuals are naturally infected by only one or a very limited number of viruses and that these viruses undergo substantial variation in their genomic sequences over time. That host factors, including immunologic responses, may exert selective pressures for certain variants over others is a hypothesis under study.

DISCUSSION

Previous studies (6-14) have highlighted the variable nature of the AIDS virus genome and have shown the outer envelope glycoprotein, in particular, to be highly mutable. The data presented herein indicate that the preponderance of genetic divergences that have been identified in virus isolates from different patients (6-12,14) and from individual patients at different time points in their disease course reflect changes that have occurred in vivo, and are not due to artifacts of in vitro cultivation. Furthermore, the data summarized in Table 1 indicate that the degree of genotypic diversity of HIV-1 even within individual patients, is striking and heretofore has generally been underestimated.

These data have several implications regarding HIV-1 biology. The striking degree of genetic variation that occurs in vivo during natural infection suggests that host factors, immunologic or otherwise, may produce rather strong selective pressures on the virus. Such pressures could select for variants that are able to evade immunologic defenses, infect or persist in specific cell types, interact preferentially with certain major histocompatibility antigens, etc. The possibility that immune pressures may be important in viral selection is supported by the rapid genotypic changes that occur in vivo but not in vitro, and by the observation that even individuals having innumerable contacts to HIV-1 infected individuals appear to be infected with only a single group of highly related, yet distinguishable, viruses. A case in point is patient RJS (Table 1, and ref. 13) who had more than 1,000 different homosexual partners from HIV-1 endemic regions between 1980 and 1985. Despite these multiple exposures, repeated virus isolations from this patient over a two-year period yielded cultures consisting of many viral genotypes. Although distinguishable, these isolates were much more closely related to each other than to independent virus isolates (from different people) and had thus clearly evolved in the immediate past from a common progenitor virus -- probably within this patient (ref. 13; M. Saag, in preparation). The model for HIV-1 genotypic variation shown in Figure 5 is consistent with these experimental observations.

An important question concerning the pathophysiology of AIDS concerns the nature and significance of the immunologic response generated against the virus. Our demonstration here (Table 1) that "isolates" of HIV-1 from individual patients are actually comprised of complex mixtures of genotypically-distinct viruses may provide an explanation for the previous failure of neutralization assays to detect high titre, type-specific antibodies in autologous and heterologous assay systems (16). Studies are currently underway using transfection-derived and genetically-defined AIDS virus isolates to reassess the biological significance of type-specific immunity to HIV-1 in man.

In light of the above discussion, it is worthwhile to consider the picornavirus "Canyon Hypothesis" (17) as a possible model for HIV-1 pathogenesis. The picornaviruses are a group of positive-sense, single-stranded RNA viruses that cause a number of medically important diseases in man and animals, including poliomyelitis, hepatitis, the common cold, foot-and-mouth disease, myocarditis, and encephalitis. The atomic structures of two of these viruses, human rhinovirus 14 (HRV-14) and Mengo virus, have recently been determined by x-ray crystallography, and from these structures, the putative viral capsid binding sites specific for target cell receptors have been identified (18,19). The "Canyon Hypothesis" obtains from the x-ray crystallographic demonstration of "canyon" or "pit" regions within the capsid structures of HRV-14 and Mengo virus. According to this model, critical peptide sequences deep in canyons, or pits, would be inaccessible to antibody yet would be accessible to smaller cellular receptor sequences. This would allow for receptor specificity and at the same time permit the evolution of new viral serotypes by altering amino acid sequences around the rim of the canyon or pit. Considerable experimental evidence supports this model for picornaviruses (17). With the identification of the CD-4 molecule and gp120 molecule as the cellular-viral receptor binding complex for HIV-1 (20-22), it should be possible to combine the techniques of x-ray crystallography, site-directed mutagenesis, and targeted peptides and antibodies to delineate the HIV-1 envelope region involved in receptor binding and immune interaction. Such information will likely be useful in the development of effective vaccines and possibly novel treatment modalities.

REFERENCES

1. Fauci AS (1986). Current issues in developing a strategy for dealing with the acquired immunodeficiency syndrome. Proc Natl Acad Sci USA 83:9278.
2. National Academy Press (1986). "Confronting AIDS: Directions for Public Health, Health Care, and Research." Washington, DC.
3. Wong-Staal F, Gallo RC (1985). Human T-lymphotropic retroviruses. Nature 317(6036):395.
4. Haase AT (1986). Pathogenesis of lentivirus infections. Nature 322:130.
5. Gallo RC (1987). "The AIDS Virus." Scientific American, New York: W H Freeman and Company, 256(1): 46.
6. Shaw GM, Hahn BH, Arya SK, Groopman JE, Gallo RC, Wong-Staal F (1984). Molecular characterization of human T-cell leukemia (lymphotropic) virus type III in the acquired immune deficiency syndrome. Science 226:1165.
7. Wong-Staal F, Shaw GM, Hahn BH, Salahuddin SZ, Popovic M, Markham P, Redfield R, Gallo RC (1985). Genomic diversity of human T-lymphotropic virus type III (HTLV-III). Science 229:759.
8. Starcich BR, Hahn BH, Shaw GM, McNeely PD, Modrow S, Wolf H, Parks ES, Parks WP, Josephs SF, Gallo RC, Wong-Staal F (1986). Identication and characterization of conserved and variable regions in the envelope gene of HTLV-III/LAV, the retrovirus of AIDS. Cell 45:637.
9. Alizon M, Wain-Hobson S, Montagnier L, Sonigo P (1986). Genetic variability of the AIDS virus: Nucleotide sequence analysis of two isolates from African patients. Cell 46:63.
10. Willey RL, Rutledge RA, Dias S, Folks T, Theodore T, Buckler CE, Martin MA (1986). Identification of conserved and divergent domains within the envelope gene of the acquired immunodeficiency syndrome retrovirus. Proc Natl Acad Sci USA 83:5038.
11. Desai SM, Kalyanaraman VS, Casey JM, Srinivasan A, Andersen PR, Devare SG (1986). Molecular cloning and primary nucleotide sequence analysis of a distinct human immunodeficiency virus isolate reveal significant divergence in its genomic sequences. Proc Natl Acad Sci USA 83:8380.

12. Hahn BH, Gonda MA, Shaw GM, Popovic M, Hoxie JA, Gallo RC, Wong-Staal F (1985). Genomic diversity of the acquired immune deficiency syndrome virus HTLV-III: Different viruses exhibit greatest divergence in their envelope genes. Proc Natl Acad Sci USA 82:4813.
13. Hahn BH, Shaw GM, Taylor ME, Redfield RR, Markham PD, Salahuddin SZ, Wong-Staal F, Gallo RC, Parks ES, Parks WP (1986). Genetic variation in HTLV-III/LAV over time in patients with AIDS or at risk for AIDS. Science 232:1548.
14. Benn S, Rutledge R, Folks T, Gold J, Baker L, McCormick J, Feorino P, Piot P, Quinn T, Martin M (1985). Genomic heterogeneity of AIDS retroviral isolates from North America and Zaire. Science 230:949.
15. Coffin JM (1986). Genetic variation in AIDS viruses. Cell 46:1.
16. Weiss RA, Clapham PR, Weber JN, Dalgleish AG, Lasky LA, Berman PW (1986). Variable and conserved neutralization antigens of human immunodeficiency virus. Nature 324:572.
17. Smith TJ, Kremer MJ, Luo M, Vriend G, Arnold E, Kamer G, Rossmann MG, McKinlay MA, Diana GD, Otto MJ (1986). The site of attachment in human rhinovirus 14 for antiviral agents that inhibit uncoating. Science 233:1286.
18. Rossmann MG, Arnold E, Erickson JW, Frankenberger EA, Griffith JP, Hecht H-J, Johnson JE, Kamer G, Luo M, Mosser AG, Rueckert RR, Sherry B, Vriend G (1985). Nature 317:145.
19. Luo M, Vriend G, Kamer G, Minor I, Arnold E, Rossmann MG, Boege U, Scraba DG, Duke GM, Palmenberg AC (1987). The atomic structure of Mengo virus at 3.0 Å resolution. Science 235:182.
20. Dalgleish AG, Beverley PCL, Clapham PR, Crawford DH, Greaves MF, Weiss RA (1984). The CD4 (T4) antigen is an essential component of the receptor for the AIDS retrovirus. Nature 312:763.
21. McDougal JS, Kennedy MS, Sligh JM, Cort SP, Mawle A, Nicholson JKA (1986). Binding of HTLV-III/LAV to T4$^+$ T cells by a complex of the 110K viral protein and the T4 molecule. Science 231:382.
22. Maddon PJ, Dalgleish AG, McDougal JS, Clapham PR, Weiss RA, Axel R (1986). The T4 gene encodes the AIDS virus receptor and is expressed in the immune system and the brain. Cell 47:333.

Human Retroviruses, Cancer, and AIDS:
Approaches to Prevention and Therapy, pages 115–122

Expression Directed by the Long Terminal Repeat of the Human Immunodeficiency Virus is Enhanced in Activated T-cells[1]

Paul A. Luciw[2], Sandra Tong-Starksen[3], and B. Matija Peterlin[3]

[2]Department of Medical Pathology, University of California, Davis, California 95616
[3]Howard Hughes Medical Institute, University of California, San Francisco, California 94143

ABSTRACT An enhancer element was functionally identified in the long terminal repeat (LTR) of the human immunodeficiency virus (HIV-1). This enhancer, contained within a 30 base pair sequence, was found to be necessary and sufficient for regulating gene expression directed by the HIV-1 LTR in activated T-cells. Thus, T-cell activation may be a critical step in converting a latent and asymptomatic HIV infection to pathogenic sequelae characteristic of the acquired immunodeficiency syndrome (AIDS).

INTRODUCTION

T-cell activation refers to the regulated set of events occurring in T-lymphoid cells responding to external signals (1,2). Under physiological conditions, an antigen presented by a macrophage interacts with the T-cell receptor on the surface of lymphoid cells, and together with interleukin I, stimulates T-cells to divide and express lymphokines and new membrane proteins. Any of several treatments can activate T-cells including exposure to lectins, phorbol myristic acid, calcium ionophores, and antibodies to certain T-cell surface proteins (1). Following these treatments, phosphodiesterase is stimulated to generate inositol triphosphate and diacylglycerol; the former increases intracellular calcium levels and the latter activates protein kinase C (1). These events culminate in induction of

---

[1]This work was supported by grants to P.A.L. and B.M.P. from the California Universitywide Task Force on AIDS.

interleukin 2 (IL2), gamma-interferon, IL2 receptor, and several other genes, presumably at the transcriptional level (1).

Several observations stress the importance of the physiological state of T-cells with respect to replication of the human immunodeficiency virus (HIV-1). The original isolation of HIV-1, identified as the lymphadenopathy-associated virus (LAV), was achieved after stimulation of human peripheral blood lymphocytes with lectins (3). Subsequent studies have shown that quiescent T4-cells in preparations of peripheral blood lymphocytes are infectable with HIV-1 but activation is required for efficient virus production and cytopathology (4-6). Treatment of human T-lymphoid tumor lines harboring HIV-1 proviruses with T-cell activating agents enhances virus release (7,8). Presented here are investigations on the transcriptional mechanism by which activated T-cells affect HIV-1 replication. The enhancer element in the promoter within the HIV-1 long terminal repeat (LTR) was shown to respond to T-cell activation signals (9).

LTR-DIRECTED GENE EXPRESSION IN ACTIVATED T-CELLS

Regulation of the IL2 promoter in T-cells has been analyzed by DNA transfection and transient expression assays in the Jurkat T-cell line (10). This human lymphoid T-cell line is permissive for HIV-1 replication (8,11) and can be stimulated in tissue culture by a variety of T-cell activating agents (1). The Jurkat cell line was chosen as a system for analyzing HIV gene regulation.The HIV-1 LTR contains sequences which are required for transcription and which function as the target (tar) for the viral transactivator (TAT) gene (12-15). Interestingly, the sequence between -302 and -246 in the U3 portion of the HIV-1 LTR shows some homology to sequences in the promoter region of the IL2 gene; the region between -125 and -109 in the LTR has some homology with the promoter of the gamma-interferon gene (9,16,17). To analyze HIV-1 expression, the LTR was positioned upstream form the bacterial chloramphenicol transacetylase (CAT) gene to produce the plasmid pTAR-1 (9,15,18). The promoters of several other viruses were also attached to the CAT gene to assess the specificity of T-cell activation events. Table 1 compares the levels of CAT in unstimulated and stimulated Jurkat cells transfected with plasmids containing various viral promoters. CAT levels were measured after transfection of Jurkat cells with these plasmids. Only the HIV-1 LTR responds to T-cell activation signals. Gene expression directed by the Rous sarcoma virus (RSV) LTR (19), the herpes simplex virus type 1 thymidine kinase (HSV TK) gene (20), or the human T-lymphotropic virus type I (HTLV-I) LTR (21) are not affected by stimulation of Jurkat cells (Table1). Co-transfection of pTAR-1 with a plasmid containing the HIV-1 TAT gene (pTAT-1) revealed that the effects of T-cell activation and TAT-mediated transactivation were multiplicative (9); this outcome suggests that the targets in the HIV-1 LTR for these two regulatory mechanisms are different.

To determine which sequences in the HIV-1 LTR are required for responding to T-cell activation events, mutations were made in the LTR and hybrid promoters were constructed and tested (9). Table 2 shows that sequences downstream from position -156 are sufficient. The U3 region in the HIV-1 LTR that has homology with the IL2 gene (-302 to -246) was positioned upstream from the HSV TK promoter; this hybrid promoter is not responsive to T-cell activation signals (Table 2). The observation that the native HSV TK promoter does not respond suggests that SP1 sites are not the targets of T-cell activation events. The remaining regulatory features in the HIV-1 LTR are the direct repeats (10 base pairs each) located between -105 to -85 that show homology to the immunoglobulin light chain gene enhancer (9,22,23). Previous studies have assigned enhancer activity to the region of the HIV-1 LTR between -134 and -17 (14). To assess the function of the region with homology to the immunoglobulin gene enhancer, an oligonucleotide encompassing sequences between -105 to -85 was synthesized and inserted in either of two orientations upstream from the enhancerless HSV TK promoter. Transfections with these two plasmids revealed that indeed the region between -105 and -85 in the HIV LTR has properties consistent with a transcriptional enhancer (Table 2). In addition, the promoters in each of these plasmids respond to T-cell activation signals (Table 2). Clustered site mutations in the HIV-1 enhancer yield promoters which are not affected by T-cell stimuli (data not shown). Thus, the HIV-1 enhancer element is necessary and sufficient for responding to T-cell activation signals.

TABLE 1

EXPRESSION OF VIRAL PROMOTERS IN ACTIVATED T-CELLS [a]

Promoter	CAT activity Unstimulated T-cells	CAT activity Stimulated T-cells	Fold activation
HIV-1 LTR	0.79	3.9	4.9
RSV LTR	5.7	4.3	0.75
HSV TK	0.11	0.13	1.2
HTLV-I LTR	0.19	0.27	1.4

[a] Jurkat cells were treated with 1 ug/ml phytohemagglutinin and 50 ng/ml phorbolmyristic acid at 48 hours after transfection, incubated for an additional 16 hours,and cell extracts were assayed for CAT enzyme activity (9,15,18,19).

TABLE 2
THE HIV-1 ENHANCER RESPONDS TO T-CELL ACTIVATION SIGNALS [a]

Promoter	CAT activity Unstimulated T-cells	Stimulated T-cells	Fold activation
HIV-1 LTR [b]	0.79	3.9	4.9
HIV-1 LTR (-156) [c]	0.33	1.6	4.8
HSV TK [d]	0.11	0.13	1.2
HSV TK + [-463 to -156] [e]	0.53	0.45	0.87
HSV TK + [-105 to -85] [f]	0.49	6.6	14
HSV TK + [-85 to -105] [g]	0.43	2.8	6.6

[a] See footnote in Table 1.

[b] The region from -463 to +80 in the HIV-1 LTR (9,17) has been positioned upstream from the CAT gene.

[c] The region from -156 to +80 in the HIV-1 LTR (9,17) has been positioned upstream from the CAT gene.

[d] The HSV TK promoter (20) has been cloned upstream from the CAT gene; this promoter does not have enhancer activity.

[e] The region from -463 to -156 in the HIV-1 LTR (9,17)has been cloned upstream from the HSV TK promoter in d above.

[f] A synthetic oligonucleotide corresponding to position -105 to -185 in the HIV-1 LTR (9,17) has been cloned in the sense orientation upstream of HSV TK promoter.

[g] The synthetic oligonucleotide in f above has been cloned in the anti-sense orientation upstream from the HSV TK promoter.

DISCUSSION

Further studies will be directed at identifying the transacting component(s) elaborated in activated T-cells that interacts with the HIV-1 enhancer element. Stimulation of murine B-cells has been shown to result in increases of a factor, designated NF-kappa B, that interacts with the enhancer sequence of immunoglobulin light chain genes (23); this sequence is similar to the enhancer element in the LTR of HIV-1 (9, 23). Whether or not the functional equivalent of NF-kappa B acts on the enhancer element in the HIV-1 LTR in activated T-cells remains to be established. Since HIV-1 also infects monocytes/macrophages, it will be necessary to determine if activation of these cells affects the level of gene expression directed by the HIV-1 LTR (24,25). In addition to induction of expression of new genes, mitogenesis is another outcome of T-cell activation (1). Regulation of HIV-1 gene expression in resting and growing cells remains to be examined. HIV-2 and simian T-lymphotropic virus type III/simian immunodeficiency virus (STLV-III/SIV) are two closely related T-cell tropic retroviruses associated with immunodeficiency in humans and rhesus macaque monkeys, respectively (26-30). The LTRs of each of these viruses have a sequence which has a high degree of homology to the enhancer element of HIV-1 (31,32). It remains to be determined if T-cell activation signals regulate expression of HIV-2 and STLV-III/SIV in a fashion similar to that of HIV-1. The STLV-III/SIV system offers an opportunity to evaluate the consequences of T-cell activation in an animal model.

T-cell activation may have significance with respect to the clinical onset of AIDS in an individual infected with HIV-1. In many instances, exposure to this virus is followed by an asymptomatic period lasting months to years (33,34). HIV-1 appears to establish a latent infection (or a low-level persistent infection) in T-cells, monocytes/macrophages, and perhaps other cell types. Infection of an individual with another virus (e.g., cytomegalovirus) (35) or with a variety of other agents can stimulate the immune system. If T-cells harboring silent proviruses are activated by these antigenic stimuli, then HIV-1 gene expression will be activated and, subsequently, viral transactivators will further escalate HIV-1 replication. Loss of a sufficient number of T4-helper/inducer lymphoid cells will immunocompromise the host. With respect to therapy, it may be proposed that inhibition of T-cell activation at appropriate times may prevent HIV-1 gene expression and may thus limit progression to AIDS.

REFERENCES

1. Weiss A, Imboden J, Hardy K, Manger B, Terhorst C, and Stobo J (1986). The role of T3/antigen receptor complex in T-cell activation. Ann. Rev. Immunol. 4:593.
2. MacDonald HR and Nabholz M (1986). T-cell activation. Ann. Rev. Cell Biol. 2:231.
3. Barre-Sinousi F, Chermann JC, Rey F, Nugeyre MT, Chamaret S, Gruest J, Dauguet C, Axler-Blin C, Vezinet-Brun F, Rouzioux C, Rosenbaum W, and Montagnier L (1984). Isolation of a T-lymphotropic retrovirus from a patient at risk for acquired immnue deficiency syndrome (AIDS). Science 22:868.
4. MacDougal JS, Mawle A, Cort SP, Nicholson JKA, Cross CD, Scheppeler-Campbell JA, Hicks D, and Sligh J (1985). Cellular tropism of the human retrovirus HTLV-III/LAV. I. Role of T-cell activation and expression of the T4 antigen. J. Immunol.

135:3151.
5. Folks T, Kelley J, Benn S, Kinter A, Justement J, Gold J, Redfeied R, Sell KW, and Fauci AS (1986). Susceptibility of normal human lymphocytes to infection with HTLV-III/LAV. J. Immunol. 136:4049.
6. Levy JA, Kaminsky LS, Morrow WJW, Steimer K, Luciw P, Dina D, Hoxie J, andOshiro L (1985). Infection by the retrovirus associated with the acquired immunodeficiency syndrome. Clinical, biological, and molecular features. Ann. Int. Med. 103:694.
7. Harada S, Koyanagi Y, Nakashima H, Kobayashi N, and Yamamoto N (1986). Tumor promoter TPA enhances replication of HTLV-III/LAV. Virology 154:249.
8. Zagury D, Bernard J, Leonard R, Cheynier R, Feldman M, Sarin PS, and Gallo RC (1986). Long-term cultures of HTLV-III-infected T-cells: a model of cytopathology of T-cell depletion in AIDS. Science 231:850.
9. Tong-Starksen SE, Luciw PA, and Peterlin BM (1987) The HIV LTR responds to T-cell activation signals. Submitted Proc. Natl. Acad. Sci. USA.
10. Fujita T, Shibuya H, Ohashi T, Yamanishi K, and Taniguchi T (1986) Regulation of human interleukin-2 gene: functional DNA sequences in the 5'flanking region for the gene expression in activated T lymphocytes. Cell 46:401.
11. Lifson JD, Reyes GR, McGrath MS, Stein BS and Engelman EG (1986) AIDS retrovirus incuced cytopathology: giant cell formation and involvement of CD4 antigen. Science 232:1123.
12. Arya SK, Guo C, Josephs SF, and Wong-Staal F (1985) Transactivator gene of human T-lymphotropic virus type III (HTLV-III). Science 229:69.
13. Sodroski J, Patarca R, Rosen C, Wong-Staal F, and Haseltine W (1985). Location of the trans-acting region of human T-cell lymphotropic virus type III. Science 229:74.
14. Rosen CA, Sodroski JG and Haseltine W (1985). The location of cis-acting regulatory sequences in the human T-lymphotropic virus type III (HTLV-III/LAV). Cell 41:813.
15. Peterlin BM, Luciw PA, Barr PJ, and Walker MD (1986). Elevated levels of mRNA can account for the transactivation of human immunodeficiency virus (HIV). Proc. Natl. Acad. Sci. USA 83:9734.
16. Starcich B, Ratner L, Josephs SF, Okamoto T, Gallo RC, and Wong-Staal F (1984) Characterization of long terminal repeat sequences of HTLV-III. Science 227:538.
17. Sanchez-Pescador R, Power MD, Barr PJ, Steimer KS, Stempien MM, Brown-Sheimer SL, Gee WW, Renard A, Randolph A,

Levy JA, Dina D, and Luciw PA (1985). Nucleotide sequence and expression of an AIDS-associated retrovirus (ARV-2). Science 227:484.
18. Gorman CM, Moffat LF and Howard BH (1982) Recombinant genomes which express chloramphenicol acetyltransferase in mammalian cells. Mol. Cell. Biol. 2:1044.
19. Gorman CM, Merlino GT, Willingham MC, Pastan I, and Howard BH (1982). The Rous sarcoma virus long terminal repeat is a strong promoter when introduced into a variety of eukaryotic cells by DNA-mediated transfection. Proc. Natl. Acad. Sci. USA 79:6777.
20. Walker MD, Edlund T, Boulet AM and Rutter WJ (1983) Cell-specific expression controlled by the 5'-flanking region of insulin and chymotrypsin genes. Nature 306:557.
21. Shah NP, Wachsman W, Cann AJ, Souza L, Slamon DJ, and Chen ISY (1986). Comparison of the trans-activation capabilities of the human T-cell leukemia virus type I and II X proteins. Mol. Cell. Biol. 6:3626.
22. Gluzman Y and Shenk T (1983) "Enhancers and Eucaryotic gene expression" Cold Spring Harbor: New York.
23. Sen R and Baltimore D (1986) Multiple nuclear factors interact with the immunoglobulin enhancer sequences. Cell 48:705.
24. Nicholson JKA, Cross GD, Callaway CS and McDougal JS (1986). In vitro infection of human monocytes with human T lymphotropic virus type III/lymphadenopathy-associated virus (HTLV-III/LAV). J. Immunol. 137:323.
25. Gartner S, Markovits P, Markovitz DM, Kaplan MH, Gallo RC, and Popovic M. (1986) The role of mononuclear phagocytes in HTLV-III/LAV infection. Science 237:215.
26. Clavel F, Guetard D, Brun-Vezinet F, Chamaret S, Rey MA, Santos-Ferreira MO, Laurent AG, Dauguet C, Katlama C, Rouzioux C, Klatzmann D, Champalimaud JL, and Montagnier L (1986). Isolation of a new human retrovirus from West African patients with AIDS. Science 233:343.
27. Kanki PJ, McLane MF, King NW, Letvin NL, Hunt RD, Sehgal P, Daniel MD, Desrosiers RC and Essex M (1985). Serologic identification and characterization of a macaque T-lymphotropic retrovirus closely related to HTLV-III. Science 228:1199.
28. Letvin NL, Daniel MD, Seghal PK, Desrosiers RC, Hunt RD, Waldron LM, Mackey JJ, Schmidt DK, Chalifoux LV and King NW (1985) Induction of AIDS-like disease in macaque monkeys with T-cell tropic retrovirus STLV-III. Science 230:71.
29. Gardner MB, Luciw PA, Lerche N, anf Marx P (1987). Non-human primate retrovirus isolates and AIDS. In Perk K (ed) "Immunodeficiency Disorders and Retroviruses" New York:

Academic Press, in press.
30. Hirsch V, Reidel N, Kornfeld H, Kanki PJ, Essex M and Mullins JI (1986). Cross-reactivity of human T-lymphotropic virus type III/lymphadenopathy associated virus and molecular cloning of simian T-cell lymphotropic virus type 3 from African green monkeys. Proc. Natl. Acad. Sci. USA 83:9754.
31. Kornfeld H, Reidel N, Viglianti G, Hirsch V, and Mullins JI (1987). Cloning of HTLV-4 and its relation to simian and human immumodeficiency viruses. Nature 326:610.
32. Guyador M, Emmerman M, Sonigp P, Clavel F, Montagnier L, and Alizon M (1987). Organization and transactivation of the human immunodeficiency virus type 2. Nature 326:662.
33. Fauci AS (1986). Current issues in developing a strategy for dealing with the acquired immunodeficiency syndrome. Proc. Natl. Acad. Sci. USA 83:9278.
34. Klatzmann D and Gluckman JC (1986). Immunology Today 7:291.
35. Rando RF, Pellet PE, Luciw PA, Bohan CA, and Srinivasan A (1987). Transactivation of human immunodeficiency virus by herpesviruses. Oncogene, in press.

Human Retroviruses, Cancer, and AIDS:
Approaches to Prevention and Therapy, pages 123–132

CELL SURFACE MAJOR HISTOCOMPATIBILITY COMPLEX CLASS II ANTIGEN EXPRESSION IS ALTERED BY HIV BINDING AND INFECTION

Dean L. Mann, Suzanne Gartner, Frances LeSane, William A. Blattner, and Mikulas Popovic

Laboratory of Human Carcinogenesis, Laboratory of Tumor Cell Biology and Environmental Epidemiology Branch, National Cancer Institute, Bethesda, MD 20892

ABSTRACT Human immunodeficiency virus (HIV) infection is mediated by the interaction of the large envelope protein (gp120) with the CD4 molecule on the target cell surface. Infection can be blocked with monoclonal antibody to CD4 and also some monoclonal antibodies to major histocompatibility (MHC) class II antigens. We investigated the possible involvement of the MHC molecules in the HIV receptor by flow cytometric analysis of CD4 and MHC class II antigens on PHA stimulated peripheral blood lymphocytes (PBL) exposed for short time periods to virus particles and immunopurified gp120. Virus exposure for 15 minutes caused a decrease in the ability of monoclonal antibodies to detect HLA-DR and CD4a antigens. HLA-DR expression gradually returned to levels of expression equivalent to or greater than unexposed lymphocytes after 120 minutes of virus exposure while CD4 expression decreased. Other products of the MHC class II genes, HLA-DQ and HLA-DP, increased in the former or remained unchanged in the latter. Incubation of the PBL with immunopurified gp120 caused a two-fold increase in HLA-DR expression while HLA-DP and HLA-DQ remained unchanged. Monocytes isolated from PBL and infected in vitro with HIV showed an increased expression of HLA-DR, decreased CD4 and HLA-DQ and HLA-DP expression remained unchanged.

These data show that HLA-DR is involved in the HIV receptor and that expression of this MHC class II gene product increases with infection.

INTRODUCTION

HIV is tropic for cells that express the CD4 molecule (1-6). These include T-lymphocytes, monocytes, dendritic cells, and Langerhan's cells of the skin (7-11). The specific interaction of the virus with the CD4 molecule has been documented (3,4,5). This interaction takes place through the binding of the large envelope protein with the CD4 molecule as evidenced by co-precipitation of these molecules from cells exposed to the virus (6) and by inhibition of virus attachment to the cell with monoclonal antibodies directed at both the large envelope glycoprotein and epitopes on the CD4 molecule (2,4). In addition to blocking infection with monoclonal antibodies to CD4 epitopes, Dalgleish and colleagues demonstrated that some monoclonal antibodies detecting MHC class II antigens were effective in inhibiting infection (2). This observation suggested that MHC class II molecules may also be involved in the HIV receptor although the specific interaction of virus with these molecules has not heretofore been demonstrated. A common feature of cells that can be infected by HIV is the expression of MHC class II antigens. The cell types cited above all express class II antigens in their resting or activated states. Recently in vitro infection of monocytes derived from peripheral blood and from other tissues has been accomplished (7-9). We have examined the interaction of HIV viral particles with PHA-stimulated peripheral blood (PBC) lymphocytes after short time periods of exposure of the virus particles to the target cells. These studies employed monoclonal antibodies detecting the separate MHC class II gene products HLA-DR, HLA-DQ, and HLA-DP. In addition, we have examined the expression of these MHC class II antigens as well the CD4 molecule on monocytes before and after infection with HIV. The results of these studies are documented in this report.

METHODS AND MATERIALS

Blood samples were obtained from volunteers who had no history of HIV infection and whose sera were negative for HIV antibodies. The lymphocytes were prepared from whole blood and stimulated with PHA as described (12). Monocytes were isolated from the PBL and infected with HIV as previously reported (8,9).

Monoclonal antibodies detecting the CD4 epitopes OKT4 and OKT4A were obtained from Ortho Diagnostics. Monoclonal antibodies detecting the products of the MHC class II antigens are listed as follows: Tu22 detects HLA-DQ, TU43 detects HLA-DR (13) and B7/21 HLA-DP.

HIV and gp120 binding studies. PBL were stimulated with PHA for 3 days and incubated with 10^{10} viral particles concentrated from tissue culture supernatants from H9 HTLV-IIIB infected cell line. After 15, 30, 60, and 120 minutes of incubation at 37°C the cells were washed and 100 μl of saturating concentrations of monoclonal antibodies added. After an additional hour of incubation at 4° C, the cells were washed and a saturating amount of fluoresceinated goat anti-mouse immunoglobulin added. These cells were washed and fixed with glutaraldehyde prior to analysis. 10^4 cells were analyzed for fluorescence with the FACS-II (Becton Dickinson, CA). In all experiments the P3 myeloma protein which was used to control for nonspecific protein binding. Ten micrograms of the gp120, immunopurified as described,(14) were added in a volume of 100 μl to 10^6 PHA stimulated PBL. The cells were sampled at the time periods given above and prepared for analysis of expression of cell surface antigens as described above.

Infected and noninfected monocytes were removed from tissue culture flasks by washing the flasks free of media and incubation with calcium and magnesium free PBS on ice for 1 hour. The cells were gently removed with rubber policemen and washed extensively in the calcium and magnesium free PBS. The cells were labeled with the monoclonal antibodies described above and analyzed by flow cytometry.

RESULTS

The reactivity of monoclonal antibodies detecting the CD4a HLA-DR, -DQ, -DP and gp120 antigens on PHA stimulated PBL exposed for various periods to HTLV-IIIB virus particles is shown in Table 1.

TABLE I

REACTIVITY OF MONCLONAL ANTIBODIES DETECTING CD4a, HLA-DR,-DQ, -DP AND GP120 ON LYMPHOCYTES[a] AFTER VARIOUS PERIODS OF INCUBATION WITH HTLV-IIIB VIRUS[b]

	0	15 min	30 min	60 min	120 min
Antigens[c]	% MFU[d]	% MFU	% MFU	% MFU	% MFU
CD4a	48(1614)	42(895)	41(620)	32(245)	24(107)
HLA-DQ	25(165)	45(483)	44(224)	39(306)	37(301)
HLA-DR	26(191)	11(48)	15(34)	17(147)	39(286)
HLA-DP	33(141)	34(137)	47(147)	42(140)	29(137)
gp120	0 (0)	35(312)	29(181)	32(296)	27(381)

[a]Peripheral blood lymphocytes isolated and stimulated with PHA is described in text.
[b]Virus particles concentrated from supernatants from the Molt-3 cell lines infected with HTLV-IIIB.
[c]Antigens detected by monoclonal antibodies as described in text.
[d]MFU - mean fluorescence units

After 15 minutes of exposure, there was a decrease in the ability to detect CD4a antigen. This decline continued over the time periods studied. The number of the cells reacting with CD4a monoclonal antibodies decreased from 48% to 24% after 1 hour exposure. There was a considerable reduction in the mean fluorescence (1,614 to 107) over this period of time studied. HLA-DQ increased after 15 minutes of virus exposure and remained elevated. The number of cells reacting with monoclonal antibodies detecting HLA-DR decreased after 15 minutes of exposure, remained low at 30 min and 60 min then increased at 120 minutes to levels higher than that seen on unexposed lymphocytes. HLA-DP increased at 30 minutes and then gradually decreased to levels comparable to the unexposed lymphocytes after 120 minutes of virus exposure. The reaction of antibodies detecting the large envelope glycoprotein gp120 confirmed the presence of the virus on the cell surface.

Since gp120 binds directly to the CD4 molecule, we investigated the possibility that the interaction of the viral large envelope protein with CD4 also involved HLA-DR (Table 2).

TABLE 2
REACTIVITY OF MONOCLONAL ANTIBODIESDETECTING CD4a, HLA-DR, -DQ, -DP and gp120 ANTIGENS WITH LYMPHOCYTES(a) INCUBATED FOR TIME PERIODS WITH HTLV-III LARGE ENVELOPE PROTEIN, gp120(b)

	0	15 min	30 min	60 min
Antigen[c]	% MFU[d]	% MFU	% MFU	% MFU
CD4a	54(1565)	29(78)	30(95)	31(84)
HLA-DQ	19(297)	24(203)	23(221)	24(224)
HLA-DR	20(202)	42(344)	38(317)	37(324)
HLA-DP	20(163)	24(161)	28(217)	26(214)
gp120	0 (0)	36(440)	34(540)	40(498)

[a]Peripheral blood lymphocytes stimulated with PHA and cultured 3 days
[b]Immunopurified gp120
[c]Antigens detected by monoclonal antibodies as described in text.
[d]MFU = mean fluorescence units

In contrast to the observations made with whole virus particles, exposure of cells to gp120 for 15 min resulted in 2 fold increase in the numbers of cells expressing HLA-DR. The increase in HLA-DR expression persisted over the time of the experiment (60 minutes). The presence of the large envelope protein on the lymphocyte cell surface was confirmed by the positive reactions with the monoclonal antibodies detecting the gp120 and a decrease in the ability to detect the CD4 antigen. HLA-DQ increased slightly at the various time periods sampled and HLA-DP remained essentially unchanged.

A comparison of the expression of the antigens on monocytes chronically infected with HIV is shown in Figure 1.

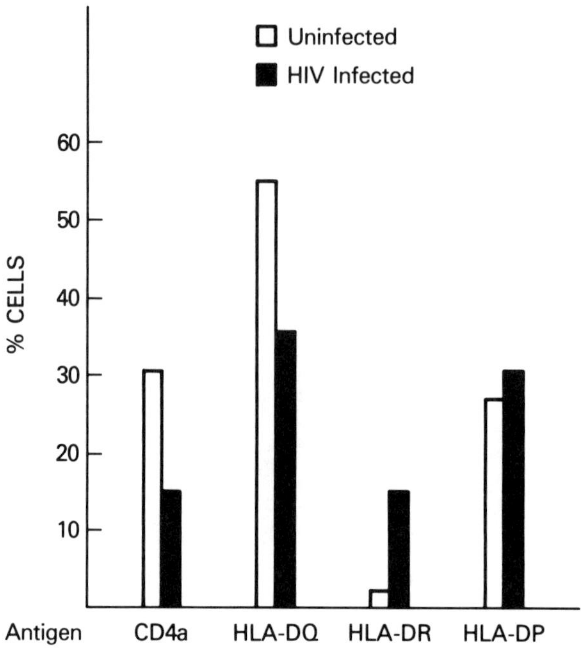

CD4 expression decreased to levels of approximately 50% of that seen on the infected monocytes. HLA-DQ was decreased and HLA-DP remained essentially unchanged in comparison of HIV infected monocytes with uninfected cells. HLA-DR increased in the infected cells compared to the numbers of uninfected cells expressing this antigen. Infection was monitored in the monocytes using antibodies to the p17 by visual indirect immunofluorescence. The number of cells infected ranged from 22 to 28%.

DISCUSSION

These observations indicate that HLA-DR is involved in the receptor site for HIV. This was demonstrated by decreased binding of monoclonal antibodies detecting HLA-DR and the CD4a antigen after short periods of exposure of PHA stimulated lymphocytes to concentrated HTLV-IIIB virus particles. These results also indicate that the interaction is restricted to only some of the products of the MHC D region. This is evidence by the fact that the numbers of the cells expressing HLA-DP and -DQ increased over the various time periods studied while HLA-DR decreased. These results may explain in part the observations made by Dalgleish *et al.* where only certain monoclonal antibodies directed against HLA class II antigens inhibited HIV infection.

Since we and others have demonstrated that the large envelope glyco- protein, gp120 binds to the CD4 molecule, we reasoned that this binding might also involve HLA-DR. The results of the studies demonstrate quite clearly that the binding of gp120 in and of itself to PHA stimulated peripheral blood lymphocytes does not directly involve MHC class II antigens. Rather an increase in the expression of HLA-DR was seen after 15 minutes of exposure of cells to gp120. These results explain the increase in the expression of HLA-DR on cells that are exposed to and subsequently infected with HIV. The results strongly indicate that perturbation of the CD4 molecule signals the cell to express increased quantities of HLA-DR. An alternative but less likely explanation is that a change in the configuration of the CD4 molecule that is effected by gp120 binding might expose the HLA-DR molecules in such a fashion that they are more accessible to reactions with these particular monoclonal antibodies. The rapid expression of HLA-DR on the cell surface after the gp120 exposure indicates that this interaction does not induce de novo expression of HLA-DR.

The infection of monocytes with HIV resulted in the loss of expression of the CD4 molecule and an increased expression of HLA-DR compared to uninfected monocytes. These results are consistent with the observations made in T-cell lines where the chronic infection of T-cells results in essentially the same phenotype, that is, a decrease in CD4 expression and an increase in HLA-DR.

The biologic significance of these results remains to be elucidated.

Both CD4 and HLA-DR molecules are important in the cellular interactions that take place in the normal immune response. HLA-DR is expressed on antigen presenting cells and plays a discriminating role in antigen presentation to CD4 positive lymphocytes. An alteration in the expression of either HLA-DR or CD4 may effect the ability of the T-cells to function in their normal role. As an example, when HIV virus or immuno-purifed gp120 is added to resting lymphocytes, PHA response is greatly diminished (12). This diminished response has also been observed when antibodies reacting with certain CD4 epitopes are added to cells when virus is not present (15). Thus, perturbation of CD4 appears to down regulate T-cell function, which, in the instance of HIV infection, may be in and of itself responsible for the immuno-suppression by mechanism other than cytolysis.

Monocytes infected with HIV showed changes in cell surface antigen expression not unlike that seen in T-cells. The results of these studies suggest that a subpopulation of monocytes might be selectively infected with HIV. We propose that this subset of monocytes are those cells that express CD4 and HLA-DR on the same cell. This conclusion is suggested by the fact that not all of the monocytes have become infected. CD4 expression decreased in a portion of the cells and a concomitant increase in HLA-DR expression also occurred in a portion of the cells. There remained, however, a population of cells that was CD4 positive, this suggests that there is a CD4 positive population that is HLA-DR negative and that these cells are not infected with HIV.

Based on these observations as well as results of other experiments, we hypothesize that the CD4 molecule binds HIV to the cell, however HLA-DR expression is necessary for virus infection to occur. The results of these studies suggest a model for the biological sequence of HIV infection. Monocytes or other antigen presenting cells (APC) are the primary target for the initial infection and serve as the virus reservior. These infected monocytes when functioning in their normal capacity as APC, present antigen together with HIV to T-cells. This results in the activation of antigen responsive CD4 T-lymphocytes and the cells become HLA-DR positive.

These cell surface molecules allow virus attachment, penetration and subsequent cell death occurs due to the cytopathic effect of the virus. As a wide spectrum of antigens are presented to the different antigen responsive T helper call clones, HIV infection occurs and the entire population is eliminated.

REFERENCES

1. Popovic M, Gallo RC, Mann DL (1984). OKT4 bearing molecule is a receptor for the human retrovirus HTLV-III. Clin Res 33:560A.

2. Dalgleish AG, Beverley PCL, Clapham PR, Crawford DH, Greaves MR, Weiss RA (1984). The CD4 (T4) antigen is an essential component of the receptor for the AIDS retrovirus. Nature 312:763-766.

3. McDougal JS, Nicholson JKA, Cross GD, Cort SP, Kennedy MS, Mawle AC (1986). Binding of the human retrovirus HTLV-III/LAV/ARV/HIV to the CD4 (T-4) molecule: Conformation dependence, epitope mapping, antibody inhibition and potential for idiotypic mimicry. J Immunol 137:2937-2944.

4. Sattentau QJ, Dagleish AG, Weiss RA, Beverley PCL (1986). Epitopes of the antigen and HIV infection. Science 234:1120-1123.

5. Maddon PJ, Dalgleish AG, McDougal JS, Clapham PR, Weiss RA, Axel R (1986). The T4 gene encodes for the AIDS virus receptor and is expressed in the immune system and the brain. Cell 47:333-348.

6. McDougal JS, Kennedy MS, Sligh JW, Cort SP, Mawle A, Nicholson KA (1986). Binding of HTLV-III/LAV to T4+ cells by a complex of 110k viral protein and the T4 molecule. Science 231:382-384.

7. Ho DD, Rota TR, Hirsch MS (1986). Infection of monocyte/macrophages by human T lymphotropic virus type III. J Clin Invest 77:1712-1715.

8. Gartner S, Markovits P, Markovitz DM, Kaplan MH, Gallo RC, Popovic M (1986). The role of mononuclear phagocytes in HTLV-III/LAV infection. Science 223:215-219.

9. Gartner S, Markovits P, Markovitz DM, Betts RF, Popovic M (1986). Virus isolation and identification of HTLV-III/LAV producing cells in brain tissue from a patient with AIDS. JAMA 256:2365-2371.

10. Koenig S, Gendelman HE, Orenstein JM, Dalcanto MC, Rezeslokpour GH, Yungbluth M, Janotta F, Akosamit A, Martin MA, Fauci AS (1986). Detection of macrophages in brain tissue from AIDS patients with encephalopathy. Science 233:1089-1093.

11. Tschachler E, Groh V, Popovic M, Mann DL, Konrad K, Safai B, Eron L, Veronese FD, Wolff K, Stingle G (1987). Epidermal Langerhans cells: A target for HTLV-III/LAV infection. J Invest Derm. (in press)

12. Mann DL, LeSane F, Popovic M, Arthur LO, Robey WG, Blattner WA, Newman MJ (in press). HTLV-III large envelope protein (gp120) suppresses PHA induced lymphocyte blastogenesis. J Immunol.

13. Ziegler A, Heinig J, Muller C, Gotz H, Thinnes FP, Uchanska-Ziegler B, Wernet P (1986). Analysis by sequential immune precipitation of the specificities of the monoclonal antibodies Tu 22, 34, 35, 36, 37, 39, 43, 58 and YD 1/63HLK directed against human HLA class II antigens. Immunobiology 171:77.

14. Robey WG, Arthur LO, Matthews TJ, Langlois A, Copeland TD, Lenche NW, Moszlan S, Bolognesi DP, Gilden RV, Fischinger PS (1986). Prospect for prevention of human immunodeficiency virus infection: Purified 120-KDa envelope glycoprotein induces meutralizing antibody. Proc Natl Acad Sci USA 83:7023.

15. Bank I, Chess L (1985). Perturbation of the T4 molecule transmits a negative signal to T cells. J Exp Med 162:1294.

III. PRODUCTS OF THE HIV GENOME

Human Retroviruses, Cancer, and AIDS: Approaches to Prevention and Therapy, pages 135–147

ANALYSIS OF PROTEINS AND PEPTIDES PURIFIED FROM SUCROSE GRADIENT BANDED HTLV-III

Louis E. Henderson, Terry D. Copeland, Raymond C. Sowder, Alan M. Schultz and Stephen Oroszlan

Laboratory of Molecular Virology and Carcinogenesis, BRI-Basic Research Program, NCI-Frederick Cancer Research Facility, Frederick, MD 21701

ABSTRACT Proteins and peptides of HTLV-III were purified by reversed phase high pressure liquid chromatography and characterized by a combination of methods including N- and C-terminal amino acid sequence analysis, phosphoamino acid analysis and fatty acid analysis. Proteins and peptides accounting for all portions of the *gag* precursor were characterized and proteolytic cleavage sites were identified. These results showed at least eight naturally occurring proteolytic cleavages in the HTLV-III *gag* precursor. The results also show that p17 is a myristylated protein and that p24 contains both phosphoserine and phosphothreonine.

Mature *env* and *pol* proteins were detected with antisera to synthetic peptides. These results showed that antisera to the C-terminal amino acid sequence of the putative viral protease detected an antigen with molecular weight of 11,500. Similarly a 13,300 dalton C-terminal fragment of reverse transcriptase and a 16,000 dalton C-terminal fragment of the *env* precursor were detected.

INTRODUCTION

Retroviruses associated with acquired immunodeficiency syndrome (AIDS) in humans are collectively designated as human immunodeficiency viruses (HIV) and include individual isolates designated human T-lymphotropic virus-III (HTLV-III) (1), lymphadenopathy-associated virus

(LAV) (2) and AID-associated retrovirus (ARV) (3). All retroviruses including HIV synthesize precursor polyproteins that subsequently undergo posttranslational modifications and proteolytic processing to produce the structural and functional proteins of the mature infectious virus. Detailed knowledge of the biosynthetic and processing events is necessary to understand the biology and pathology of HIV.

In order to define the structures of the various mature viral proteins, we have used the method of reversed phase high pressure liquid chromatography (RP-HPLC) to separate and purify proteins present in sucrose gradient-purified preparations of HTLV-III. Proteins and peptides derived from the gag polyprotein were identified by N- and C-terminal amino acid sequence analyses and comparing these data to the translated DNA sequence. Products from the pol region of the gag-pol polyprotein and products from the env polyprotein were detected and partly characterized by reaction with antisera prepared against synthetic peptides representing selected regions of the translated HTLV-III proviral DNA sequence (4). The data reported in this communication are in good agreement with previous immunological and structural studies and extend our knowledge of the proteolytic processing in HTLV-III.

MATERIALS AND METHODS

HTLV-III was grown in H-9 cells, purified by continuous flow density gradient centrifugation, and supplied by the Biological Products Laboratory, Program Resources, Inc., NCI-Frederick Cancer Research Facility, Frederick, MD. RP-HPLC was performed on a 19 x 150 mm column of μ-Bondapak C_{18} (Waters Associates Inc., Milford, MA) using volatile buffers and techniques previously described for the purification of other retroviral proteins (5-7). Purified proteins and peptides were analyzed for amino acid content with a model D-500 analyzer (Dionex Corp., Marlton, NJ). Edman degradations were performed with a model 470A gas phase sequencer and peptides were synthesized with a model 430A synthesizer (Applied Biosystems, Foster City, CA) as recommended by the manufacturer. C-terminal amino acid sequences were determined by the method of carboxypeptidase digestion as previously described (8).

RESULTS AND DISCUSSION

As a preliminary step to RP-HPLC, 50 ml of 1000x concentrated virus (in phosphate buffer at pH 7.2) containing about 50 mg of total protein was made 8.2 M in guanidium hydrochloride and 1% in 2-mercaptoethanol and allowed to stand at room temperature for 30 min. before it was adjusted to pH 2.0 with the addition of trifluoroacetic acid. The resulting clear solution was pumped into the RP-HPLC column and the retained material eluted with increasing concentrations of organic solvents. The resulting chromatogram is shown in Fig. 1. Column fractions corresponding to uv peaks in Fig. 1 were analyzed by sodium dodecyl sulfate - polyacrylamide gel electrophoresis (SDS-PAGE) and/or amino acid analysis and fractions containing highly purified proteins or peptides were taken for further structural analysis to determine N- and C-terminal amino acid sequences. Column fractions containing mixtures of proteins and/or peptides were taken for rechromatography on RP-HPLC

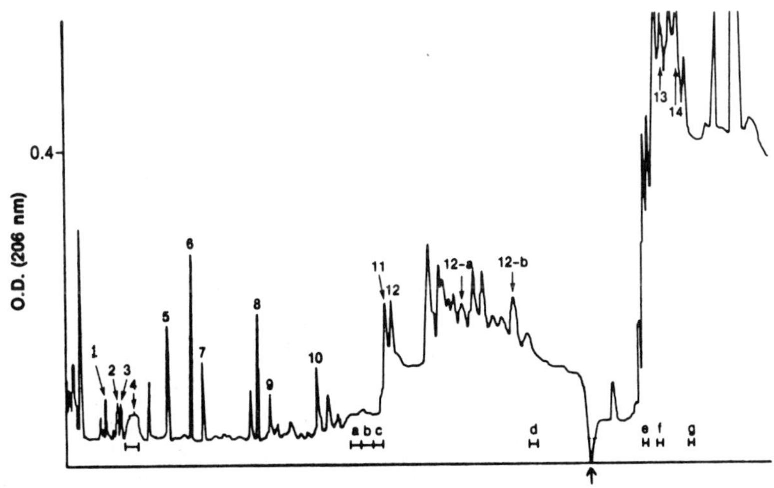

FIGURE 1. The figure shows the chromatogram obtained from the separation of proteins and peptides present in HTLV-III by the method of reversed phase high pressure liquid chromatography. Elution from a 19 x 150 mm column was accomplished at pH 2 with a flowrate of 5 ml per min. and a linear gradient of acetonitrile (0 to 60% over 10 hr, see arrow) at 23C followed by a linear gradient of 1-propanol (0 to 100% over 3 hr) at 50C. Uv peaks of eluted proteins discussed in the text are numbered in the figure. Column fractions containing antigens discussed in the text are lettered in the figure.

columns (C_{18} or diphenyl) to obtain more pure preparations for structural analysis. Amino acid sequences of purified proteins or peptides were compared to the translated proviral DNA sequence of HTLV-III (4) to determine their viral origin or to the Dayhoff Data Base for identification of cellular proteins. A summary of these results is given in Table 1 where numbered peaks in Fig. 1 are listed together with the origin and identity of the purified proteins or peptides.

The class II histocompatibility antigens (HLA-II-DR-4 alpha and beta chains; peaks 13 and 14) purified from this preparation of HTLV-III as in Fig. 1 were reported previously (10). Ubiquitin (peak 9) is a cellular protein commonly found in preparations of mammalian retroviruses (unpublished) and its association within

TABLE 1
PROTEINS AND PEPTIDES IDENTIFIED

Peak Number[a]	Origin and Identity[b]
1	HTLV-III _gag_ (367-376)
2	HTLV-III _gag_ (478-495)
3	HTLV-III _gag_ (478-495)
4	HTLV-III _gag_ (377-447), p7
5	HTLV-III _gag_ (448-447)
6	HTLV-III _gag_ (432-447)
7	HTLV-III _gag_ (496-511)
8	HTLV-III _gag_ (448-511), p6/p9
9	Cell, Ubiquitin
10	Cell, Unknown
11	HTLV-III _gag_ (1-131), p17
12	HTLV-III _gag_ (132-362), p24
13	Cell, HLA-II DR-4 alpha
14	Cell, HLA-II DR-4 beta

[a] From Fig. 1
[b] Numbers in parentheses indicate amino acid residues as shown in Fig. 2.

```
 MYR                                                        130    ↕
 /                                                         <---p17] [p24--->
GLY-ALA-ARG-ALA-SER-(...121 residues..)-SER-GLN-VAL-SER-GLN-ASN-TYR-PRO-ILE-
                                                            <-- <-] [-> -->
                        140                                             150
VAL-GLN-ASN-ILE-GLN-GLY-GLN-MET-VAL-HIS-GLN-ALA-ILE-SER-PRO-ARG-THR-LEU-ASN-
--> --> --> --> --> --> --> --> --> --> --> -->
                                                                    360
(...........200 residues..............)-GLY-GLY-PRO-GLY-HIS-LYS-ALA-ARG-VAL-
                                                                        <--
   ↕               ↕                                        ↕
p24                             370                         [p7->       380
LEU-ALA-GLU-ALA-MET-SER-GLN-VAL-THR-ASN-THR-ALA-THR-ILE-MET-MET-GLN-ARG-GLY-
<-]                [--> --> --> --> --> --(367-376) --> ->] [-> (377-431)->
                                                <-- <-- <-]
    [-> --> --> --> --> --> --> (363-???)----
                                    390
ASN-PHE-ARG-ASN-GLN-ARG-LYS-MET-VAL-LYS-CYS-PHE-ASN-CYS-GLY-LYS-GLU-GLY-HIS-
--> --> --> --> --> --> --> --> --> --> --> --> --> --> --> --> --> --> -->

400                                     410
THR-ALA-ARG-ASN-CYS-ARG-ALA-PRO-ARG-LYS-LYS-GLY-CYS-TRP-LYS-CYS-GLY-LYS-GLU-
--> --> --> --> --> --> --> --> --> --> --> --> --> --> ------(377-431)----

                                                   ↕
    420                                     430
GLY-HIS-GLN-MET-LYS-ASP-CYS-THR-GLU-ARG-GLN-ALA-ASN-PHE-LEU-GLY-LYS-ILE-TRP-
------------------------------------------- <-- <-] [-> --> --> --> --> -->

                                        ↕
        440                      <--p7] [p6-->  450
PRO-SER-TYR-LYS-GLY-ARG-PRO-GLY-ASN-PHE-LEU-GLN-SER-ARG-PRO-GLU-PRO-THR-ALA-
--> --(432-447) --> --> --> GLN --> --] [-> --> --> --> --> --> --> --> -->
                                <-- <-] [-> --> --> --> --> --> --> --> -->

            460                                     470
PRO-PRO-PHE-LEU-GLN-SER-ARG-PRO-GLU-PRO-THR-ALA-PRO-PRO-GLU-GLU-SER-PHE-ARG-
--> --> --> --> --> --> --> --> -->---------(448-477)------ <-- <-- <-- <--
--> --> --> --> --> --> --> --> --> --> --> --> --> --> --> -->--(448-511)--

       ↕        480                                     490
SER-GLY-VAL-GLU-THR-THR-THR-PRO-PRO-GLN-LYS-GLN-GLU-PRO-ILE-ASP-LYS-GLU-LEU-
<-- <-] [-> --> --> --> --> --> --> --> --> --> -->------(478-495)---------
----------------------------------------------------------------------------

   ↕
                    500                                     510
TYR-PRO-LEU-THR-SER-LEU-ARG-SER-LEU-PHE-GLY-ASN-ASP-PRO-SER-SER-GLN
--] [-> --> --> --> --> --> --> --> --> --> --> -->----(496-511)--]
------------------------------------------------------------------]
```

FIGURE 2: The amino acid sequence of HTLV-III Pr55-gag deduced from the DNA sequence of the BH10 provirus (4) is shown with 121 residues in the p17 and 200 residues in the p24 domains omitted. Numbers above residues refer to the location of residues in the sequence of Pr55-gag. Proteolytic cleavage sites are indicated by vertical arrows (↕). Peptides or proteins derived by proteolysis and purified as in Fig. 1 and Table 1 are indicated by brackets ([ ]), amino acid residues determined by N-terminal sequencing are underlined with an arrow to the right (-->), residues determined by C-terminal sequencing are underlined with arrows to the left (<--), residues indicated by amino acid composition are underlined (--). Numbers in brackets ( ) indicate the residue number in the sequence of Pr55-gag of the first and last residue of the underlined peptide. MYR indicates a myristyl group.

the virion is currently under study (T. Copeland, in preparation). The cellular protein in peak 10 is at present unidentified but has the following N-terminal amino acid sequence: Ile-Thr-Arg-Thr-.

All of the other numbered peaks (Fig. 1 and Table 1) are products derived from proteolysis of the HTLV-III gag precursor (Pr55) and are located in the structure of Pr55 as indicated in Table 1 and as shown in Fig. 2 where the results of amino acid sequence analysis of peptides and proteins are also summarized. These data are in complete agreement with previously reported N-terminal sequence analysis of p24 (4,11) and C-terminal analysis of p17 and p24 (4,11). The more extensive data reported here are also in complete agreement with the translated DNA sequence (4) except for residue 445 where the protein has a glutamine instead of the predicted glycine. The tetrapeptide (Ala-Glu-Ala-Met) residues (363-366) predicted by the DNA sequence and the cleavage sites shown in Fig. 2 was not isolated. However, a minor fraction of the protein eluting in peak 4 together with p7 gave the N-terminal sequence beginning at Ala-363 as indicated in Fig. 2. Taken together, the data reveal proteolytic cleavage sites in Pr55 and show that the entire predicted structure of the precursor can be accounted for by proteins and peptides found in the mature virus.

In many other retroviruses the gag precursor is posttranslationally modified by proteolytic removal of the initiator methionine residue and covalent attachment of a myristyl (Myr) group to the newly formed N-terminal glycine residue (12-14). In the case of Moloney murine leukemia virus (15) and Mason-Pfizer monkey virus (16) a N-terminal glycine residue is required for attachment of the Myr group that was shown to be essential for budding. Since the HTLV-III gag gene begins with Met-Gly-, it was of interest to analyze the purified p17 for the presence of a Myr group. The purified p17 was hydrolyzed (acid hydrolysis) and quantitatively analyzed by a HPLC method (A. Schultz, unpublished) and found to contain one mole of myristic acid per mole of protein. This is in agreement with the observation that HTLV-III Pr55 can be labeled with radioactive myristic acid in the culture medium (F di Marzo Veronese et al., in preparation).

Phosphorylation is another posttranslational modification often observed in other retroviral gag precursors.

To investigate this possibility the proteins and derived from HTLV-III Pr55 (listed in Table 1) were analyzed for phosphoamino acids by a method employing mild acid hydrolysis and anion exchange chromatography (17). Analysis of p24 showed peaks eluting in the positions of both phosphoserine and phosphothreonine, whereas all other proteins and peptides analyzed gave negative results. These results suggest that p24 is phosphorylated on both serine and threonine hydroxyl groups and are supported by the finding that p24 incorporates ^{32}P *in vivo* (F di Marzo Veronese, et al., in preparation).

HTLV-III p24 exhibited considerable chromatographic heterogeneity in the separation shown in Fig. 1. Peak 12 contained p24 and a small contamination of p17 from peak 11 but many of the peaks eluting after peak 12 in the acetonitrile gradient contained additional amounts of p24. All of these p24-containing column fractions were shown to contain a 24 KDa component that reacted with a monospecific antisera to equine infectious anemia virus p26 (7). Each of three column fractions containing peaks with substantial amounts of p24 (labeled 12, 12-a, and 12-b in Fig. 1) were rechromatographed and in each case the p24 component retained its unique chromatographic mobility. These chromatographically distinct p24s were indistinguishable by N-terminal and C-terminal sequence analysis and by amino acid composition but did show slightly different mobilities in SDS-PAGE when run side by side on the same gel. The observed differences in mobility were no greater than 0.2 KDa equivalents and most likely reflect differences in posttranslational modification. Each of the repurified p24s appeared to contain both phosphoserine and phosphothreonine, but did show different ratios of the phosphoamino acids. This observation suggests but does not prove that the apparent heterogeneity of p24 may be due to differences in the extent of phosphorylation.

Protein products derived from the *pol* and *env* genes were also partly purified and are present in column fractions shown in Fig. 1. In order to search for these products, antisera to synthetic peptides that correspond to predicted amino acid sequences for selected regions of the *pol* gene were used. The synthetic peptides were as follows: putative protease C-terminal (pro-CT) peptide predicted in the *pol* reading frame in a previous study (18); a peptide contained within the reverse transcriptase C-terminal region (RT-CT); a peptide representing the C-terminal end of the env precursor (env-CT) (4). Proteins and peptides in column fractions (Fig. 1) were separated by SDS-PAGE, transferred to diazo paper, allowed to react with the antisera to the synthetic peptide and antigen-antibody complexes detected by radioautography after reaction with 125-I protein A (7). The molecular weight of the reactive antigen was estimated by comparing its mobility in SDS-PAGE to molecular weight standards.

The pro-CT peptide is identical to the amino acid sequence predicted from the pol reading frame directly preceding the known N-terminal residue of reverse transcriptase (RT) (18). By analogy to other retroviruses this region of pol may code for the C-terminal end of the viral protease (19). Antisera to pro-CT detected bands of about 11.5 KDa in fractions c and f and an additional weaker band of about 10.2 KDa in fraction a (Fig. 1). Following reduction (2-mercaptoethanol) and rechromatography of fraction f the 11.5 KDa antigen eluted from the column in about the same concentration of acetonitrile as for fraction c in Fig. 1. This observation suggests that the antigen detected in fraction f may have been present in the form of disulfide complexes that were not completely dissociated in the first reduction step prior to chromatography. The specificity of the antiserum (pro-CT) makes the 11.5 KDa antigen a reasonable candidate for the mature viral protease and the 10.2 KDa antigen may be a minor truncated product.

It is known that antibody to HTLV-III RT precipitates two proteins (p66-pol and p51-pol) and results of N-terminal sequence analysis suggested that p51-pol may be a N-terminal proteolytic fragment of p66-pol (18). Thus the existence of a C-terminal proteolytic fragment of p66-pol was suggested. The RT-CT synthetic peptide contains 14 residues in a sequence identical to a predicted amino acid sequence that should be within the putative C-terminal fragment of p66-pol. A 13.3 KDa band (fraction d, Fig. 1) reacted with the antisera shown to recognize RT. This data supports the suggestion that p66-pol is cleaved to p51-pol and the 13.3 KDa protein described here.

The data presented here extends our knowledge of the proteolytic cleavage events that lead to viral proteins derived from the pol gene as summarized in Fig. 3. Pr145-gag-pol is a polyprotein synthesized by initiation at the gag initiator and shift in the reading frame within the region where the gag and pol reading frames overlap. The site of the frameshift is unknown for HTLV-III. If frameshifting in HTLV-III occurs upstream near to the gag terminator as in mouse mammary tumor virus (19) and Rous sarcoma virus (20) then it is possible that N-terminal sequence analysis of the 11.5 KDa putative protease may show it to be a transframe protein.

Column fractions containing gp120 (fraction c, Fig. 1) and gp41 (fraction g, Fig. 1) were identified by immunoblot analysis using patient antisera (G. Robey, personal communication). The fractions containing gp120 were rechromatographed, and the N-terminal amino acid sequence of the repurified protein was determined and found to be in complete agreement with the previously reported N terminus determined by radioactive amino acid sequencing (21). Column fractions containing partly purified gp41 (22) were further purified by SDS-PAGE and the band was cut from the gel and used for immunizations to prepare anti-gp41 rabbit antisera. The remaining column fractions were analyzed for antigens reacting

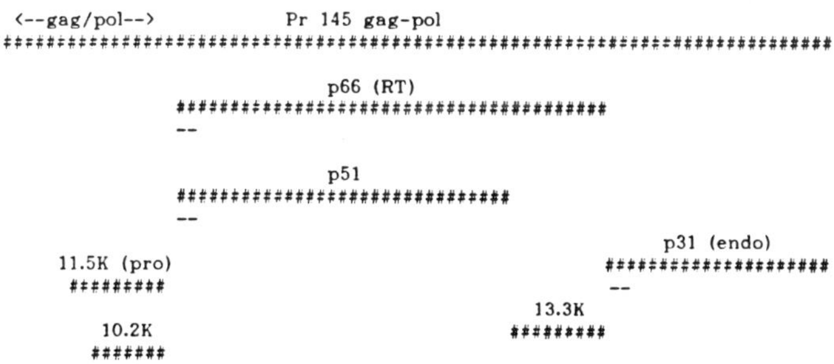

FIGURE 3: PROTEOLYTIC CLEAVAGE MAP OF HTLV-III POL GENE PRODUCT: Underlines (--) indicate that the N-terminal amino acid sequence is known. Cleavage products with known or suspected enzymic function are indicated; reverse transcriptase (RT); protease (prot); endonuclease (endo).The N-terminal amino acid sequence of p31 (putative endonuclease) was determined by M. Lightfoote and coworkers (25).

with antisera to the env-CT synthetic peptide. This analysis revealed a 16 KDa band in column fraction b (Fig. 1) that is an extreme C-terminal fragment of gPr160-*env*.

The data provided here extends our knowledge of the proteolytic cleavages that can occur in HTLV-III. The various peptide bonds that are currently known to be cleaved in HTLV-III proteins are listed in Table 2 and grouped according to sequence homology at and or around the cleavage site. In other retroviruses maturation cleavages in the *gag* and *gag-pol* precursors have been shown to be catalyzed by a single virus-encoded protease (23,24). It remains to be seen whether all the cleavage sites for HTLV-III, as summarized in Table 2, represent maturation cleavages and are catalyzed by a single protease.

TABLE 2

Peptide Bonds Cleaved in HTLV-III

Peptide Bond Cleaved (-:-)	Location of Peptide Bond
-Ser-Gln-Asn-Tyr-↓:-Pro-Ile-Val-Gln-	Pr55-*gag* (131-132)
-Lys-Glu-Leu-Tyr-:-Pro-Leu-Thr-Ser-	Pr55-*gag* (495-496)
-Thr-Leu-Asn-Phe-:-Pro-Ile-Ser-Pro-	Pr145-*gag-pol* (*pol* 167-168)
-Ala-Glu-Ala-Met-:-Ser-Gln-Val-Thr-	Pr55-*gag* (366-367)
-Ala-Thr-Ile-Met-:-Met-Gln-Arg-Gly-	Pr55-*gag* (376-377)
-Ala-Arg-Val-Leu-:-Ala-Glu-Ala-Met-	Pr55-*gag* (362-363)
-Arg-Lys-Ile-Leu-:-Phe-Leu-Asp-Gly-	Pr145-*gag-pol* (*pol* 727-728)
-Pro-Gln-Asn-Phe-:-Leu-Gln-Ser-Arg-	Pr55-*gag* (447-448)
-Arg-Gln-Ala-Asn-:-Phe-Leu-Gly-Lys-	Pr55-*gag* (431-432)
-Phe-Arg-Ser-Gly-:-Val-Glu-Thr-Thr-	Pr55=*gag* (477-478)

REFERENCES

1. Gallo RC, Salahuddin SZ, Popovic M, Shearer GM, Kaplan M, Hayes BF, Parker TJ, Redfrield R, Oleske J, Safai, B, White G, Foster P, Markham PD (1984). Frequent detection and isolation of cytopathic retroviruses (HTLV-III) from patients with AIDS and at risk for AIDS. Science 224: 500-503.
2. Barre-Sinoussi F, Chermann JC, Rey F, Nugeybe MT, Chamaret S, Gruest J, Dauguet C, Axlar-Blin C, Vezinet-Brun F, Rouzioux C, Rozenbaum, W, Montagnier L (1983). Isolation of T-lymphotropic retrovirus from a patient at risk of acquired immune deficiency syndrome (AIDS). Science 220: 868-870.
3. Levy JA, Hoffman AD, Kramer SM, Lanois JA, Shimabukuro JM, Oskiro LS (1984). Isolation of lymphocytopathic retroviruses from San Francisco patients with AIDS. Science 225:840-842.
4. Ratner L, Haseltine W, Patarca R, Livak J, Starcich B, Josephs SF, Doran ER, Rafalski JA, Whitehorn EA, Baumeister K, Ivanoff L, Petteway SR, Jr., Pearson ML, Lautenberger JA, Papas TS, Ghrayeb J, Chang NT, Gallo RC, Wong-Staal F (1985). Complete nucleotide sequence of the AIDS virus, HTLV-III. Nature (London) 313:277-283.
5. Henderson LE, Sowder RC, Smythers G, Benveniste RE, Oroszlan S (1985). Purification and N-terminal amino acid sequence comparisons of structural proteins from retrovirus-D/Washington and Mason-Pfizer monkey virus. J. Virol 55:778-787.
6. Henderson LE, Sowder RC, Copeland TD, Smythers G, Oroszlan S (1984). Quantitative separation of murine leukemia virus proteins by reversed-phase high-pressure liquid chromatography reveals newly described gag and env cleavage products. J. Virol. 52:492-500.
7. Henderson LE, Sowder RC, Smythers GW, Oroszlan S (1987). Chemical and immunological characterizations of equine infectious anemia virus gag-encoded proteins. J. Virol 61:1116-1124.
8. Oroszlan S, Henderson LE, Stephenson JR, Copeland TD, Long CW, Ihle JN, Gilden RV. (1978). Amino- and carboxyl-terminal amino acid sequences of proteins coded by gag gene of murine leukemia virus. Proc. Natl. Acad. Sci. USA 75:1404-1408.

9. Laemmli UK. Cleavage of structural proteins during the assembly of the head of bacteriophage T4. Nature (London) 227:680-685.
10. Henderson LE, Sowder R, Copeland TD, Oroszlan S, Arthur LO, Robey WG, Fischinger PJ (1987). Direct identification of class II histocompatibility DR proteins in preparatins of human T-cell lymphotropic virus type III. J. Virol 61: 629-632.
11. Sanchez-Pescador R, Power MD, Barr PJ, Steimer KS, Stemfeien MM, Brown-Shimer SL, Gee WW, Bernard A, Randolph A, Levy JA, Dina D, Luciw PA (1985). Nucleotide sequence and expression of an AIDS-associated retrovirus (ARV-2). Science 227:484-492.
12. Henderson LE, Krutzch HC, Oroszlan S (1983). Myristyl amino termination acylation of murine retroviral proteins: a new posttranslational protein modification. Proc. Natl. Acad. Sci. USA 80:339-343.
13. Schultz AM, Henderson LE, Oroszlan S (1983). Myristylation of gag polyproteins of type B, C, and D retroviruses and also of retroviral transforming proteins. In Rich A (ed): "Leukemia Review International" vol 1, New York, Marcell Dekker, Inc, p. 304-305.
14. Schultz AM, Oroszlan S (1983). In vivo modification of retroviral gag gene-encoded polyproteins by myristic acid. J. Virol 46:355-361.
15. Rein A, McClure MR, Rice NR, Luftig RB, Schultz AM (1986). The myristylation site in Pr65gag is essential for virus particle formation by Moloney MuLV. Proc. Natl. Acad. Sci. USA 83:7246-7250.
16. Rhee SS, Hunter E (1987). Myristylation is required for intracellular transport but not for assembly of D-type retrovirus capsids. J. Virol 61:1045-1053.
17. Yang JC, Fujitaki JM, Smith RA (1982). Separation of phosphohydroxyamino acids by high performance liquid chromatography. Anal. Biochem. 122:360-363.
18. Veronese FdM, Copeland TD, DeVico AL, Rahman R, Oroszlan S, Gallo RC, Sarngadharan MG (1986). Characterization of highly immunogenic p66/51 as the reverse transcriptase of HTLV-III/LAV. Science 231:1289-1291.
19. Hizi A, Henderson LE, Copeland TD, Sowder RC, Hixson CV, Oroszlan S (1987). Characterization of mouse mammary tumor virus gag-pro gene products and the ribosomal frameshift site by protein sequencing. Proc. Natl. Acad. Sci. USA, submitted.

20. Jacks T, Varmus HE (1985). Expression of the Rous sarcoma virus pol gene by ribosomal frameshifting. Science 230:1237-1242.
21. Robey WG, Arthur LO, Matthews TJ, Langlois A, Copeland TD, Lerche NW, Oroszlan S, Bolognesi DP, Gilden RV, Fischinger PJ (1986). Prospect for prevention of human immunodeficiency virus infection: Purified 120-kDa envelope glycoprotein induces neutralizing antibody. Proc. Natl. Acad. Sci. USA 83:7023-7027.
22. Veronese F diMarzo, DeVico AL, Copeland TD, Oroszlan S, Gallo RC, Sarngadharan MG (1985). Characterization of gp41 as the transmembrane protein coded by the HTLV-III/LAV envelope gene. Science 229:1402-1405.
23. Yoshinaka Y, Katoh I, Copeland TD, Oroszlan S (1985). Murine leukemia virus protease is encoded by the gag-pol gene and is synthesized through suppression of an amber termination codon. Proc. Natl. Acad. Sci. 82:1618-1622.
24. Oroszlan S, Copeland TD (1985). Primary structure and processing of gag and env gene products of human T-cell leukemia viruses HTLV-I_{CR} and HTLV-I_{ATK}. Curr. Top. Microbiol. Immunol. 115: 221-233.
25. Lightfoote MM, Coligan JE, Folks TM, Fauci AS, Martin MA, Venkatesan S (1986). Structural characterization of reverse transcriptase and endonuclease polypeptides of the acquired immunodeficiency syndrome retrovirus. J. Virol 60:771-775.

Research sponsored by the National Cancer Institute, DHHS, under contract No. N01-CO-23909 with Bionetics Research, Inc.

Human Retroviruses, Cancer, and AIDS:
Approaches to Prevention and Therapy, pages 149–159

HIV NEUTRALIZING ANTIBODIES ELICITED BY RECOMBINANT ENVELOPE PROTEINS

Scott Putney,[1] James Rusche,[1] Thomas Matthews,[2] Kai Krohn,[3] Helen Carson,[1] Debra Lynn,[1] Jennifer Jackson,[1] W. Gerard Robey,[4] Annamari Ranki,[3] Marjorie Robert-Guroff,[3] Robert Gallo,[3] and Dani Bolognesi,[2]

[1]Repligen Corporation, Cambridge, MA 02139
[2]Department of Surgery Duke University Medical School Durham, NC 27710
[3]Laboratory of Tumor Cell Biology NCI/NIH Bethesda, MD 20205
[4]National Cancer Institute - FCRF Frederick, MD 21701

ABSTRACT The HTLV-III_B envelope primary translation product (gp160) was expressed in insect cells using a baculovirus expression vector encoding the HTLV-III_B envelope. This protein (denoted r160) is glycosylated and has the same apparent molecular weight as gp160 from virus infected cells. Antibodies from animals immunized with r160 neutralize the HTLV-III_B virus and block fusion of virus infected H9 cells. Titers of this antisera in both of these assays is five to ten-fold higher than that of antisera to native gp120 isolated from the virus. PB1, a fragment from the carboxyl-terminal half of HTLV-III_B gp120 also elicits HTLV-III_B neutralizing antibodies and completely eliminates the cell fusion blocking activity of anti-r160 sera. This indicates that major neutralizing epitopes and cell fusion epitopes are located in this region. Anti-r160 and anti-PB1 sera efficiently neutralize the homologous HIV isolate, HTLV-III_B, but not the divergent isolate, HTLV-III_{RF}. This indicates that envelope directed antisera is HIV type specific.

INTRODUCTION

Important proteins to consider as HIV vaccine candidates are those associated with the viral envelope. These are derived from a precursor, gp160, that is proteolytically cleaved to generate the external envelope glycoprotein gp120 and the transmembrane envelope glycoprotein gp41 (Figure 1) (1-5). Several lines of evidence support the notion that gp120 is involved in important biological processes related to the virus life cycle and that a subunit vaccine based on gp120 may be possible. 1) Antibodies that neutralize HIV infection have been found in sera of people with AIDS and ARC as well as asymptomatic individuals infected with the virus (6,7) and antibodies exist in such sera that bind to purified gp120 (8); 2) purified gp120 elicits production of neutralizing antibodies (9) as does a large segment of gp120 produced in E. coli and mammalian cells (10,11); and 3) direct binding of gp120 to the T4 receptor has been demonstrated (12,13) and monoclonal antibodies recognizing certain epitopes of the virus receptor prevent viral infection (13).

We describe here production and properties of two recombinant HIV subunit vaccine candidates. One, PB1, is produced in E. coli and is a segment of gp120 (10). The other, r160, is expressed in an S. frugiperda insect cell line and is the entire envelope primary translation product. Both of these proteins elicit HIV neutralizing antibodies.

RESULTS AND DISCUSSION

Figure 1 shows the gp120 and gp41 regions of the envelope and we focused our efforts on the envelope protein to develop HIV vaccine candidates. To determine which region of the envelope would best elicit HIV neutralizing antibodies, numerous recombinant fragments of the HTLV-III$_B$ envelope (14) were expressed and purified.

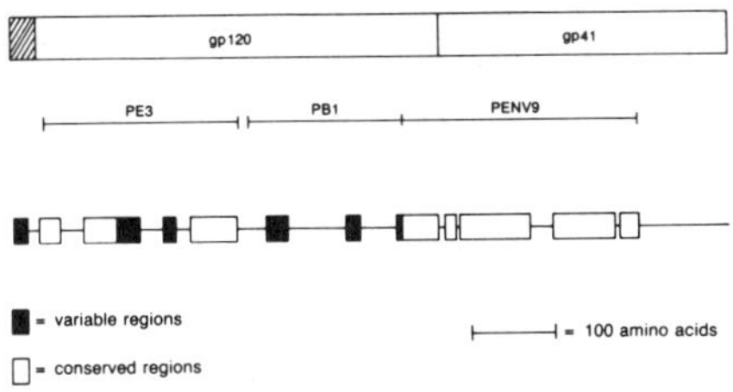

FIGURE 1. Location of proteins PB1, PB3, and PENV9 in relation to gp120 and gp41. The envelope is synthesized as a precursor, gp160, that is cleaved to give gp120 and gp41. The secretion signal sequence is hatched. The location of the variable and conserved regions (5) are shown as darkened or open boxes, respectively, PE3 and PENV9 were constructed by John Ghrayeb and Stephen Petteway at Centocor and DuPont, respectively. These three recombinant proteins extend over 84% of the envelope.

One of these, PB1, is expressed as approximately 15% of total cellular protein and is purified using a single carboxy-methyl Sepharose column. Approximately 300 milligrams of purified PB1 are obtained per liter of cell culture. Several animals including mice, rabbits, goats, rhesus monkeys, and chimpanzees have been immunized with PB1 and the work described here was done with goats. Two milligrams initial dose and one milligram boosts in complete freunds adjuvant were used as immunogen. Immune sera was analyzed for its ability to immunoreact with HIV envelope proteins and to neutralize HIV infection <u>in vitro</u>.

Two HIV neutralization assays were used in these studies. 1) Infection of H9 cells was assayed by the appearance of viral specific proteins including reverse transcriptase and p24 (6,9) and 2) HIV mediated cytolysis of the HTLV-I infected cell line ATH8 was assayed by thymidine incorporation (K. Krohn, et. al., PNAS, in press). Additionally, the ability of antisera to prevent HIV mediated cell fusion was assayed by mixing infected and uninfected cells with sera and measuring blockade of giant cell formation after 48 hours.

Goat sera to native gp120 isolated from HTLV-III_B infected H9 cells or enzymatically deglycosylated gp120 shows effective virus neutralization with approximately equivalent titers. PB1 elicits neutralizing titers approximately ten-fold higher than native gp120. These results show that the extensive glycosylation of gp120 is unnecessary to elicit neutralizing antibodies and additionally localizes major neutralizing epitopes to the PB1 region of gp120.

Blockade of multinucleated cell formation can occur by several mechanisms. As cell fusion is believed to occur following the interaction between the CD4 protein and gp120 expressed on the surface of the infected cell, this interaction can be blocked by proteins that bind the regions responsible for this interaction. gp120 blocks this interaction (10) as do particular CD4 directed monoclonal antibodies (13). Cell fusion can also be blocked by antibodies to regions of the envelope. Virus spread through cell-cell contact could potentially be prevented by such gp120 directed antibodies. It has been shown that although gp120 completely blocks syncitia formation, PB1, even at a 50-fold higher molar concentration, does not block fusion (10). This suggests that PB1 is unable to bind CD4. Its apparent lack of association with human T4 cells suggests that it may be a more attractive vaccine candidate than a viral subunit which interacts with CD4 and hence may have negative influences on T4 cell functions.

While PB1 protein does not inhibit cell fusion, PB1 directed antisera blocks fusion of HTLV-III_B infected CEM cells at a dilution of approximately 1 to 50 (Table 1). In contrast, gp120 specific sera also blocks cell fusion at a lower titer, and this is consistent with the lower neutralizing titer elicited by gp120 relative to PB1. We have found that although the titers measured by the cell fusion blockade assay are lower than those measured by virus neutralization, the results of the anti-HTLV-III effect of antisera measured in these two ways correlate and all proteins that elicit cell fusion blocking antibodies also elicit virus neutralizing antibodies.

TABLE 1
HIV VARIANT SPECIFIC NEUTRALIZATION
BY ANTI-ENVELOPE SERA

	H9 Infectivity*			Cell Fusion Blocking**		
	III_B	MN	RF	III_B	MN	RF
PB1-III_B	1000	0	0	60	0	0
PB1-RF	0	N.T.	20	0	0	10
r160-III_B	1000	0	0	60	0	0
gp120-III_B	100	0	0	<10	0	0
ARC sera	300	200	250	10	<10	<10

* Titer is the dilution at which HIV ineffectivity is 50% of preimmune sera.

**Titer is the highest dilution at which no multinucleated cells form.

In addition to producing envelope proteins in *E. coli*, we also expressed the complete envelope in insect cells using the bacculovirus expression vector. This expression system is capable of producing multiple milligram amounts of recombinant protein per liter of culture media (15-17), and the sequence encoding HTLV-III gp160 including the secretion signal sequence which was reconstructed using synthetic oligonucleotides was cloned into a baculovirus transfer vector.

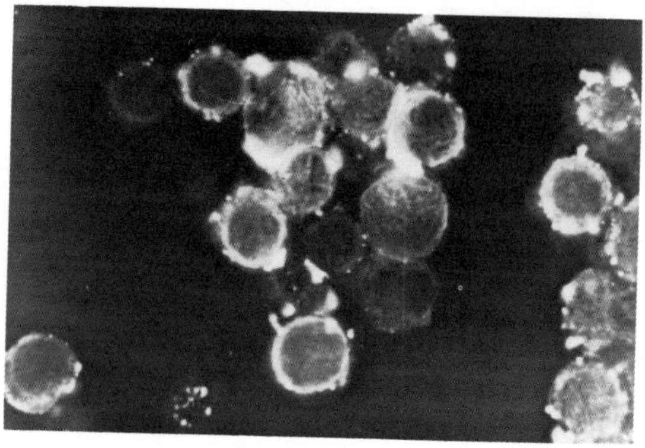

FIGURE 2. Immunofluorescence of insect cells expressing r160 on their surface. Cells were labeled with gp120 specific goat antisera and fluorescein thiocyanate conjugated rabbit anti-goat antisera.

Figure 2 is an immunofluorescene micrograph of r160 expressing insect cells labeled with gp120 specific goat antisera and fluorescene thiocyanate conjugated rabbit anti-goat sera. Predominant staining is at the cell surface, and this is expected because r160 contains the transmembrane region of the envelope. r160 is extensively glycosylated and treatment of r160 with endoglycosidase F (not shown) reduces its apparent molecular weight to about 100kD, which is slightly larger than that expected for the non-glycosylated polypeptide. This result is similar to such treatment of native gp120 which reduces the molecular weight to about 58,000 (10).

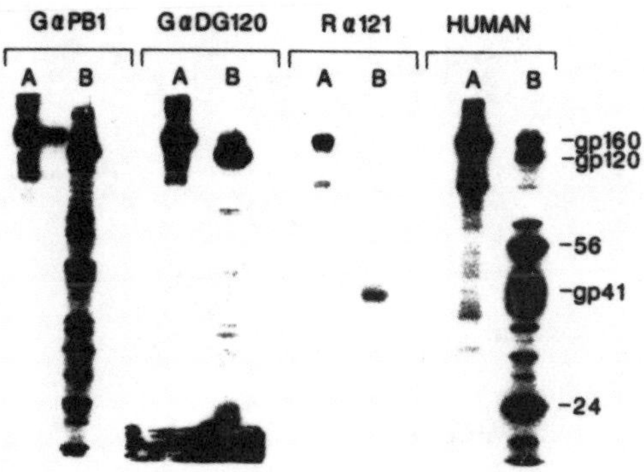

FIGURE 3. Western blot of r160 and lysates of HIV infected cells (lanes A and B, respectively). Blots were probed with antisera to PB1, gp120, peptide 121 (which is a recombinant segment of gp41 (18) and human AIDS sera. Each of these antisera binds r160.

Figure 3 is a Western Blot showing specific immunoreactivity with r160 using envelope directed antisera. Lane A in each panel is r160 and Lane B is a lystate from HTLV-III infected cells. The first and second panels are probed with gp120 directed antisera and both the r160 and the gp120 and gp160 react, whereas the third panel is probed with sera to peptide 121 which is a segment from the amino terminal half of gp41 (18). In this case, r160, gp160 and gp41 are immunoreactive, whereas gp120 is not. When probed with human AIDS sera, all three glycoproteins react. This shows that r160 has the same apparent molecular weight as gp160 and that it is not cleaved to gp120 and gp41 as it is in mammalian cells (19,20).

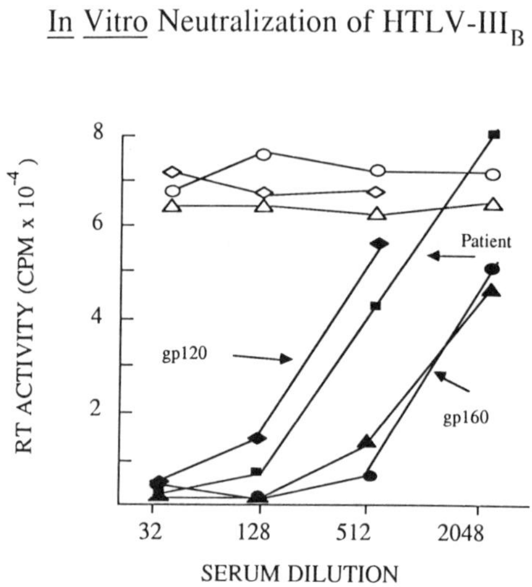

FIGURE 4. Neutralization of HTLV-III$_B$ infection with r160 immune goat sera. Sera to gp120, r160 (indicated as gp160 here) or patient sera were diluted and assayed for HTLV-III$_B$ virus neutralization. Preimmune sera (◊, △, ○) and immune sera (♦, ▲, ●, ■) were from goats immunized with gp120 and r160 (two goats) or an AIDS patient. Diluted sera was mixed with the virus and incubated 30 minutes at 37°C and the mixture was added to H9 cells. After 7 to 10 days in culture, virus was measured by reverse transcriptase activity.

r160 was purified from infected cells using a series of solvent extraction procedures and SDS gel electrophoresis. Goats were immunized and boosted with 200 micrograms of protein in complete Freunds adjuvant and immune sera was assayed for its ability to neutralize HTLV-III$_B$ infection. Figure 4 shows that the neutralization titers of r160 are approximately ten fold higher than those to gp120. r160 antisera also blocks infected cell fusion (Table 1 and Figure 4).

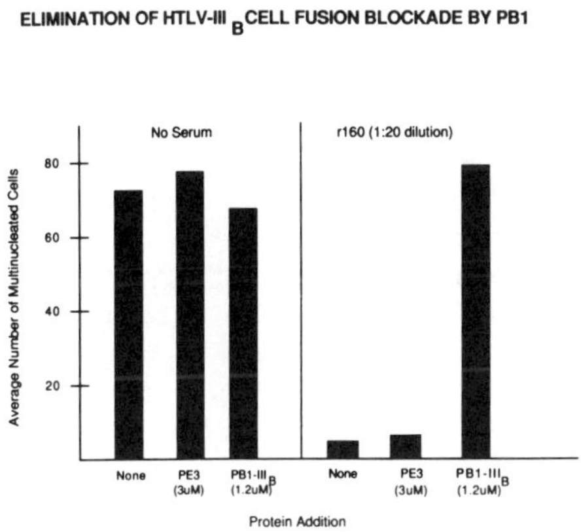

FIGURE 5 Blocking of HIV mediated cell fusion by anti-r160 sera and elimination of blocking by PB1-III_B.

To determine to which region of the envelope these neutralizing antibodies are directed, we investigated whether PB1 could prevent the HTLV-III_B cell fusion blockade with anti r160 sera. Figure 5 shows that r160 antisera is efficient in blocking cell fusion, and that PE3 does not interfere with this process. On the other hand, 1.2 micromolar PB1-III_B completely eliminates this cell fusion blockade thus indicating that PB1 has all of the epitopes recognized by cell fusion blocking antibodies.

Another issue addressed was the HIV variant cross neutralization properties of PB1-III_B, r160-III_B, and gp120-III_B antisera. The variants we chose to study other than HTLV-III_B were the HTLV-III_{MN} and RF viruses (21). The variability of the amino acid sequence within the envelope is substantial (21,22) (M. Reitz, unpublished) and HTLV-III_B differs from MN and RF by 17.9 and 20.8% in gp120. The PB1 region contains even more variability and in the PB1 region, PB1-III_B differs from MN and RF by 32.3 and 25.2%, respectively. These studies also addressed the question of whether antisera to the PB1 region of another HIV isolate would also neutralize the homologous virus, thus bolstering the evidence that the PB1 region indeed contains the neutralizing epitopes.

Table 1 shows the results of these experiments. Although PB1-III_B and r160-III_B sera neutralize the homologous isolate with a titer of 1,000 and a titer of 60 in the H9 infectivity and cell fusion blocking assays respectively, no neutralization of either the MN or the RF variants is observed. This result is also true for sera to native gp120-III_B. On the other hand, the PB1 region from the RF isolate, which was expressed and purified in a manner similar to the III_B variant, elicits antibodies capable of neutralizing RF but not III_B or MN infected cells. These experiments were performed with early bleeds from the $PB1_{RF}$ immunized animals and hence the neutralizing titers are lower than titers of PB1-III_B sera. In contrast, sera from an HIV sero positive individual is capable of neutralizing all three variants with approximately equal titers, and it is generally true that such sera has antibodies capable of broad neutralization. This result indicates that HIV neutralizing antibodies elicited by a single envelope variant of virus type specific. This suggests that a subunit vaccine based on the envelope may have to be composed of a cocktail which would elicit neutralizing antibodies to a broad spectrum of virus types.

ACKNOWLEDGEMENTS

This work was supported in part by NIH contract number NO1-AI-62558 awarded to Repligen by NIAID. We thank W. Herlihy, T. Fraser and K. Javaherian for useful discussions and C. Dennis for excellent technical assistance. We also thank M. Reitz for the sequence of the HTLV-III_{MN} envelope gene.

REFERENCES

1. Robey WG, et al., (1985) Science, 228:593.
2. Barin F, et al., ibid, p. 1094.
3. Allan JS, et al., ibid., p. 1091.
4. Starcich BR, et al., (1986) Cell, 45:637.
5. Veronese FD, et al., (1985) Science, 229:1402.
6. Robert-Guroff M, Brown M, Gallo RC, (1985) Nature (London), 316:72.
7. Weiss RA, et al., ibid, p. 69.
8. Matthews TJ, et al., (1986) Proc. Natl. Acad. Sci. U.S.A., 83:9709.
9. Robey WG, et al., (1986) ibid, 83:7023.
10. Putney SD, et al., (1986) Science, 234:1392-95.
11. Lasky L, et al., (1986) Science, 223:209.
12. Seligmann M, et al., (1984) N. Engl. J. Med., 311:1286.
13. McDougal JS, et al., (1986) Science, 231, 382.
14. Ratner L, et al., Nature (1985) (London), 313, 277.
15. Pennock GD, Shoemaker C and Miller LK, (1983) Molecular and Cellular Biology, 4:399-406.
16. Smith GE, Ju G, Erickson BL, Moschera J, Lahm H-W, Chizzonite R and Summers MD (1985), Proc. Natl. Acad. Sci. USA, 82:8404-08.
17. Miyamoto C, et al., (1985) Molecular and Cellular Biology, 5:2860-65.
18. Chang T-W, Kato I, McKinney S, Chanda P, Barone AD, Wong-Staal F, Gallo RC and Chang NT (1985) Bio/Technology, 3:905-09.
19. Chakrabarti S, Robert-Guroff M, Wong-Staal F, Gallo RC & Moss B, (1986) Nature, 320:535-37.
20. Shiu-Lok H, Kosowski SG, Dalrymple JM, (1986) Nature, 320:537-40.
21. Starcich BR, (1986) Cell, 45:637-48.
22. Hahn BH, et al., (1986) Science, 232:1548.

Human Retroviruses, Cancer, and AIDS:
Approaches to Prevention and Therapy, pages 161–174

MAPPING OF IMMUNOGENIC AND IMMUNODOMINANT EPITOPES OF HUMAN IMMUNODEFICIENCY VIRUS GP120 WITH ENV-ENCODED SYNTHETIC PEPTIDES

Thomas J. Palker, Thomas J. Matthews, Michael E. Clark, George J. Cianciolo[1], Richard R. Randall[1], Alphonse J. Langlois, Gilbert C. White[2], Bijan Safai[3], Ralph Snyderman[1], Dani P. Bolognesi, and Barton F. Haynes

Duke University Medical Center, and Howard Hughes Medical Institute[1], Durham, North Carolina 27710, Department of Medicine[2], University of North Carolina, Chapel Hill, North Carolina 27514, Memorial Sloan-Kettering Cancer Center[3], New York, New York 10021

ABSTRACT Synthetic peptides with amino acid sequences from hydrophilic regions of human immunodeficiency virus (HIV) HTLV-III$_B$ gp120 envelope glycoprotein were used to map the antibody response of HIV seropositive patients. A highly immunogenic epitope from a conserved C-terminal region of HTLV-III$_B$ gp120 was identified with antisera from HIV+ subjects and a synthetic peptide (SP-22) containing an amino acid sequence from this region. Peptide SP-22 absorbed up to 100% of anti-gp120 antibody reactivity from HIV+ patient sera in immunoblot assays and up to 79% of anti-gp120 reactivity in competition radioimmunoassays (RIA). Human anti-SP-22 antibodies obtained by affinity chromatography reacted with gp120 in RIA and immunoblot assay but did not neutralize HTLV-III$_B$ nor react with the surface of HIV infected cells. An additional synthetic peptide (SP-10) containing an amino acid sequence from a central region of gp120 defined by recombinant protein PB1 (Putney et al, Science, 234:1392, 1986) bound antibodies that reacted with native gp120 and with the surface of HIV-infected cells. Results presented here indicate that it is possible to evaluate the topological distribution and functional importance of epitopes on gp120 using human anti-gp120 antibodies obtained by affinity chromatography with HIV env-encoded synthetic peptides.

INTRODUCTION

Retroviral envelope glycoproteins have been shown to be important in evoking virus-neutralizing antibody responses. Envelope antigens of murine (1,2), bovine (3), feline (4,5), and human (6) retroviruses have been identified that will serve as targets for killing of virus infected cells or that, as immunogens, will elicit a neutralizing antibody response to the virus. Recent studies have shown that either the native gp120 envelope protein of the Human Immunodeficiency Virus (HIV) (7,8) or genetically engineered portions of this molecule (9,10) can be used to raise antibodies that will neutralize HIV in a strain specific manner. However, little is known regarding the precise location of epitopes on the 120kd envelope protein of HIV that are either immunogenic in HIV+ patients or that give rise to neutralizing antibodies. We describe here the use of HIV env-encoded synthetic peptides as antigens for mapping the host antibody response to gp120 and as immunoadsorbants for evaluating the functional importance of antibodies to discrete epitopes on gp120.

MATERIALS AND METHODS

Synthetic Peptides and Recombinant Proteins.

Synthetic peptides containing hydrophilic amino acid sequences from $HTLV-III_B$ gp120 (11) were synthesized on an Applied Biosystems 430A peptide synthesizer using chemical and program cycles supplied by the manufacturer. Peptides were conjugated to bovine serum albumin (BSA) (molar ratio of 30:1 peptide to BSA) with M-maleimidobenzoyl-N-hydroxysuccinimide ester (MBS) according to Green et al. (12). Conjugation of peptides to BSA was monitored by subjecting conjugates to SDS-PAGE under non-reducing conditions and by measuring the increase in apparent molecular weights over that of BSA treated with MBS and BSA. Coupling efficiencies also monitored by trace iodination of peptides varied from 10-30% depending on the peptide. Recombinant protein PENV9 (14) containing the C-terminal region of gp120 and the N-terminus of gp41 [Bgl II to Bam H1 sites, (11)] was obtained from Dr. S. Petteway, Dupont, Wilmington, DE. Recombinant protein PE3 containing an amino-terminal region of gp120 (Kpn I to Pvu II sites) was obtained from Dr. N. Chang, Centecor Inc. Malvern, PA.

HIV-infected Cells.

H-9 T-cell lines infected with HIV isolates $HTLV-III_B$ (14), $HTLV-III_{MN}$ (15) and $HTLV-III_{RF}$ (14) were obtained from Dr. R. Gallo, NCI, NIH Bethesda, MD.

Immunoassays and HIV Neutralization Assays.

Antibodies in HIV+ patient sera were screened in radioimmunoassay (RIA) for reactivity to synthetic peptide-BSA conjugates bound to Immulon (Dynatech) microtiter wells as described (16). Peptide-BSA conjugates or purified $HTLV-III_B$ gp120 (7) were also iodinated and subjected to immunoprecipitation with HIV+ patient antibodies and fixed *Staphylococcus aureus* (Pansorbin, Calbiochem) as described (16). Competitive immunoblot assays were performed by pre-incubating HIV+ patients sera (100ul) with synthetic peptide-BSA conjugates (100ul of 1mg/ml solution) prior to incubation with blotted lysates of $HTLV-III_B$+ H-9 cells or with purified gp120. For affinity chromatography of HIV+ patient sera, synthetic peptide-BSA conjugates were covalently linked to CNBr-activated Sepharose 4B (Pharmacia) and bound antibodies were eluted with 4M $MgCl_2$. HIV neutralization and syncytium inhibition assays were performed as previously described (8,10).

RESULTS

Shown in Figure 1 is a diagram of synthetic peptides and recombinant proteins (PE3, PENV9) used in this study that were derived from amino acid sequences of $HTLV-III_B$ gp120. Recombinant proteins PE3, PB1 and PENV9 have been described elsewhere (10,13). Synthetic peptide SP-1 was derived from an amino acid sequence contained in PE3 at the amino-terminal region of gp120. Peptides SP-10, 10A, 11, 14, and 15 contain amino acid sequences from the central region of gp120 that are also present in PB1, while peptide SP-22 contains an amino acid sequence at the C-terminus of gp120 adjacent to the predicted cleavage site (11) between gp120 and gp41. Peptides SP-73 and SP-70A (16), containing amino acid sequences from the N- and C-terminal regions of human T-cell leukemia virus type I (HTLV-I) respectively, were used as negative controls. The amino acid sequences of HIV env-encoded synthetic peptides used in this study are shown in Table 1.

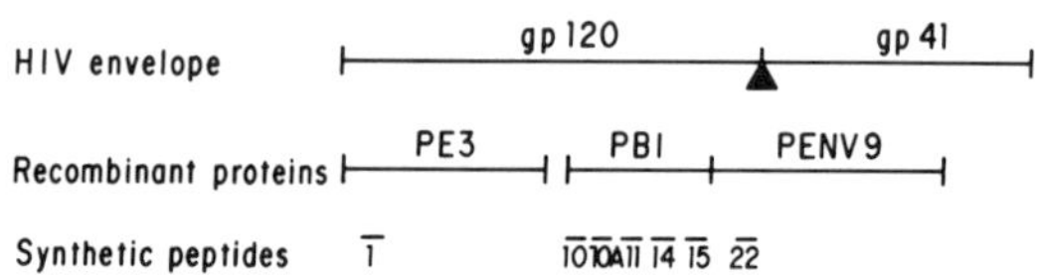

Figure 1. Recombinant proteins and synthetic peptides used in study (see text and Table 1).

TABLE 1
SYNTHETIC PEPTIDES WITH HYDROPHILIC AMINO ACID SEQUENCES OF $HTLV-III_B$ USED IN STUDY

Synthetic Peptide	Amino Acid Number[a]	Sequence[b]
SP-1	80-91	ACVPTDPNPQEV(Y)
10	303-321	CTRPNNNTRKSIRIQRGPG(Y)
10A	328-344	(Y)GKIGNMRQAHCNISRAK
11	341-363	(Y)SRAKWNNTLKQIDSKLREQFGNN(C)
14	393-421	(Y)NSTQLFNSTWFNSTWSTKGSNNTEGSDTI(C)
15	461-475	(Y)LTRDGGNSNNESEIF(C)
22	504-518	APTKAKRRVVQREKR(C)

[a]According to Ratner et. al., Nature, 313:277, 1985.
[b]Amino acids in parentheses were added for iodination of peptide (Y) and coupling to carrier protein (C).

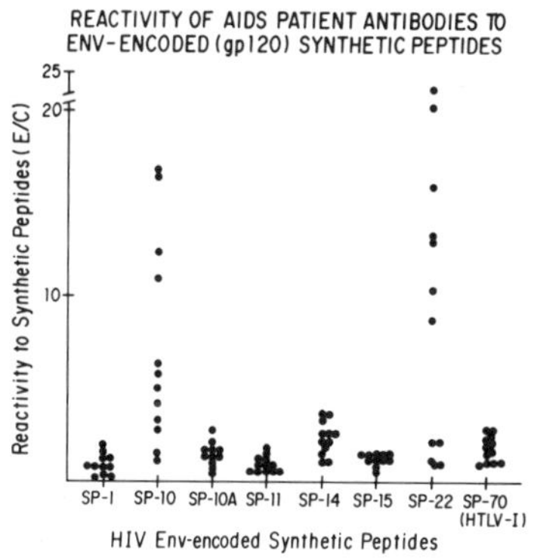

Figure 2. Reactivity of AIDS patient antibodies to env-encoded synthetic peptides. Synthetic peptides (Table 1) were coupled to BSA and used as antigens in radioimmunoassay with AIDS patient sera (N=12) and normal serum controls (N=4). Results are expressed as a ratio (E/C) of duplicate cpm values obtained with experimental (E) AIDS sera and control (C) serum samples. E/C > 3.0 = positive.

Synthetic peptides derived from hydrophilic regions of gp120 were coupled to bovine serum albumin (BSA) and used as antigens in radioimmunoassay (RIA) to evaluate the HIV+ patient antibody response to epitopes on gp120 (Figure 2). The majority of AIDS patient sera reacted with two synthetic peptides, SP-10 (9/12, 75%) and SP-22 (8/12, 67%), while little or no antibody reactivity was found with these sera to the remaining peptides. To evaluate further the reactivity of HIV+ patient antibodies to SP-22, competitive immunoblot assays (Figure 3) and radioimmunoassays (Figure 4) were performed. When pre-incubated with SP-22-BSA and then tested in immunoblot assays, HIV+ patient antibodies were inhibited from binding either to purified gp120 (Figure 3A) or to gp120 in lysates of $HTLV-III_B$ infected H-9 cells (Figure 3B). However, when the same HIV+ patient serum used in Figure 3A was tested for reactivity to ^{125}I-labelled gp120 in competition RIA, only 60% of antibody reactivity to gp120 could be inhibited by SP-22-BSA (not shown). From these data, it was postulated that some antigenic sites on gp120 used in RIA were

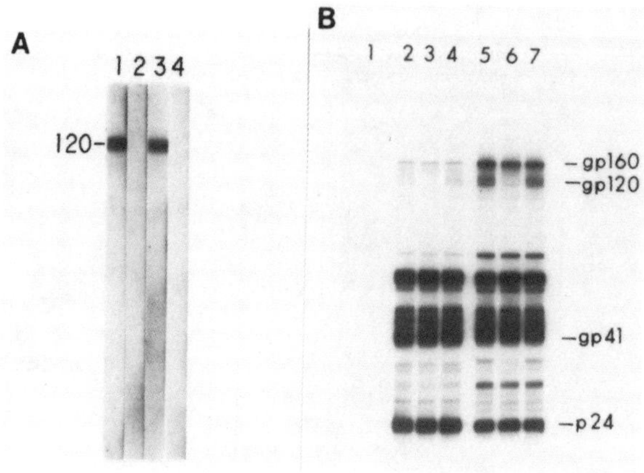

Figure 3: Inhibition by peptide SP-22 of HIV+ patient antibody reactivity to gp120 in immunoblot assays. HIV+ patient antibodies or a normal human serum control was preincubated with peptide-BSA conjugates and reactivity was tested to purified gp120 (3A) or to gp120 in lysates of HIV+ infected cells (3B) as described in Methods. Figure 3A shows the inhibition of HIV+ patient serum #3 antibody binding to purified gp120 by SP-22-BSA (lane 2), whereas equivalent amounts of BSA treated with coupling agent MBS (lane 1) or peptide conjugate SP-73-BSA (lane 3) containing an amino acid sequence from HTLV-I gp45 did not inhibit antibody binding to gp120. Lack of reactivity of normal human serum to purified gp120 in shown in lane 4. Figure 3B shows that antibodies in HIV+ patient serum #3 (lanes 2-4) and serum #12 (lanes 5-7) were specifically inhibited from binding to gp120 by prior incubation with SP-22 (BSA) (lanes 3 and 6) but not with equivalent amounts of SP-73-BSA (lanes 2 and 5) or BSA-MBS (lanes 4 and 7). Nearly complete inhibition of antibody binding to gp120 by SP-22-BSA was achieved in Western blot assay. Lane 1 shows the lack of reactivity of antibodies in normal human serum to HIV infected cell lysates.

destroyed when subjected to denaturation with sodium dodecyl sulfate and 2-mercaptoethanol in immunoblot assays. In other RIAs not shown, HIV+ patient antibodies were inhibited in the presence of SP-22-BSA from binding to gp120 by up to 79%. In the converse experiment, HIV+

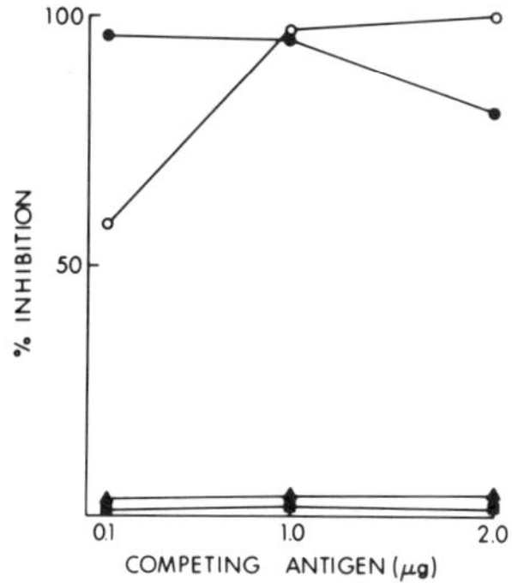

Figure 4. Inhibition of HIV+ patient antibody binding to ^{125}I-labelled SP-22 conjugates in competition RIA. HIV+ patient serum was pre-incubated with HIV gp120 (○), Friend Leukemia Virus (FLV) gp71 (■), recombinant protein PENV9 from the C-terminus of HIV gp120 (●) or recombinant protein PE3 from the N-terminus of gp120 (▲) and then tested for the ability to precipitate ^{125}I-labelled SP-22-BSA. Antibodies were inhibited from binding to SP-22-BSA by HIV gp120 and recombinant protein PENV9 that contains the amino acid sequence of peptide SP-22 but not by equivalent amounts of FLV gp71 or recombinant protein PE3 that lacks the C-terminal amino acid sequence of SP-22.

patient antibodies were also inhibited from binding to ^{125}I-labelled SP-22-BSA complexes when pre-incubated either with gp120 or with recombinant protein PENV9 containing the amino acid sequence of SP-22 (Figure 4). Thus, a highly conserved C-terminal region of HTLV-III$_B$ gp120 contains an immunodominant epitope that is the predominant antigen on gp120 detected in immunoblot assays.

To evaluate the functional importance of antibodies directed to the C-terminus of gp120, anti-SP-22 antibodies were purified from HIV patient sera by passage over an affinity column containing SP-22-BSA conjugates covalently linked to CNBr-activated Sepharose. Bound and unbound antibody fractions were collected and tested for reactivity to SP-22 and gp120, and for the ability to neutralize HTLV-III$_B$ *in vitro*. When HIV+ patient serum was passed over the SP-22 affinity column and tested for reactivity to

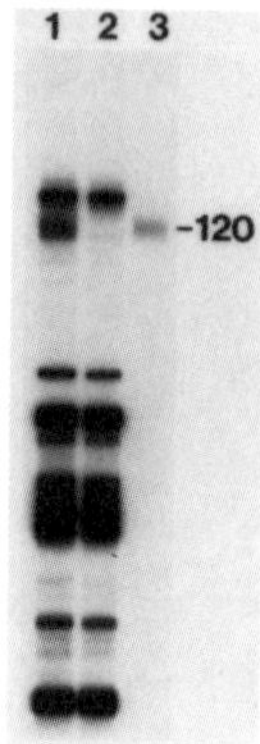

Figure 5. Isolation of anti-gp120 antibodies reactive to SP-22 by affinity chromatography. Serum from an HIV seropositive patient #12 was passed over an SP-22-BSA affinity column and the bound and unbound fractions were collected and tested in immunoblot assays against lysates of HIV+ H-9 cells. Lane 1: Antibody reactivity of untreated HIV+ patient serum #12. Lane 2: Antibody reactivity of #12 serum after passage over affinity column. Lane 3: Reactivity of antibodies to gp120 that were bound to the SP-22-BSA column and eluted with 4M $MgCl_2$. Bound antibodies were further tested for the ability to inhibit syncytium formation and neutralize HIV *in vitro*.

HIV proteins in immunoblot assay (Figure 5), antibodies to gp120 were selectively removed (lane 2) and could be recovered by eluting the column with 4M $MgCl_2$ (lane 3). When tested in RIA and neutralization assays (Table 2), anti-SP-22 antibodies were identified exclusively in the fraction that bound to the SP-22 affinity column. These antibodies also reacted with ^{125}I-labelled gp120 in RIP assay and accounted for approximately 70% of all antibodies to gp120 in the test serum. Although not detected in immunoblot assay, SP-22 non-reactive anti-gp120 antibodies were found in the unbound fraction by RIP assay and accounted for the remaining 30% of antibody reactivity to gp120. In neutralization assays, only the SP-22 non-reactive (unbound) antibodies inhibited $HTLV-III_B$

TABLE 2

Effect of Affinity Purified Anti-gp120 Human Antibodies on HTLV-III_B Replication *In Vitro*

Affinity Column[a]	HIV+ Patient Serum Fraction[b]	Reactivity[c] to SP-22	Reactivity[c] to gp120	Neutralization of HTLV-III_B as Measured by[d]: Reverse Transcriptase Production (cpm)	Neutralization of HTLV-III_B as Measured by[d]: Production of Viral P24 (ng/ml)
SP-22 (BSA)	Bound	15,031	88,904	225,692	20
	Unbound	104	33,259	2,697	<0.3
SP-70A (BSA)	Bound	44	1,110	206,775	20
	Unbound	5,963	12,312	9,504	<0.3
gp120[e]	Bound	ND[f]	44,730	4,000	1.2
	Unbound	ND	1,467	2,228	<0.3

a Synthetic peptide - bovine serum albumin (BSA) conjugates or purified HIV gp120 were coupled to CNBr-activated Sepharose and used as affinity columns for purification of antibodies from HIV+ patient serum. Peptide SP-22 is derived from the C-terminus of HIV gp120; peptide SP-70A contains sequences from the C-terminus of HTLV-I gp45 (see Materials and Methods). Data shown are representative of two experiments performed with SP-22 (BSA) and SP-70 (BSA) affinity columns.

b HIV+ patient serum was passed over affinity columns and the bound and unbound fractions were collected as described in Materials and Methods.

c Data are expressed as Δ cpm obtained in radioimmunoprecipitation (RIP) assays using sera passed over affinity columns and ^{125}I-labelled SP-22 (BSA) or ^{125}I-labelled gp120.

d The serum fractions were tested at a dilution of 1 to 32 for their ability to neutralize infection of HTLV-III_B and described in Materials and Methods. Virus infection was monitored on the basis of both reverse transcriptase activity and viral p24 core antigen (competition RIA) released into the supernatant of challenged H9 cells. The untreated serum completely blocked infection at a dilution of up to 1 to 100.

e The unbound fraction of HIV+ patient serum from an SP-22 affinity column was additionally passed over a gp120 affinity column and both bound and unbound serum fractions were collected.

f ND = Not done.

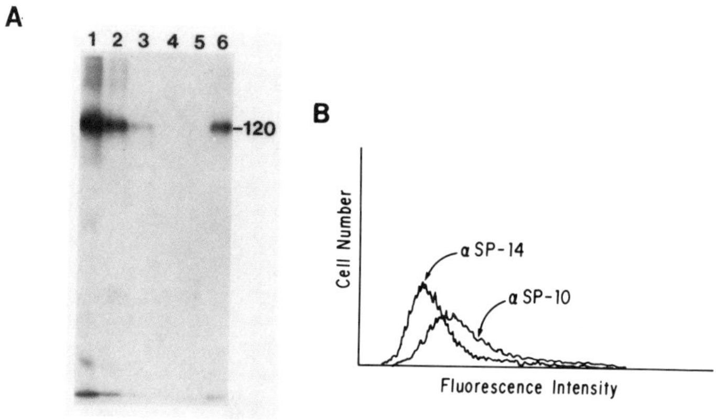

Figure 6: Reactivity to gp120 of HIV+ patient antibodies purified over synthetic peptide affinity columns. For preparation of affinity columns synthetic peptides containing amino acid sequences from HTLV-III$_B$ gp120 (SP-10, 10A,11,14,15,22, see Figure 1) were coupled to BSA and then covalently linked to CNBr-activated Sepharose. Serum aliquots (2ml) from an HIV seropositive patient were then passed over each column and the antibodies that bound to the affinity columns were then tested for reactivity to purified ^{125}I-labelled HIV gp120 in RIP assay (A) and for reactivity to the surface of H-9 cells infected with HTLV-III$_B$ in indirect immunofluorescence assays (B). A) In RIP assay, bound antibodies from the SP-10 (lane 1), SP-10A (lane 2), SP-11 (lane 3), and SP-22 (lane 6) affinity columns reacted with gp120 in RIP assay, with antibodies from the SP-10 column showing the greatest reactivity to gp120. B) Antibodies reactive with synthetic peptide SP-10 bound to the surface of HIV-infected cells, while binding of affinity purified antibodies to SP-14 or to SP-10A,11, 15 or 22 (not shown) was not detected. These data suggest that the antigenic site(s) defined by SP-10 are accessible to antibody binding when gp120 is present on the surface of HIV+ cells.

infection of H-9 cells. To evaluate the ability of SP-22 non-reactive, anti-gp120 antibodies to neutralize HTLV-III$_B$

in vitro, the unbound antibody fraction from the SP-22 column was also passed over a gp120 affinity column, and both bound and unbound antibody fractions were collected and tested as described above. Both bound and unbound antibody fractions from the gp120 affinity column neutralized HIV. These results further supported the hypothesis that, although the C-terminus of gp120 is highly immunogenic, it does not contain antigens that elicit a neutralizing antibody response in man. Further, in immunoblot assays, affinity purified anti-SP-22 antibodies reacted with gp120 in lysates of H-9 cells infected with $HTLV-III_{MN}$ and $HTLV-III_{RF}$, indicating that the antigens at the C-terminus of $HTLV-III_B$ were also present on gp120 from disparate isolates of HIV (not shown).

To begin to evaluate other regions of $HTLV-III_B$ gp120 for the presence of neutralizing epitopes, 2ml aliquots of AIDS patient serum containing a high titer of neutralizing antibodies (>1/125) were passed over affinity columns containing each of 5 synthetic peptides (SP-10, 10A,11,14 and 15) derived from a central portion of gp120 that is also present in recombinant protein PB1 (Figure 1). Antibodies to PB1 have previously been shown to neutralize $HTLV-III_B$ *in vitro* (10). Bound antibody fractions from the 5 affinity columns were recovered and tested for reactivity to ^{125}I-labelled gp120 in RIP assay. As shown in Figure 6A, affinity purified antibodies that bound to affinity columns containing peptides SP-10, 10A and 11 also reacted with gp120 in RIP assay (lanes 1-3). As a positive control, patient antibodies purified over an SP-22 affinity column were also found to react with gp120 in RIP assay (lane 6). When tested in FACS analysis, anti-SP-10 antibodies reacted with the surface of $HTLV-III_B$ infected H-9 cells (Figure 6B). Reactivity of other affinity purified antibodies to the surface of HIV+ cells could not be detected in this assay (not shown).

Using techniques described above, we are currently evaluating the functional importance of antibodies directed to synthetic peptide SP-10.

DISCUSSION

In studies described here, we have used synthetic peptides derived from hydrophilic amino acid sequences of $HTLV-III_B$ gp120 to map the host antibody response to an immunodominant epitope at the C-terminus of gp120 and to a second epitope contained within the central region of gp120 defined by recombinant protein PB1. With sera from some HIV+ patients, up to 100% of total antibody reactivity to gp120 in immunoblot assay and as much as 79% of antibody reactivity in RIP assay was mapped to the C-terminus of gp120 by using peptide SP-22 in competitive binding studies. Despite this predominant antibody response, anti-SP-22 antibodies did not neutralize $HTLV\text{-}III_B$ *in vitro*. This result is consistent with the observation that antibodies to recombinant protein PENV9 containing the C-terminal amino acid sequence of gp120 also fail to neutralize $HTLV\text{-}III_B$ *in vitro* (10). Moreover, in preliminary studies, affinity purified antibodies to SP-22 did not react with the surface of virus infected cells, suggesting that the C-terminal region of gp120 is not accessible to antibody binding when gp120 is associated with the envelope of the virus. Studies designed to address this question are underway. In contrast, antibodies that were affinity purified by absorption with synthetic peptide SP-10 reacted with gp120 in RIP assay and also with the surface of H-9 cells infected with $HTLV\text{-}III_B$. This is significant in that: 1) the amino acid sequence of SP-10 is derived from a central region of gp120 also defined by recombinant protein PB1 that is known to elicit a neutralizing antibody response in goats and 2) neutralizing epitopes of non-human retroviruses are present on the surface of virus-infected cells (3,5). Studies are underway to evaluate the homologous region of gp120 for the presence of neutralizing epitopes by using affinity purified anti-SP-10 antibodies in neutralization assays.

ACKNOWLEDGEMENTS

The authors acknowledge the expert secretarial assistance of Ms. Joyce Lowery and Ms. Kim McClammy and the expert technical assistance of Ms. M. McAdams and Ms. C. McDanal.

REFERENCES

1. Nowinski RC, Pickering R, O'Donnell PV, Pinter A, Hammerling U (1981). Selective neutralization of ecotropic murine leukemia virus by monoclonal antibodies: localization of a site on the gp70 protein associated with ecotropism. Virology 111:84.
2. Fischinger PJ, Dunlop NM, Schwarz H, Ihle JN, Weinhold KJ, Bolognesi DP and Schafer W (1982). Properties of mouse leukemia viruses. XVIII. Effective treatment of AKR leukemia with antibody to gp71 eliminates the neonatal burst of ecotropic AKR virus producing cells. Virology 119:68.
3. Bruck C, Portetelle D, Burny A, Zavada J (1982). Topographical analysis by monoclonal antibodies of BLVgp51 epitopes involved in viral functions. Virology 122:353.
4. De Noronha F, Schafer W, Essex M, Bolognesi DP (1978). Influence of antisera to oncornavirus glycoprotein (gp71) on infections of cats with feline leukemia virus. Virology 85:617.
5. Grant CK, Ernisse BJ, Jarrett O, Jones FR (1983). Feline leukemia virus envelope gp70 of subgroups B and C defined by monoclonal antibodies with cytotoxic and neutralizing functions. J Immunol 131:3042.
6. Kiyokawa T, Yoshikura H, Hattori S, Seiki M, Yoshida M (1984). Envelope proteins of human T-cell leukemia virus: expression in Escherichia coli and its application to the studies of env gene functions. Proc Natl Acad Sci USA 81:6202.
7. Robey WG, Arthur LO, Matthews TJ, Langlois A, Copeland TD, Lerche NW, Oroszlan S, Bolognesi DP, Gilden RV, Fischinger PJ (1986). Prospect for prevention of human immunodeficiency virus infection: purified 120kDa envelope glycoprotein induces neutralizing activity. Proc Natl Acad Sci USA 83:7023.
8. Matthews TJ, Langlois AJ, Robey WG, Chang NT, Gallo RC, Fischinger PJ, Bolognesi DP (1986). Restricted neutralization of divergent HTLV-III/LAV isolates by antibodies to the major envelope glycoprotein. Proc Natl Acad Sci USA 83:9709.
9. Laskey LA, Groopman JE, Fernie CW, Benz PM, Capon DJ, Dowbenko DJ, Nakamura GR, Nunes WM, Renz ME, Berman PW (1986). Neutralization of the AIDS retrovirus by

antibodies to a recombinant envelope glycoprotein. Science 233:209.

10. Putney SD, Matthews TJ, Robey WG, Lynn DL, Robert-Guroff M, Mueller WT, Langlois AJ, Ghrayeb J, Petteway SR, Weinhold KJ, Fischinger PJ, Wong-Staal F, Gallo RC, and Bolognesi DP (1986). HTLV-III/LAV neutralizing antibodies to an E. coli. produced fragment of the virus envelope. Science 234:1392.
11. Ratner L, Haseltine W, Patarca R, Livak KJ, Starcich B, Josephs SF, Doran ER, Rafalski JA, Whitehorn EA, Baumeister K, Ivanoff L, Petteway SR, Pearson ML, Lautenberger JA, Papas TS, Grayeb J, Chang NT, Gallo RC, Wong-Staal F (1985). Complete nucleotide sequence of the AIDS virus, HTLV-III. Nature 313:277.
12. Green N, Alexander H, Olson A, Alexander S, Shinnick TM, Sutcliffe JG, Lerner RH (1982). Immunogenic structure of the influenza virus hemagglutinin. Cell 28:477.
13. Petteway SR, Reed D, Reagen K, Matthews T, Tritch R, Ivanoff L, Tribe D, Chamberlain M, Cybulski R, Bolognesi DP, Keneally W (1986). Immunological characterization of HTLV-III recombinant proteins: potential as diagnostics and vaccine candidates. In Gallo RC, Haseltine W, Klein G, Zur-Hausen H (eds): "Viruses and Human Cancer: UCLA Symposia on Molecular and Cellular Biology," New York: Alan R Hess, in press.
14. Popovic M, Sarngadharan MG, Read D, Gallo RC (1984). Detection, isolation and continuous production of cytopathic retroviruses (HTLV-III) from patient with AIDS and pre-AIDS. Science 224:497.
15. Shaw GM, Hahn BH, Arya SK, Groopman JE, Gallo RC, Wong-Staal F (1984). Molecular characterization of human T-cell leukemia (lymphotropic) virus type III in the acquired immmune deficiency syndrome. Science 226:1165.
16. Palker TJ, Matthews TJ, Clark ME, Cianciolo GJ, Randall RR, Langlois AJ, White GC, Safai B, Snyderman R, Bolognesi DP, Haynes BF (1987). A conserved region at the COOH terminus of human immunodeficiency virus gp120 envelope protein contains an immunodominant epitope. Proc Natl Acad Sci USA, in press.

Human Retroviruses, Cancer, and AIDS:
Approaches to Prevention and Therapy, pages 175–184

EXPRESSION OF HIV ENVELOPE PROTEIN IN YEAST

Richard Kramer[1], Michael Schaber[1], Kathleen Fargnoli[1], E.P. Reddy[2,3], Flossie Wong-Staal[4] and Robert Gallo[4]

[1]Department of Molecular Genetics
Roche Research Center
and
[2]Department of Molecular Oncology
Roche Institute of Molecular Biology
Hoffmann-La Roche, Inc.
Nutley, NJ 07052

[4]Laboratory of Tumor Cell Biology
National Cancer Institute
Bethesda, MD 20205

ABSTRACT The HIV env gene was engineered for expression in yeast either with or without its signal peptide. The expression of different regions of env as well as env/gag fusions was examined. The presence of the signal peptide resulted in glycosylation of the env proteins.

INTRODUCTION

The retrovirus HIV is the etiological agent of a variety of immunological abnormalities including acquired immune deficiency syndrome (AIDS) (1-3). Molecular cloning and nucleotide sequence analysis of HIV and its variants have demonstrated that this viral genome exhibits many of the structural features of the avian and mammalian retroviruses (4-7). The viral genome contains information coding

[3]Present Address: Wistar Institute, Philadelphia, PA 19104.

for the three structural proteins (gag, pol and env) characteristic of retroviruses and, in addition, has two short open reading frames of apparent regulatory function and two of unknown function.

The need for sensitive and rapid methods for the detection of individuals exposed to or infected with HIV and a vaccine to curtail the global spread of this disease is clear. Toward this end, we have expressed various segments, including the entire coding region, of the HIV env glycoprotein gene in the yeast Saccharomyces cerevisiae. Glycosylated env protein as well as unmodified species were obtained that could prove useful in the development of diagnostics and/or a vaccine.

METHODS

Construction of Plasmids

The 4.5 kb EcoR I fragment with the HIV env gene was from λHXB-3 (8). This fragment was inserted into the EcoR I site of the yeast expression vector PYE7 (9) that utilizes the promoter/regulatory region from the PHO5 gene of yeast. The resulting plasmid with the env gene in the correct orientation relative to the promoter was designated pYE7/env. Since the first ATG codon in the env open reading frame is 478 bp downstream from the EcoR I site, it was necessary to delete these extra sequences to obtain expression. This was accomplished by in vitro deletion mutagenesis (10) directed by the synthetic oligonucleotide, GCAAGCAAATTCGAATTCATGAGAGTGAAG. This yielded a plasmid, pENV1, with the EcoR I site directly before the initial ATG of the env reading frame, as well as a deletion of the 5 bp before the EcoR I site of pYE7 (9), that codes for the entire env polyprotein including the putative signal sequence (amino acids 1-30). Portions of the env coding region were removed by deleting DNA sequences downstream of the Hind III, Alu I, and Dpn I sites (Fig.1).

To remove the putative signal peptide coding region, pYE7/env was cut with Asp 718 (Boehringer-

Mannheim) that recognizes the same sequence as KpnI, but leaves a 4-base 5' overhang. This overhang was "filled-in" with the Klenow fragment of E. coli DNA polymerase and the DNA cut with BamH I to yield a 2.0 kb fragment (Fig. 1). This fragment was blunt-end ligated to the 560 bp BamH I/Aha III fragment from PHO5 (11) that has the promoter as well as the first two codons from PHO5. The ligation mix was digested with BamH I and the resulting 2.6 kb BamH I fragment inserted into BamH I cut pYE7/env vector to restore the COOH-terminal coding region of env to yield pENV2. Deletion mutants coding for truncated proteins were then prepared as for the signal sequence containing plasmids.

An XmnI to Hpa II restriction fragment coding for part of the p24 gag protein was inserted in the env deletions in which sequences downstream of the Alu I and Dpn I sites were removed. In both cases the env and gag genes are in frame, resulting in a plasmid coding for an env/gag fusion protein.

Growth and Induction of Yeast Strains

The env expression plasmids were transformed into the yeast strain 20B-12 (12). Cultures were grown and induced by transfer to phospate-free medium as described (9). Where indicated, tunicamycin (Sigma) was added at 2.5 ug/ml one hr after transfer to the phospate-free medium. About 6 hrs after transfer, cells were collected by centrifugation and spheroplasts prepared and collected (9). Spheroplasts were usually stored at -20°C prior to analysis.

Sample Preparation and Immunoblot Analysis

Spheroplast pellets were resuspended in 2x sample buffer (13), incubated in a boiling water bath for 10 min and subjected to SDS-PAGE (13). The fractionated proteins were electrophoretically transferred to nitrocellulose membranes and the blot developed as described (14, 15). The antibodies used were either from rabbit serum raised against a synthetic peptide made to a region of gag or an AIDS patient's serum.

Plasmid	Amino Acids env/gag
ENV8/p24	1-466/163-299
ENV7/p24	1-517/163-299
ENV6/p24	42-466/163-299
ENV5/p24	42-517/163-299
ENV4	1-640
ENV3	42-640
ENV2	42-856
ENV1	1-856

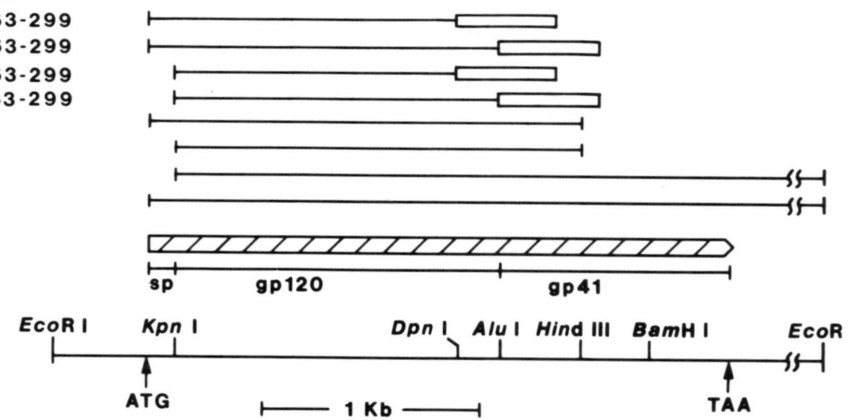

FIGURE 1. Map of HIV env gene and plasmid inserts. The positions of relevant restriction sites, the start and stop codons in the env gene and the regions coding for the signal peptide (SP), gp120 and gp41 are indicated. The part of the env gene (solid line) and, where applicable, the gag p24 region (open box) for each of the expression plasmids is shown with the amino acids coded by that plasmid. Amino acids are numbered from the first methionine encoded in the env and gag open reading frames.

RESULTS

Expression of the env gene in yeast

A number of different HIV envelope expression plasmids were made that contain the various env coding regions shown in Fig. 1. All are driven by the promoter/regulatory region from the yeast gene for an inducible acid phosphatase, PHO5 (9). The details of the plasmid construction are given in Methods.

The plasmid pENV1 contains the coding region for amino acids 1-856, the entire env coding sequence from the first methionine codon in the env open reading frame. If this methionine codon represents the actual translation initiation site, the information for the env signal peptide should be included in this plasmid. The plasmid pENV2 encodes the first two amino acids of PHO5 followed by amino acids 42-856 of env. Other plasmids contain truncated versions of the env gene as shown in Fig. 1. In addition, part of the p24 gag coding region was fused to some of the env gene constructs.

The PHO5 promoter in the env expression plasmids was induced by growth in phosphate-free medium, and extracts of the cells were analyzed for the presence of env specifc proteins by immuno-blot analysis with serum from an AIDS patient. In each case, the induced cells were grown with or without tunicamycin, an inhibitor of glycosylation. As can be seen in Fig. 2, the pENV1, pENV2, and pENV3 plasmids directed the synthesis of immuno-reactive material. Yeast cells with vector but not inserts gave no detectable reactivity (Fig. 3).

The env protein made from pENV1 (Fig. 2, panel 1) appeared as a heterogenous "smear" with the major immunoreactive material in the 140-160 kd size range. The same cells treated with tunicamycin yielded material at around 90 kd, with several smaller species. Thus, the high molecular weight material observed in the induced cells with pENV1 appears to by glycosylated HIV env protein. The plasmid pENV4 yielded similar material of 120-150 kd (not shown).

Induction of cells with pENV2 also yielded heterogenous material, but much less high molecular

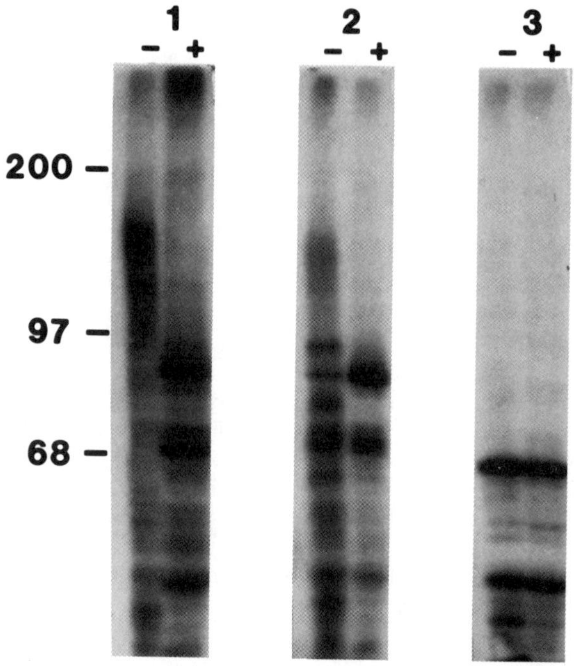

FIGURE 2. Immunoblot analysis of env proteins made in yeast. Lysates of induced yeast cells with (1) pENV1, (2) pENV2, or (3) pENV3 were fractionated by SDS-PAGE and electroblotted onto nitrocellulose filters. The env proteins were detected with an AIDS patient's serum. The samples in lanes marked + were from cells induced in the presence of tunicamycin. The position and sizes (in kd) of molecular weight markers are indicated.

weight species than with pENV1 were observed. The high molecular weight material that is observed is not seen with tunicamycin and presumably represents glycosylated material. Thus, the removal of the first 42 amino acids, containing the putative signal peptide, from the env protein appears to decrease but not eliminate the glycosylation relative to pENV1.

The plasmid pENV3 directed the synthesis of much more homogeneous immunoreactive material than the previous plasmids. A major band was detected at about 68 kd, the size expected for the entire amino acid 44-640 protein. Another band about 45 kd and several minor bands were also observed. The similarity of the sample from cells grown in the presence of tunicamycin suggests that there is no glycosylation of this protein. Thus, the region from amino acids 640-856 appears to be responsible for the glycosylation observed in the ENV2 protein.

When plasmids were constructed that coded only for the gp120 region of *env* (pENV5-8, Fig.1), no immunoreactive proteins could be detected on Western blots with the same AIDS patient's serum used previously. This indicated that either much less stable *env* protein was being made from these plasmids or that the serum only recognized epitopes in the gp41 region. In order to facilitate the detection of these proteins, a part of the p24 *gag* gene was fused to the *env* coding region as shown in Fig. 1. Western blot analysis of the hybrid proteins made from these plasmids revealed immunoreactive proteins with the expected migrations (Fig. 3) with either the AIDS serum or polyclonal antibodies to p24 peptides. As before, the presence of the putative signal peptide resulted in a large increase in apparent molecular weight, presumably due to extensive glycosylation.

DISCUSSION

We expressed various forms of the HIV *env* gene in yeast, although none were to a level high enough for detection by Coomassie blue staining of the SDS-polyacrylamide gel. Kuga *et al*. (16) reported the expression of the HTLV-I gp62 *env* protein in yeast as heterodisperse, glycosylated material at a level of less than 0.1% of total cell protein (16). We did not attempt to quantitate the HIV *env* proteins. While the glycosylated material from the *env/gag* fusions appears to be reduced relative to that lacking the signal sequence, it is likely that the transfer of the higher molecular weight species is less efficient.

While we do see extensive modification of the *env* gene products when the NH_2-terminal region is present, no apparent processing at the gp120/gp41 site is observed, even with the full *env* gene in

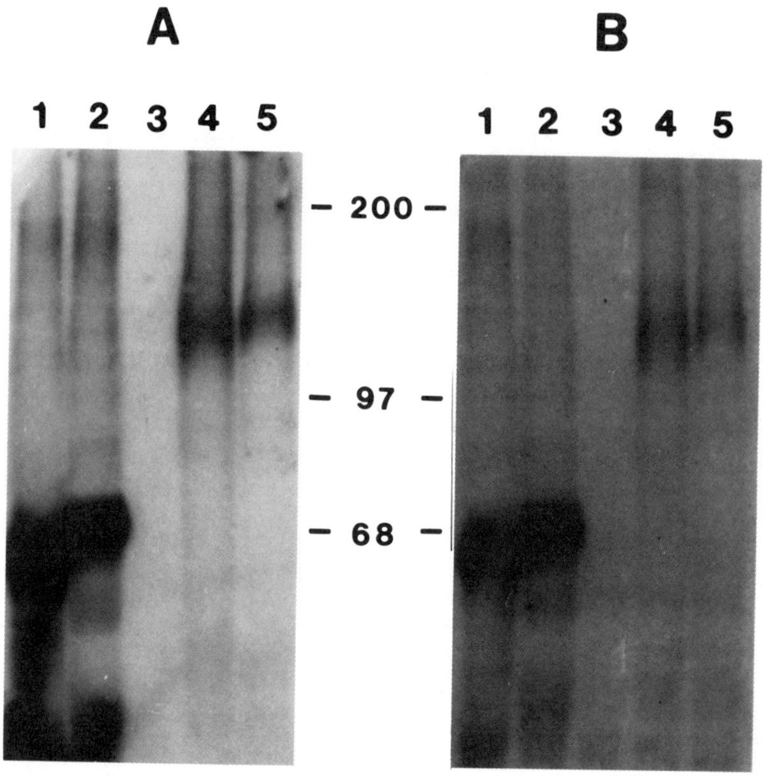

FIGURE 3. Immunoblot analysis of *env/gag* fusion proteins. Lysates of induced cells with (1) pENV5/p24, (2) pENV6/p24, (3) pYE7, (4) pENV7/p24, or (5) pENV8/p24 were fractionated by SDS-PAGE and electroblotted onto nitrocellulose filters. The *env/gag* fusion proteins were detected with (A) an AIDS patient's serum or (B) rabbit antibodies raised against p24 synthetic peptides. The position and sizes (in kd) of molecular weight markers are indicated.

pENV1. If correct processing did occur, an immunoreactive species of about 40kd should be produced but none is observed. Thus, either cleavage does not occur or, if it does, the product is unstable.

It is interesting to note that the expression of *env* amino acids 42-856 results in the appearance of some glycosylated material (Fig. 2, lane 2), while that of 42-640 does not (Fig. 2, lane 3). This suggests that part of the 640 to 856 region may act as an internal signal sequence. This region contains the highly hydrophobic transmembrane portion (amino acids 666-705) of gp41 that could provide a signal-like function.

REFERENCES

1. Barre-Sinoussi F, Chermann JC, Rey F, Nugeyre MT, Chamaret S, Gruest J, Dauguet C, Axler-Blin C, Vezinet-Brun F, Rouzioux C, Rozenbaum W, Montagnier L (1983). Isolation of a T-lymphotropic retrovirus from a patient at risk of acquired immune deficiency syndrome (AIDS). Science 220:868.
2. Popovic M, Sarngadharan MG, Read E, Gallo RC (1984). Detection, isolation and continuous production of cytopathic retroviruses (HTLV-III) from patients with AIDS and pre-AIDS. Science 224:497.
3. Levy JA, Hoffman AD, Kramer SM, Landis JA, Shimabukuro JM, Oshiro LS (1984). Isolation of lymphocytopathic retroviruses from San Francisco patients with AIDS. Science 225:840.
4. Ratner L, Haseltine W, Patarca R, Livak KJ, Starcich B, Josephs SF, Doran ER, Rafalski JA, Papas TS, Ghrayeb J, Chang NT, Gallo RC, Wong-Staal F (1985). Complete nucleotide sequence of the AIDS virus, HTLV-III. Nature 313: 227.
5. Sanchez-Pescador, R, Power, MD, Barr PJ, Steimer K.S, Stempien MM, Brown-Shimer SL, Gee WW, Renard A, Randolph A, Levy JA, Dina D, Luciw PA (1985). Nucleotide sequence and expression of an AIDS-associated retrovirus (ARV-2). Science 227, 484.
6. Muesing MA, Smith DH, Cabradilla CD, Benton CV, Lasky LA, Capon DJ (1985). Nucleic acid structure and expression of the human AIDS/lymphadenopathy retrovirus. Nature 313: 450.
7. Wain-Hobson S, Sonigo P, Danos O, Cole S, Alizon M (1985) Nucleotide sequence of the AIDS virus, LAV. Cell 40: 9.

8. Shaw GM, Hahn BH, Arya SK, Groopman JE, Gallo RC, Wong-Staal F (1984). Molecular characterization of human T-cell leukemia (lymphotrophic) virus type III in the acquired immune deficiency syndrome. Science 226: 1165.
9. Schaber MD, DeChiara TM, Kramer RA (1986). Yeast vectors for production of interferon. In Pestka S(ed): "Methods in Enzymology, vol 119: Interferons, Part C," Orlando: Academic Press, p. 416.
10. Morinaga Y, Franceschini T, Inouye S, Inouye M (1984). Improvements of oligonucleotide-directed site-specific mutagenesis using double-stranded plasmid DNA. Bio/Technology 2: 636.
11. Thill GP, Kramer RA, Turner JT, Bostian KA (1983). Comparative analysis of the 5'-end regions of two repressible acid phosphatase genes in Saccharomyces cerevisiae. Mol. Cell. Biol. 3: 570.
12. Jones E (1977), Proteinase mutants of Saccharomyces cerevisiae. Genetics 85: 23.
13. Laemmli UK (1970). Clevage of structural proteins during the assembly of the head of bacteriophage T4. Nature 227: 680.
14. Towbin H, Staehelin T, Gordon J (1979) Electrophoretic transfer of proteins from polyacrylamide gels to nitrocellulose sheets: procedure and some applications. Proc. Natl. Acad. Sci. USA 76: 4350.
15. Burnette NW (1981). "Western blotting": electrophoretic transfer of proteins from sodium dodecyl sulfate-polyacrylamide gels to unmodified nitrocellulose and radiographic detection with antibody and radioiodonated protein A. Anal. Biochem. 112: 195.
16. Kuga T, Seisuke H, Yoshida M, Taniguchi T (1986). Expression of human T-cell leukemia virus type I envelope protein in Saccharomyces cerevisiae. Gene 44: 337.

IV. VIRAL PATHOGENESIS

Human Retroviruses, Cancer, and AIDS:
Approaches to Prevention and Therapy, pages 187–196

IMMUNOPATHOGENIC MECHANISMS OF HUMAN IMMUNODEFICIENCY VIRUS (HIV) INFECTION

Anthony S. Fauci, M.D.

National Institute of Allergy and Infectious Diseases
Bethesda, Maryland 20892

ABSTRACT There are a number of proven and potential mechanisms whereby HIV exerts its pathogenic effects on the CD4+ helper/inducer subset of T4 lymphocytes. This paper focuses on two of the major pathogenic mechanisms in HIV infection: selective impairment of antigen-responsive T4 cells and induction of virus from latent, chronically infected target cells. Although the defect in antigen responsiveness in HIV infections can occur as a result of selective depletion of CD4+ cells, it is now clear that viable CD4+ cells can be functionally impaired as a result of prior HIV exposure and/or a low-level, perhaps latent or chronic, infection. Induction of HIV from latently or chronically infected cells can occur following mitogenic or antigenic stimuli, transfection of DNA from heterologous viruses, and exposure to a variety of cytokines. Upregulation of HIV expression was shown to be associated with the induction of expression of IL-1 messenger RNA and protein in a chronically infected, cloned promonocyte cell line. Dissection of the mechanisms of induction of HIV expression will play a major role in understanding the progression of HIV infection from an asymptomatic state to full-blown AIDS.

INTRODUCTION

It has been well established that the common denominator of the immunopathogenic mechanisms of HIV infection is specific binding of HIV to the CD4 molecule of the T4 lymphocyte via the envelope region of the virus leading to internalization of the virus and subsequent functional impairment and/or destruction of the target CD4+ lymphocyte (1-4). The precise mechanisms whereby the T4 cell is eliminated are uncertain at present, but a number of theories have been described and are discussed elsewhere in this conference. It should also be pointed out that a number of other cells that express the CD4 molecule are also susceptible to infection with HIV (5). However, not all infected cells undergo a cytopathic effect and this lack of cytopathicity may well be related to the relative paucity of expression of CD4 molecules on these alternative target cells. Such cells include the monocyte/macrophages (6-8), endothelial cells (9), Langerhans cells (10), colorectal cells (11), and others (12).

We have pointed out previously that the broad scope of immunologic defects in patients with HIV infection is very likely related to the fact that a wide variety of immunologic functions in man require an intact T4 cell inductive signal in order to fully express their immunologic competence (13). This is true both for the induction of immunoglobulin secretion, the induction of other lymphoid cell functions such as natural killer cell activity, cytotoxic T cell activity, suppressor cell activity, and a variety of other lymphoid and nonlymphoid functions. For the purpose of the present discussion, we will focus on two major aspects of the HIV pathogenic effect. The first is the selective impairment of the antigen-responsive T4 cell, and the second is the mechanisms whereby a latent, chronically infected target cell can be induced to express the virus at high levels.

ANTIGEN-RESPONSIVE T4 LYMPHOCYTE

The most obvious defect of T4 lymphocytes in individuals with HIV infection is a quantitative deficiency of the CD4+ subset (14, 15). The lack of these cells strongly suggests that there is a specific in vivo cytopathic effect that parallels the well-documented in vitro cytopathic effect of the virus on T4 cells. However, it is also quite clear that there is a qualitative defect in certain T4 lymphocyte functions and that the antigen-responsive T4 cell is selectively deficient in AIDS patients; this deficiency occurs early in the course of the disease. This was first reported by our group when we noted that in individuals with HIV infection, the defective mitogen responsiveness could generally be reconstituted in vitro by separately culturing equivalent numbers of T4 cells from normal controls and from patients with HIV infection (16). In other words, if the reversed T4 to T8 ratio could be normalized in vitro, there was generally a normal responsiveness to mitogens. However, this was not the case with antigen-specific responsiveness such as the response to the soluble antigen tetanus toxoid. Even if purified T4 populations were cultured in the presence of adequate numbers of macrophages, there was still a marked decrease in the antigen-specific responses. This could not be explained by a monocyte defect in patients with HIV infection since we had the opportunity to perform syngeneic coculture experiments with normal macrophages (Koenig et al., unpublished observation). In these latter experiments, highly purified monocytes from HIV seronegative identical twins of AIDS patients were cocultured with purified T4 cells from the AIDS patients to determine the competency of the T4 cell responsiveness to soluble antigen. Even in the presence of normal monocyte/macrophages, the response to soluble antigen was decreased.

In addition, we had noted that in a large group of healthy HIV seropositive homosexual men, even individuals who had normal total numbers of T4 lymphocytes early on in their disease, several still had remarkable diminution in their response to soluble antigens (Lane et al., unpublished observations). This suggested to us that the functional impairment in antigen responsiveness within the CD4+ T cell subset was due either to selective depletion of antigen-responsive CD4+ cells or to a functional impairment of the antigen-responsive cell that was still present and viable in the body.

The suggestion that the virus itself could induce a functional impairment or even perhaps a desensitization or tolerance of T4+ cells came from studies by Margolick et al. (17). They demonstrated that prior exposure of peripheral blood mononuclear cells to the virus itself without obvious infection resulted in the inability of those cells to respond to antigen stimulation, although response to mitogens was also somewhat decreased (Table 1). Based on these experiments, it was concluded that at least two possibilities exist for the selective defect in antigen responsiveness. The first is a quantitative defect of all

Table 1[1]

Inhibition of Proliferative Responses of PBMNC[2] by Exposure to HIV[3]

	Exp. 1							Exp. 2	Exp. 3
Primary stimulus (day 0)	KLH			TT		No antigen		No antigen	
Secondary stimulus (days 17-21)	PHA[4]	KLH[5]	PHA	TT	PHA	TT	KLH	PHA	PHA
Virus (day 3)									
0	51,182[5]	29,349	52,449	19,126	23,447	12,700	6,712	36,918	77,255
10^{-4}	8,767	392	6,598	341	7,815	97	0	8,751	35,215
10^{-5}	27,979	14,804	24,101	10,959	30,409	2,863	2,436	36,389	49,416

[1]Adapted from reference 17.

[2]PBMNC - peripheral blood mononuclear cells.

[3]PBMNC were incubated either with antigen (tetanus toxoid (TT) - 10 μg/ml; keyhole limpet hemocyanin (KLH) - 100 μg/ml) or media alone on day 0, were exposed to live virus on day 3, and were maintained in the culture until restimulation.

[4]PHA - phytohemagglutinin.

[5]The data are presented as Δcpm compared with cells restimulated with medium (including irradiated autologous PBMNC) alone.

lymphocytes and perhaps even a selective defect of the antigen-responsive CD4+ cells. The second is a functional impairment of T4 cells related to prior exposure to virus and/or a low-level infection, perhaps even a latent or chronic infection of the CD4+ cell. This could result in a variety of potential abnormalities of antigen responsiveness including the inability to interact in a major histocompatibility complex-restricted manner with monocyte/macrophages or a post-antigen receptor signal transduction defect.

THE CONVERSION OF A LATENT OR CHRONIC INFECTION TO A FULLY EXPRESSED VIRAL INFECTION

It has been well established that activation signals are required for HIV to infect lymphocytes (18, 19). If resting lymphocytes are exposed to virus, syncytia form but reverse transriptase cannot be measured in the supernatant. In addition, the question arose whether or not cells which were chronically or latently infected with the virus also required an activation signal to fully express the virus. This led us to perform a series of experiments aimed at determining the mechanisms involved in converting a latent or chronic HIV infection to a productive infection. Folks et al. first observed that in cells in the A3.01 (ALEX) cell line, which were chronically or latently infected with the virus, there was no spontaneous reverse transcriptase in the supernatant of these cultures (20). However, when these cells, which had survived an initial infection, were exposed to IUdR or azacytidine, virus was fully expressed (Fig. 1). In addition, we subsequently demonstrated, as did others (18, 19), that mitogen or antigenic stimuli were able to convert a latent infection to a full-blown infection. In order to mimic the potential clinically and physiologically relevant situation of other microbes inducing the expression of HIV, a series of experiments were performed by Gendelman et al. (21). SW480 colorectal carcinoma cells, which were chronically infected with HIV, were simultaneously cotransfected with a variety of viral constructs. Cells either received a construct containing the long terminal repeat (LTR) of HIV together with the chloramphenicol acetyltransferase (CAT) gene and/or the *tat* gene and/or heterologous DNAs such as the immediate early genes of herpes simplex virus. In these experiments it was demonstrated that the DNAs of these heterologous

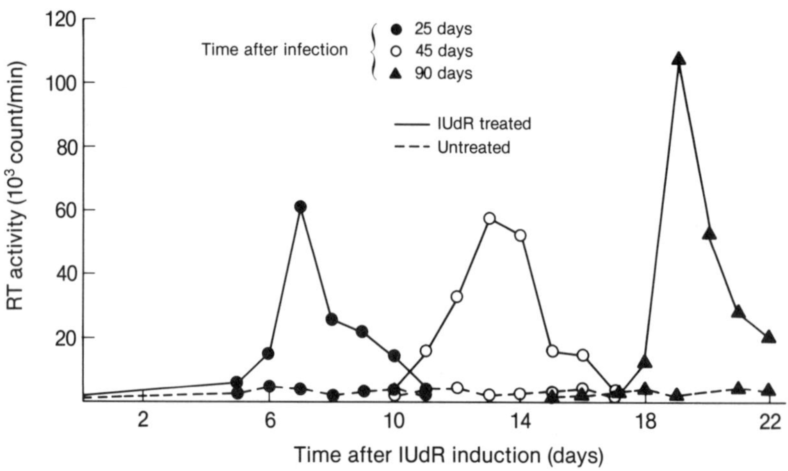

FIGURE 2. Inducibility of HIV after treatment with IUdR. Aliquots (1×10^6) were treated with IUdR (100 micrograms/ml) for 24 hr, washed three times in medium and cocultured with 1×10^6 A3.01 cells. Supernatants were tested daily for reverse transcriptase activity. Untreated survivor cells were also cocultured with A3.01 cells and monitored for reverse transcriptase activity. Adapted from reference 20.

viruses together with the <u>tat</u> gene of HIV when cotransfected with the LTR-CAT construct markedly upregulated the expression of CAT activity (21). These studies strongly suggest that other heterologous viruses that may coinfect HIV-infected cells could be responsible for the upregulation of expression of HIV. In fact, in recent experiments, Gendelman et al. have transfected an entire infectious clone of HIV and have demonstrated that cotransfection with heterologous DNAs resulted in the upregulation of expression of virus that could be measured by reverse transcriptase in the supernatant (21). Similar types of cotransfection studies with other heterologous viruses have been performed (22, 23).

In order to approximate a more physiologic situation in which immune stimuli might induce the expression of virus in latently infected cells, we developed a series of clones derived from chronically infected U937 cells. One in particular was a clone called U1 that was persistently infected with HIV but which did not spontaneously produce virus in detectable amounts (Folks et al., manuscript submitted). The U1 cell contains two integrated copies of the retrovirus and was shown to be induced to express virus by a variety of cytokines including a phytohemagglutinin supernatant, granulocyte-macrophage/colony stimulating factor, and a low molecular weight cytokine derived from macrophages (Dinarello et al., unpublished observations). Recombinant interferon-gamma, recombinant interleukin (IL)-1 beta, recombinant IL-1 alpha, recombinant IL-2, or recombinant tumor necrosis factor did not induce expression of virus. Associated with the latent infection of U1 was a marked upregulation of the expression of messenger RNA and protein of IL-1, indicating that infection with HIV can markedly upregulate the expression of certain cellular genes. Furthermore, these series of experiments strongly suggest that physiologic signals delivered during the course of a normal immune response or upon exposure to a variety of microbes could induce the expression of virus in an otherwise latently or chronically infected cell. Current studies are in progress to determine the precise mechanisms whereby the IL-1 gene or its products and the integrated provirus in the U1 cell or its products interact to result in upregulation of viral expression.

SUMMARY

The present study has reviewed a variety of the immunopathogenic mechanisms of HIV infection. In particular, we have focused on the real and potential mechanisms whereby there is a selective defect in antigen-responsive T cells early in HIV infection. In addition, we have established a model for the induction of expression of virus in chronically infected promonocyte cell lines by a variety of cytokines. Hopefully, these studies will increase our understanding of the total scope of immunopathogenic mechanisms of HIV infection.

ACKNOWLEDGMENTS

I wish to recognize the contributions of Drs. H. Clifford Lane, Thomas Folks, Scott Koenig, Howard E. Gendelman, Malcolm A. Martin, Arnold Rabson, and Zeda Rosenberg, and the editorial assistance of Ms. Ann C. London.

REFERENCES

1. Bowen DL, Lane HC, Fauci AS (1985). The immunopathogenesis of the acquired immunodeficiency syndrome. Ann Intern Med 103:704.
2. Fauci AS, Lane HC (1986). Antiretroviral therapy and immunologic reconstitution in AIDS. In Gluckman JC, Vilmer E (eds): "Acquired ImmunoDeficiency Syndrome," Paris: Elsevier, p 229.
3. Dalgleish AG, Beverley PCL, Clapham PR, Crawford DH, Greaves MF, Weiss RA (1984). The CD4 (T4) antigen is an essential component of the receptor for the AIDS retrovirus. Nature 312:763.
4. Klatzmann D, Champagne E, Chamaret S, Gruest J, Guetard D, Hercend T, Gluckman JC, Montagnier L (1984). The T4 molecule behaves as the receptor for human retrovirus LAV. Nature 312:767.
5. Maddon PJ, Dalgleish AG, McDougal JS, Clapham PR, Weiss RA, Axel R (1986). The T4 gene encodes the AIDS virus receptor and is expressed in the immune system and the brain. Cell 47:333.
6. Ho DD, Rota TR, Schooley RT, Kaplan JC, Allan JD, Groopman JE, Resnick L, Felsenstein D, Andrews CA, Hirsch MS (1985). Isolation of HTLV-III from cerebrospinal fluid and neural tissues of patients with neurologic syndromes related to the acquired immunodeficiency syndrome. N Engl J Med 313:1493.
7. Koenig S, Gendelman HE, Orenstein JM, Dal Canto MC, Pezeshkpour GH, Yungbluth F, Jannotta F, Aksamit A, Martin MA, Fauci AS (1986). Detection

of AIDS virus macrophages in brain tissue from AIDS patients with encephalopathy. Science 233:1089.

8. Gartner S, Markovits P, Markovitz DM, Kaplan MH, Gallo RC, Popovic M (1986). The role of mononuclear phagocytes in HTLV-III/LAV infection. Science 233:215.
9. Wiley CA, Schreier RD, Nelson JA, Lampert PW, Oldstone MB (1986). Cellular localization of human immunodeficiency virus infection within the brains of acquired immune deficiency syndrome patients. Proc Natl Acad Sci USA 83:7089.
10. Tschachler G, Groh V, Popovic M, Mann DL, Konrad K, Safai B, Eron L, diMargo Veronese F, Wolff K, Stinzl G (1987). Epidermal Langerhans cells - a target for HTLV-III/LAV infection. J Invest Dermatol 88:233.
11. Adachi A, Koenig S, Gendelman H, Dougherty D, Gattoni-Celli S, Fauci AS, Martin MA (1987). Productive persistent infection of human colorectal cell lines with the AIDS retrovirus. J Virol 61:209.
12. Funke I, Hahn A, Rieber EP, Weiss E, Riethmuller G (1987). The cellular receptor (CD4) of the human immunodeficiency virus is expressed on neurons and glial cells in human brain. J Exp Med 165:1230.
13. Fauci AS (1985). Immunologic abnormalities in the acquired immunodeficiency syndrome (AIDS). Clin Res 32:491.
14. Lane HC, Fauci AS (1985). Immunologic reconstitution in the acquired immunodeficiency syndrome. Ann Intern Med 103:714.
15. Margolick JB, Lane HC, Fauci AS (1987). Immunopathogenesis of HTLV-III/LAV infection. In Gallo RC, Haseltine W, Klein G, zur Hausen H (eds): "Viruses and Human Cancer (UCLA Symposia on Molecular and Cellular Biology, New Series)," New York: Alan R. Liss, p 59.
16. Lane HC, Masur H, Edgar LC, Whalen G, Fauci AS (1983). Abnormalities of B cell activation and immunoregulation in patients with the acquired immune deficiency syndrome. N Engl J Med 309:453.
17. Margolick JB, Volkman DJ, Folks TM, Fauci AS (1987). Amplification of HTLV-III/LAV infection by antigen-induced activation of T cells and

direct suppression by virus of lymphocyte blastogenic responses. J Immunol 138:1719.
18. McDougal JS, Mawle A, Cort SP, Nicholson JKA, Cross GD, Scheppler-Campbell JA, Hicks D, Sligh J (1985). Cellular tropism of the human retrovirus HTLV-III/LAV. I. Role of T cell activation and expression of the T4 antigen. J Immunol 135:3151.
19. Folks TM, Kelly J, Benn S, Kinter A, Justement J, Gold J, Redfield R, Sell KW, Fauci AS (1986). Susceptibility of normal human lymphocytes to infection with HTLV-III/LAV. J Immunol 136:4049.
20. Folks T, Powell DM, Lightfoote MM, Benn S, Martin MA, Fauci AS (1986). Induction of HTLV-III/LAV expression from a nonvirus-producing T cell line: implications for latent infection in man. Science 231:600.
21. Gendelman HE, Phelps W, Geigenbaum L, Ostrove JM, Adachi A, Howley PM, Khoury G, Ginsberg HS, Martin MA (1986). Trans-activation of the human immunodeficiency virus terminal repeat sequence by DNA viruses. Proc Natl Acad Sci USA 83:9759.
22. Pagano J (1987). Data presented at the UCLA Symposium on Molecular and Cellular Biology, Keystone Colorado, April 1987.
23. Luciw P (1987). Data presented at the UCLA Symposium on Molecular and Cellular Biology, Keystone Colorado, April 1987.

Human Retroviruses, Cancer, and AIDS:
Approaches to Prevention and Therapy, pages 197–212

HEMATOLOGIC MANIFESTATIONS OF THE HUMAN IMMUNE DEFICIENCY VIRUS (HIV)

Jerome E. Groopman*
Robert E. Donahue+
Steven C. Clarke+
Margaret M. Johnson*
Leonard I. Zon *&

*Division of Hematology/Oncology
Department of Medicine
New England Deaconess Hospital
+Genetics Institute, Inc.
87 Cambridge Park Drive
Cambridge, Massachusetts 02140
&Division of Medical Oncology
Dana-Farber Cancer Institute
Harvard Medical School
Boston, Massachusetts, 02215

INTRODUCTION

In 1983 Spivak et al. first reported pancytopenia associated with AIDS (1). Anemia, granulocytopenia, and thrombocytopenia have subsequently been described in all clinical stages of HIV infection (2). Several studies of the pathogenesis of these abnormalities have been confounded by the high frequency of coexistent infectious and neoplastic disorders and the myelosuppressive drugs used in these populations. We have reviewed the hematologic findings in well characterized cohorts of patients with AIDS, AIDS-related complex (ARC), and asymptomatic homosexual men at risk for HIV. Bone marrow aspirates and biopsies were also studied. Further investigations using *in vitro* cultures of adherence depleted bone marrow mononuclear cells has yielded a better understanding of the pathophysiology of these hematologic alterations.

RESULTS

One hundred and two patients were studied. This included 25 patients with AIDS manifest as Kaposi's sarcoma, 23 patients with AIDS without Kaposi's sarcoma who had had a prior but not current opportunistic infection, 25 patients with ARC, and 29 asymptomatic healthy male homosexuals. Using the enzyme-linked immunosorbent assay (ELISA) and Western blot techniques for the detection of serum antibodies to HIV, all patients tested positive except for 17 out of the 29 healthy homosexual males.

Hemoglobin, hematocrit, white blood count, and platelet counts were examined on the patients first visit to the hospital. The frequency of decreased peripheral blood counts for each of the cohorts studied is shown in Table 1. The frequency of hematologic abnormalities in the populations studied were statistically significant as asymptomatic HIV infection progressed to ARC and AIDS.

Thrombocytopenia occurred occasionally as an isolated hematologic finding. Anemia and granulocytopenia tended to occur simultaneously. 88 percent of granulocytopenic patients with AIDS were anemic and 69 percent of anemic patients had granulocytopenia. However less than half of the granulocytopenic patients and only one-third of the anemic patients were thrombocytopenic.

Forty-one bone marrow aspirates and biopsies were reviewed from 34 HIV seropositive individuals. This included 8 patients with AIDS and Kaposi's sarcoma, 15 patients with AIDS with prior or coincident opportunistic infection, 10 patients with ARC, and one healthy asymptomatic homosexual man. Table 2 shows the bone marrow characteristics of the group studied. Twenty patients (59%) had hypercellular marrows, 12 patients (35%) had normocellular marrows, and two patients (6%) had hypocellular marrows. Marrow dysplasia was noted in half of the patients. Dysplasia was prominent in the erythroid and myeloid series with megaloblastoid and maturational abnormalities. Plasmacytosis was present in the majority of cases. Twenty one percent of patients had lymphoid aggregates or infiltrates. Three patients had eosinophilia. Increased bone marrow reticulin was common. All samples had increased or adequate iron staining.

TABLE 1

	HGB 14.0 g/dl	HCT 41.0 %	WBC 4000 /mm^3	SEG 1600 /mm^3	LYMPH 800 /mm^3	PLT 150000 /mm^3
HH-	0/17 (0)	1/17 (6)	0/17 (0)	0/15 (0)	1/15 (7)	0/16 (0)
HH+	1/12 (8)	2/12 (17)	1/12 (8)	3/10 (30)	0/10 (0)	1/8 (13)
ARC	5/25 (20)	4/25 (16)	5/25 (20)	1/20 (5)	3/20 (15)	2/19 (11)
AIDS/KS	15/24 (63)	16/25 (64)	10/25 (40)	10/25 (40)	7/25 (28)	6/24 (25)
AIDS	15/21 (71)	16/23 (70)	15/23 (65)	11/23 (48)	16/23 (70)	9/23 (43)
p value	6.4×10^{-9}	1.8×10^{-7}	1.5×10^{-7}	.004	3.7×10^{-7}	.0004

Table 1: Frequency of low peripheral blood counts in populations studied. HGB = hemoglobin. HCT = hematocrit. WBC = total white blood count. SEG = absolute segmented neutrophil count. LYMPH = absolute lymphocyte count. PLT = platelet count. Numbers in parentheses represent percentage. The p-value tested the trend of frequencies of low blood counts in the populations HH- to AIDS in the order listed on this table.

TABLE 2

MARROW CHARACTERISTICS	NUMBER OF PATIENTS	PERCENT
HYPERCELLULAR	20	59
NORMOCELLULAR	12	35
HYPOCELLULAR	2	6
DYSPLASIA	17	50
ERYTRHOID DYSPLASIA	16	47
MYELOID DYSPLASIA	10	29
PLASMACYTOSIS	18	53
INCREASED MEGAKARYOCYTES	17	50
ADEQUATE MEGAKARYOCYTES	17	50
INCREASED IRON	18	53
ADEQUATE IRON	16	47
LYMPHOID AGGREGATES/INFILTRATES	7	21*
EOSINOPHILIA	3	9
INCREASED RETICULIN	7	21
HISTIOCYTOSIS	3	9
GRANULOMAS	2	6
ACID FAST ORGANISMS	2	6
RINGED SIDEROBLASTS	1	3

Table 2: Bone marrow morphologic characteristics in 34 patients with HIV infection. Dysplasia = total number of patients with either erythroid or myeloid dysplasia. (* = one patient did not have a bone marrow biopsy; therefore, lymphoid aggregates or infiltrates could not be detected).

Thirteen patients (Group A) had evidence of active opportunistic infection or were receiving drug therapy for an infection or tumor. The bone marrow characteristic of this group was compared to the 21 patients (Group B) who did not have current infections and were not receiving drugs (Table 3). Seventy-seven percent of Group A had hypercellular marrows, while in Group B, only half of the marrows were hypercellular. The two hypocellular marrows occurred in Group A. The findings of dysplasia, plasmacytosis, increased megakaryocytes, and lymphoid aggregates/infiltrates were prominent characteristics of both groups.

Anemia, granulocytopenia, and thrombocytopenia were noted in 90%, 55%, and 33% of patients respectively with hypercellular marrows compared to 58%, 50% and 33% of patients with normocellular marrows. In the anemic patients, 67% had hypercellular marrows, 26% had normocellular marrows and 7% had hypocellular marrows. The absolute segmented neutrophil count was decreased in 9 of 19 patients with hypercellular marrows and 4 of 11 normocellular marrows. The two patients with hypocellular marrows had pancytopenia.

All 17 patients with dysplasia of the bone marrow were anemic, while 11 were granulocytopenic and five were thrombocytopenic (Table 3). All patients with erythroid dysplasia were anemic. Nine of 10 patients with myeloid dysplasia were granulocytopenic. Nine of 17 patients with marrow dysplasia had low absolute segmented neutrophil counts.

Table 4 and 5 show the relationship of the bone marrow characteristics to peripheral blood counts for Groups A and B. There was no difference between the two groups for the marrow correlation with anemia and granulocytopenia. However, the prevalence of thrombocytopenia in patients with marrows showing hypercellularity, dysplasia, lymphoid aggregates/infiltrates, and increased megakaryocytes is much lower in Group A than in Group B.

In vitro cultures of adherence depleted bone marrow mononuclear cells from patients with HIV infection were studied, particularly observing the effects of recombinant granulocyte-macrophage colony- stimulating factor and erythropoietin on proliferation of bone marrow progenitor cells (3,4). In the presence of HIV seronegative serum, colony formation from the bone marrow of patients with HIV infection was quantitatively and qualitatively similar

TABLE 3

MARROW CHARACTERISTIC	LOW HCT	LOW WBC	LOW PLT
HYPERCELLULAR	18/20 (90%)	11/20 (55%)	6/18 (33%)
NORMOCELLULAR	7/12 (58%)	6/12 (50%)	4/12 (33%)
HYPOCELLULAR	2/2 (100%)	2/2 (100%)	1/2 (50%)
DYSPLASIA OF ANY TYPE	17/17 (100%)	11/17 (65%)	5/16 (31%)
ERYTHROID DYSPLASIA	16/16 (100%)	10/16 (63%)	5/15 (33%)
MYELOID DYSPLASIA	10/10 (100%)	9/10 (90%)	3/10 (30%)
PLASMACYTOSIS	16/18 (89%)	13/18 (72%)	5/18 (28%)
LYMPHOID AGGREGATES/INFILTRATES	4/7 (57%)	5/7 (71%)	3/7 (43%)
INCREASED OR ADEQUATE IRON	27/34 (79%)	N.A.	N.A.
INCREASED MEGAKARYOCYTES	N.A.	N.A.	6/17 (35%)
ADEQUATE MEGAKARYCOTYES	N.A.	N.A.	5/15 (33%)

Table 3: Frequency of anemia, granuocytopenia, and thrombocytopenia in patients with specific bone marrow characteristics. Anemia is defined as hematocrit 41.0 percent. Granulocytopenia was defined as total white blood count 4,000 cells/mm^3. Thrombocytopenia was defined as platelet count 150,000 cells/mm^3.

TABLE 4

MARROW CHARACTERISTIC	GROUP A 13 PATIENTS NUMBER	PERCENT	GROUP B 21 PATIENTS NUMBER	PERCENT
HYPERCELLULAR	10	77	10	48
NORMOCELLULAR	1	8	11	52
HYPOCELLULAR	2	15	0	0
DYSPLASIA OF ANY TYPE	8	62	9	43
ERYTRHOID DYSPLASIA	7	54	9	43
MYELOID DYSPLASIA	5	38	5	24
PLASMACYTOSIS	10	77	8	38
INCREASED MEGAKARYOCYTES	8	62	9	43
ADEQUATE MEGAKARYOCYTES	5	38	12	57
INCREASED IRON	7	54	11	52
ADEQUATE IRON	6	46	10	48
LYMPHOID AGGREGATES/INFILTRATES	3	23	4	20*
EOSINOPHILIA	1	8	2	10
INCREASED RETICULIN	4	31	3	14
HISTIOCYTOSIS	1	8	2	10
GRANULOMAS	2	15	0	0
ACID FAST ORGANISMS	2	9	0	0
RINGED SIDEROBLASTS	1	5	0	0

Table 4: Bone marrow morphologic characteristic in Group A and Group B. Group A represents 13 HIV seropositive patients with active opportunistic infection or ongoing drug therapy. Group B represents 21 HIV seropositive patients with no concurrent infection or therapy.

compared to the marrow from HIV seronegative donors. However, in the presence of serum containing HIV antibodies, bone marrow progenitor cultures showed suppression of both granulocyte-macrophage colony forming units (CFU-GM) and burst forming units (BFU-E) in the patients with HIV infection, but not in marrow cultures of seronegative donors. Suppression of multi-lineage colonies (CFU-Mix) could not be demonstrated because of the low number of these colonies found normally in progenitor cultures.

In three patients, the effect on bone marrow cultures of sera derived before and after infection with HIV was studied. While sera obtained before HIV infection had no effect on CFU-GM or BFU-E colony formation, sera obtained subsequent to HIV infection markedly suppressed in vitro myelopoiesis and erythropoiesis. Therefore a specific marrow suppressive effect was present when marrow from patients with AIDS or ARC was cultured in the presence of serum from the same HIV-infected population.

To determine whether the immunoglobulin fraction of the sera of HIV-infected patients contained marrow suppressive activity, the immunoglobulin fraction was isolated and purified from a patient with ARC. When bone marrow from HIV seropositive patients was cultured in the presence of purified immunoglobulin significant suppression of the formation of CFU-GM and BFU-E occurred. Purified immunoglobulin from HIV negative sera had no effect on in vitro hematopoiesis.

We attempted to demonstrate active HIV infection in the progenitor population. HIV was isolated in vitro from pooled marrow progenitor colonies from one of four patients with AIDS. We also demonstrated that adherence depleted bone marrow from a seronegative donor could be infected with HIV. HIV has also been detected in myeloid precursors in bone marrow from AIDS patients by in situ hybridization. The cellular targets of HIV in marrow are still undetermined.

Rabbit heteroantiserum directed to recombinant gp130 was obtained. This had previously been shown to neutralize HTLV-3b infection of target H9 cells (5). When bone marrow was cultured in the presence of the rabbit heteroantiserum, significant suppression of CFU-GM was observed compared to pre-immune serum.

Circulating levels of all hematopoietic elements may be affected following HIV infection. The majority of patients

TABLE 5

MARROW CHARACTERISTICS		LOW HCT		LOW WBC		LOW PLT	
HYPERCELLULAR	GROUP A	9/10	(90%)	6/10	(60%)	1/9	(11%)
	GROUP B	9/10	(90%)	5/10	(50%)	5/9	(56%)
NORMOCELLULAR	GROUP A	0/1	(0%)	1/1	(100%)	1/1	(100%)
	GROUP B	7/11	(64%)	5/11	(45%)	3/11	(27%)
HYPOCELLULAR	GROUP A	2/2	(100%)	2/2	(100%)	1/2	(50%)
	GROUP B	0/0		0/0		0/0	
DYSPLASIA OF ANY TYPE	GROUP A	8/8	(100%)	5/8	(63%)	0/7	(0%)
	GROUP B	9/9	(100%)	6/9	(67%)	5/9	(56%)
ERYTHROID DYSPLASIA	GROUP A	7/7	(100%)	4/7	(57%)	0/6	(0%)
	GROUP B	9/9	(100%)	6/9	(67%)	5/9	(56%)
MYELOID DYSPLASIA	GROUP A	5/5	(100%)	4/5	(80%)	0/5	(0%)
	GROUP B	5/5	(100%)	5/5	(100%)	3/5	(60%)
PLASMACYTOSIS	GROUP A	9/10	(90%)	8/10	(80%)	3/10	(30%)
	GROUP B	7/8	(88%)	5/8	(63%)	2/8	(25%)
LYMPHOID AGGREGATES/ INFILTRATES	GROUP A	2/3	(67%)	2/3	(67%)	0/3	(0%)
	GROUP B	2/4	(50%)	3/4	(75%)	3/4	(75%)
INCREASED OR ADEQUATE IRON	GROUP A	11/13	(85%)	N.A.		N.A.	
	GROUP B	16/21	(76%)	N.A.		N.A.	
INCREASED MEGAKARYOCYTES	GROUP A	N.A.		N.A.		1/8	(13%)
	GROUP B	N.A.		N.A.		5/9	(56%)
ADEQUATE MEGAKARYOCYTES	GROUP A	N.A.		N.A.		2/4	(50%)
	GROUP B	N.A.		N.A.		3/11	(27%)

Table 5: Frequency of anemia, granulocytopenia, and thrombocytopenia in patients of Group A and Group B with specific bone marrow characteristics.

TABLE 6

AUTHOR	Spivak	Franco	Abrams	Osborne	Geller	Castella	Schneider	Shendy	Zon
UMBER OF PATIENTS	12	17	6	32	30	35	8	55	34
YPERCELLULAR	42%	N.D.	N.D.	N.D.	53%	15%	88%	86%	59%
ORMOCELLULAR	33%	N.D.	100%	N.D.	N.D.	67%	13%	0%	35%
YPOCELLULAR	25%	N.D.	N.D.	22%	N.D.	17%	0%	14%	6%
YSPLASIA	25%	N.D.	N.D.	N.D.	N.D.	N.D.	100%	N.D.	50%
RYTHROID DYAPLASIA	N.D.	N.D.	N.D.	N.D.	N.D.	N.D.	100%	N.D.+	47%
ELOID DYSPLASIA	N.D.	N.D.	N.D.	N.D.	N.D.	N.D.	100%	N.D.	29%
ASMACYTOSIS	100%	42%	83%	31%	N.D.	83%	88%	63%	53%
CREASED MEGAKARYOCYTES	N.D.	N.D.	N.D.	N.D.	58%	37%	88%	51%	50%
EQUATE MEGAKARYOCYTES	N.D.	N.D.	N.D.	N.D.	N.D.	54%	13%	40%	50%
CREASED IRON	N.D.	N.D.	N.D.	50%*	N.D.	44%	N.D.	14%	53%
EQUATE IRON	N.D.	N.D.	N.D.	N.D.	N.D.	31%	100%	80%	47%
MPHOID AGGREGATES	33%	42%	33%	38%	N.D.	10%	50%	37%	21%
SINOPHILIA	50%	N.D.	20%	N.D.	72%	N.D.	N.D.	9%	9%
CREASED RETICULIN	91%	N.D.	80%	N.D.	78%	52%	38%	50%	21%
STIOCYTOSIS	58%	N.D.	17%	N.D.	N.D.	N.D.	N.D.	N.D.	9%
ANULOMAS	0%	N.D.	N.D	6%	N.D.	15%	0%	11%	6%
ID FAST ORGANISMS	0%	N.D.	N.D.	6%	N.D.	12%	0%	3%	6%

ble 6: Results of the studies on the bone marrow characteristcs of patients infected with HIV.

= 50% of patients in this study had decreased or absent iron.

= 6% of samples studied had megaloblastic changes in the erythroid series.

with AIDS manifest anemia and granulocytopenia, and about one third have thrombocytopenia (2). In earlier studies these abnormalities were attributed to concomitant infections, neoplasms, antibiotics and cytotoxic drugs. We studied a cohort of patients with AIDS who did not have coexistent infections or neoplasms and were not receiving drug therapy. These hematologic changes were still present. Decreased peripheral blood counts were also found in the earlier clinical stages of HIV infection, but in a lower frequency. For example, anemia, granulocytopenia, and thrombocytopenia have been found respectively in 17, 8, and 13 percent of asymptomatic HIV carriers. The frequency of these hematologic manifestations also increased with progression from asymptomatic HIV infection to AIDS.

Several studies have addressed bone marrow morphology in patients with AIDS (2,6-14). Table 6 illustrates the compilation of these studies. Prominent findings include hypercellularity, lymphoid aggregates, plasmacytosis, and dysplasia.

In patients with thrombocytopenia, the bone marrow most often has adequate megakaryocytes. Other marrow findings did not correlate with the thrombocytopenia. It is postulated that an immune mechanism causes the peripheral destruction of platelets in patients with HIV infection. The anemia and granulocytopenia, however, is related to the prominent findings of the bone marrow and appears to be due to reduced production of blood cells.

Several studies have improved our understanding of the pathophysiologic mechanism by which HIV infection leads to thrombocytopenia. Walsh et al. studied 33 homosexual males with thrombocytopenia and compared this group to 23 patients with classic autoimmune thrombocytopenia (ATP)(15). Both groups had similar platelet counts. Serum HIV antibodies were not determined in the homosexual group: however the study included 10 patients with AIDS. Platelet bound IgG and complement were quantitatively found to be three to four fold higher in the homosexual group. Using a polyethylene glycol technique, circulating immune complexes were found in 21 of 24 homosexual males. Immune complexes were absent in the ATP group. Only 1 of 10 platelet eluates from the homosexual group reacted with normal platelets compared 12 of 15 eluates from the ATP group. IgG was isolated from three homosexual males and an antiplatelet antibody could not be demonstrated. Two patients with ATP had documented antiplatelet antibodies.

Savona et al studied 70 intravenous drug addicts who had thrombocytopenia (16). Thirteen of 15 patients tested had serum antibodies to HIV. Platelet bound IgG, IgM, and complement were quantitatively increased compared to a group of patients with ATP. In addition, 11 of 18 addicts had serum platelet-reactive IgG that was a 7S IgG antibody. F(ab')2 fragments of this antibody were found to bind platelets and to specifically block the binding of positive-reacting purified IgG to platelets. The authors postulated that the mechanism of thrombocytopenia in drug addicts is due to the coating of platelets with immunoglobulin. This immunoglobulin consists of circulating immune complexes and/or a specific antiplatelet 7S IgG.

McGrath et al. have studied a cohort of 42 hemophiliacs with serum antibodies to HIV (17). Seven (18%) of these patients had thrombocytopenia. Fifty-three percent of these patients had platelet bound immunoglobulin.

Stricker et al. studied 30 thrombocytopenic male homosexuals who did not manifest symptoms of AIDS or AIDS-related illnesses, but did have serum antibodies to HIV (18). Twenty-nine of the 30 patients studied had serum antibodies directed against a 25,000 dalton platelet associated antigen. This specific antibody did not bind to other blood cells. It did, however, react with a 25,000 dalton antigen associated with cultured herpes simplex virus Types I and II and human fibroblasts. The presence of this antiplatelet antibody in serum did not uniformly lead to thrombocytopenia. The sera of 15 of 16 nonthrombocytopenic patients with AIDS and generalized lymphadenopathy also contained the antibody. In our study, AIDS patients with active infections or patients undergoing drug therapy had a lower incidence of thrombocytopenia than asymptomatic AIDS patients (2). Perhaps the normal platelet counts in this typically thrombocytopenic population represented a reactive thrombocytosis to an infection or therapy. Several studies have also reported the normalization of platelet counts in previously asymptomatic thrombocytopenic homosexual patients when they develop AIDS (19,20). Defective clearance of circulating immune complexes which are bounded to the C3b receptor of erythrocytes has been shown in the progression from asymptomatic HIV infection to development of AIDS (21). Fc-receptor mediated clearance has also been found to be defective in AIDS (22). In nonthrombocytopenic patients with AIDS who have serum antiplatelet antibodies, abnormal receptor clearance may mediate a normalization of the platelet count.

Yu et al. have documented the presence of anti-immunoglobulin antibodies in thrombocytopenic patients at risk for AIDS (23). Sevene of 16 homosexual patients had IgG anti-F(ab')2 antibody with broad reactivity against autologous, homologous, and control F(ab')2 fragments. Three homosexuals had limited reactivity against specific F(ab')2 fragments. Six of six narcotic addicts had IgG anti F(ab')2 antibody, with five of these patients having limited reactivity. Anti-F(ab')2 antibodies could not be detected in patients with classical autoimmune thrombocytopenia. These antibodies, however, have been reported in patients with autoimmune disorders such as rheumatoid arthritis and systemic lupus. Both platelet eluates and immune complexes isolated from these patients did not contain antibodies to a specific viral antigen, including EBV, CMV, HSV, rubeolla, and adenoviruses. Viral antigens could also not be detected on the platelet membrane from these patients.

Recently a patient with thrombocytopenia complicating acute HIV infection was shown to have a serum antiplatelet antibody (24). This antibody was not characterized further. It may represent the same antibody as described by Sticker et al.

Treatment of the thrombocytopenia seen in HIV infection has been similar to the standard therapy for classical autoimmune thrombocytopenia. Walsh et al. studied 33 male homosexual patients with thrombocytopenia (19). Six of these patients spontaneously developed normal platelet counts without treatment over a period from 5 to 27 months. Sixteen of seventeen patients were controlled with prednisone: 8 patients increased their platelet counts greater than $100{,}000/mm^3$ and 9 others increased their counts greater than $50{,}000/m^3$. Ten of ten patients responded to splenectomy including the one patient who did not respond to prednisone. Goldsweig et al. studied 25 male homosexual patients with thrombocytopenia (20). Eight had spontaneous recovery of their platelet count. Four did not require therapy because of stable but low platelet counts. Twelve received prednisone and seven of these twelve required splenectomy. Six of the seven splenectomized patients developed normal platelet counts.

In the series by Walsh et al., 4 of 6 patients who subsequently developed AIDS had received prednisone and had underwent splenectomy. The other two patients had not received therapy for thrombocytopenia. In the study by Goldsweig et al., two of the 25 patients developed AIDS, one of whom had received steroids and splenectomy. There is an insufficient number of patients studied to determine whether steroids or splenectomy accelerate the progression of HIV infection to AIDS. Other investigators have advocated use of anti-Rh(D) or vincristine (25-27). We attempt to avoid the use of steroids in this population, often trying danazol initially. If the patient requires further treatment, a splenectomy is undertaken.

As previously stated, the anemia and granulocytopenia found in patients with HIV infection appears to be caused by ineffective production of peripheral cells by the bone marrow. We have studied in vitro cultures of adherence depleted bone marrow mononuclear cells from patients with HIV infection, particularly observing the effects of recombinant granulocyte-macrophage colony-stimulating factor and erythropoietin on the bone marrow progenitor cells (28). In the presence of serum containing HIV antibodies, progenitor cultures showed suppression of both granulocyte-macrophage colony forming units (CFU-GM) and burst forming units (BFU-E) in the patients with HIV infection, but not in the cultures or seronegative donors.

While sera obtained before HIV infection had no effect on CFU-GM or BFU-E colony formation, sera obtained subsequent to infection markedly suppressed in vitro myelopoiesis and erythropoiesis. Therefore, a specific marrow suppressive effect is present when marrow from patients with AIDS or ARC was cultured in the presence of serum from the same population.

Purified immunoglobulin from the sera of HIV-infected individuals significantly suppressed the formation of CFU-GM and BFU-E colonies compared to a different pooled purified immunoglobulin control The immunoglobulin fraction may contain antibodies which specifically interact with the cell surface of the progenitor cells of the marrow. Since this is a specific interaction in patients who are HIV seropositive, HIV is likely to have a direct role in this process. HIV has been known to infect follicular dendritic cells and monocyte-macrophage cells in vivo (29-34) and cell lines of human B cells, monocytes, myeloblasts, and promyelocytes in vitro (30,33-38). Since these cells are derived from marrow progenitor cells, we attempted to demonstrate active HIV infection in the progenitor population. In one of four patients with AIDS, HIV was isolated in vitro from pooled marrow progenitor colonies. In these systems HIV may be difficult to isolate for technical reasons or because GM-CSF may inhibit virus production, as has been found in a monocyte cell line U937 (35). We also demonstrated that adherence depleted bone marrow from a seronegative donor can be infected with the virus. HIV has also been detected in myeloid precursors in bone marrow from AIDS patients by in situ hybridization (Sullivan J, Groopman J, et al., unpublished results).

Based on the normal progenitor proliferation of HIV-infected marrows in the presence of rGM-CSF, progenitor infection by itself is not sufficient to cause the described defect in hematopoiesis. We postulate that HIV infects progenitor cells, causing the expression viral antigens on the cell surface of these progenitors. Antibody directed against these viral determinants suppresses the normal proliferative capacity of these progenitors. When bone marrow was cultured in the presence of the rabbit heteroantiserum directed to recombinant gp130, suppression of CFU-GM colony production was present compared to the same study using pre-immune rabbit serum. This finding supports our hypothesis. Hematopoiesis, however, is not absolutely suppressed by the immunoglobulin fraction of the sera of HIV-infected individuals. This may indicate a marrow population which is not infected with the virus.

The sera of patients with HIV infection does not appear to have any colony stimulating activity as measured in our assay system with normal bone marrow. Such activity has been documented in the sera of patients with low peripheral blood counts. For instance, the sera from patients with aplastic anemia supports colony growth in the absence of rGM-CSF (Donahue, RE, Rapport JM, Nathan DG, unpublished results). Lymphokine production by T cells in HIV-infected individuals has been reported to be defective (39) and this may explain the apparent defect in hematopoietic growth factor production in HIV-infected patients. Alternatively peripheral blood mononuclear cells have been found to produce suppressor substances in patients with HIV related illnesses (41,41). Thus the anemia and granulocytopenia seen in patients with HIV infection may be the result of the release of hematopoietic suppressor substances, the inability of cells to secrete hematopoietic colony stimulating activities, and the effect of antibodies directed specifically against the hematopoietic cells in the bone marrow of HIV-infected individuals.

Despite the documented hematopoietic suppression in this patient population, GM-CSF dependent colony formation was not completely inhibited. Recently rGM-CSF has been used to stimulate hematopoiesis in an immunodeficient pancytopenic rhesus monkey (M. mulatta) which had been infected with a Type D retrovirus (42). We are currently conducting a study of the effect of rGM-CSF in pancytopenic patients with HIV infection. The initial data from this study demonstrate that recombinant GM-CSF is well tolerated by leukopenic AIDS patients and is biologically active. The circulating leukocyte count can be elevated in a dose-dependent fashion. Further studies of GM-CSF in improvement of host defense following HIV infection are warranted.

REFERENCES

1. Spivak JL, Selonick SE, Quinn TC (1983). Acquired immune deficiency syndrome and pancytopenia. JAMA 250(22):3084.
2. Zon LI, Arkin C, Groopman JE (1987). Haematologic manifestations of the human immune deficiency virus (HIV). British Jour Haematology 66:(in press).
3. Wong GG, Witek JS, Temple PA, Wilkens KM, Leary AC, Luxenberg DP, Jones SS, Brown EL, Kay RM, Orr EC, et al (1985). Human GM-CSF: Molecular cloning of the complementary DNA and purification of the natural and recombinant proteins. Science 228(4701):810.
4. Jacobs K, Shoemaker C, Rudersdorf R, Neill SD, Kaufman RJ, Mufson A, Seehra J, Jones SS, Hewick R, Fritsch EF, et al (1985). Isolation and characterization of genomic and cDNA clones of human erythropoietin. Nature 313(6005):806.
5. Lasky LA, Groopman JE, Fennie CW, Benz PM, Capon DJ, Dowbenko DJ, Nakamura GR, Nunes WM, Renz ME, Berman PW (1986). Neutralization of the AIDS retrovirus by antibodies to a recombinant envelope glycoprotein. Science 233(4760):209.
6. Spivak JL, Bender BS, Quinn TC (1984). Hematologic abnormalities in the acquired immune deficiency syndrome. Am J Med 77(2):224.
7. Franco CM, Hendrix LE, Lokey JL (1984). Bone marrow abnormalities in the acquired immunodeficiency syndrome (letter). Ann Intern Med 101(2):275.

8. Hromas RA, Murray JL (1984). Bone marrow in the acquired immunodeficiency syndrome (letter). Ann Intern Med 101(6):877.
9. Abrams DI, Chinn EK, Lewis BJ, Volberding PA, Conant MA, Townsend RM (1984). Hematologic manifestations in homosexual men with Kaposi's sarcoma. Am J Clin Pathol 81(1):13.
10. Osborne BM, Guarda LA, Butler JJ (1984). Bone marrow biopsies in patients with the acquired immunodeficiency syndrome. Hum Pathol 15(11):1048.
11. Geller SA, Muller R, Greenberg ML, Siegal FP (1985). Acquired immunodeficiency syndrome. Distinctive features of bone marrow biopsies. Arch Pathol Lab Med 109(2):138.
12. Castella A, Croxson TS, Mildvan D, Witt DH, Zalusky R (1985). The bone marrow in AIDS. A histologic, hematologic, and microbiologic study. Am J Clin Pathol 84(4):425.
13. Schneider DR, Picker LJ (1985). Myelodysplasia in the acquired immune deficiency syndrome. Am J Clin Pathol 84(2):144.
14. Shenoy CM, Lin JH (1986). Bone marrow findings in acquired immunodeficiency syndrome (AIDS). Am J Med Sci 292(6):372.
15. Walsh CM, Nardi MA, Karpatkin S (1984). On the mechanism of thrombocytopenic purpura in sexually active homosexual men. N Engl J Med 311(10):635.
16. Savona S, Nardi MA, Lennette ET, Karpatkin S (1985). Thrombocytopenic purpura in narcotics addicts. Ann Intern Med 102(6):737.
17. McGrath KM, Spelman D, Barnett M, Kellner S (1986). Spectrum of HTLV-III infection in a hemophilic cohort treated with blood products from a single manufacturer. Am J Hematol 23(3):239.
18. Stricker RB, Abrams DI, Corash L, Shuman MA (1985). Target platelet antigen in homosexual men with immune thrombocytopenia. N Engl J Med 313(22):1375.
19. Walsh C, Krigel R, Lennette E, Karpatkin S (1985). Thrombocytopenia in homosexual patients. Prognosis, response to therapy, and prevalence of antibody to the retrovirus associated with the acquired immunodeficiency syndrome. Ann Intern Med 103(4):542.
20. Goldsweig HG, Grossman R, William D (1986). Thrombocytopenia in homosexual men. Am J Hematol 21(3):243.
21. Inada Y, Lange M, McKinley GF, Sonnabend JA, Fonville TW, Kanemitsu T, Tanaka M, Clark WS (1986). Hematologic correlates and the role of erythrocyte CR1

(C3b receptor) in the development of AIDS. AIDS Res 2(3):235.
22. Bender BS, Quinn TC, Lawley TJ, Smith W, Brinkman C, Frank MM (1984). Acquired immune deficiency syndrome (AIDS): A defect in Fc-receptor specific clearance. Clin Res 32:511a.
23. Yu JR, Lennette ET, Karpatkin S (1986). Anti-F(ab')2 antibodies in thrombocytopenic patients at risk for acquired immunodeficiency syndrome. J Clin Invest 77(6):1756.
24. Lima J, Ribera A, Garcia-Bragado F, Monteagudo M, Martin-Vega C, Bastida MT (1987). Antiplatelet antibodies in primary infection by human immunodeficiency virus (letter). Ann Intern Med 106(2):333.
25. Durand JM, Harle JR, Verdot JJ, Weiller PJ, Mongin M (1986). Anti-Rh(D) immunoglobulin for immune thrombocytopenic purpura. Lancet July 5:49.
26. Biniek R, Malessa R, Brockmeyer NH, Luboldt W (1986). Anti-Rh(D) immunoglobulin for AIDS-related thrombocytopenia. Lancet September 13:627.
27. Mintzer DM, Real FX, Jovino L, Krown SE (1985). Treatment of Kaposi's sarcoma and thrombocytopenia with vincristine in patients with the acquired immunodeficiency syndrome. Ann Intern Med 102(2):200.
28. Donahue RE, Johnson MM, Zon LI, Groopman JE (1987). In vitro suppression of hematopoiesis after human immunodeficiency virus infection. Nature March 12:
29. Armstrong JA, Horne R (1984). Follicular dendritic cells and virus-like particles in AIDS-related lymphadenopathy. Lancet 2(8399):370.
30. Gartner S, Markovits P, Markovits DM, Kaplan MH, Gallo RC, Popovic M (1986). The role of mononuclear phagocytes in HTLV-III/LAV infection. Science 233(4760):215.
31. Gyorkey F, Melnick JL, Sinkovics JG, Gyorkey P (1985). Retrovirus resembling HTLV in macrophages of patients with AIDS (letter). Lancet 1(8420):106.
32. Koenig S, Gendelman HE, Orenstein JM, Dal-Canto MC, Pezeshkpour GH, Yungbluth M, Janotta F, Aksamit A, Martin MA, Fauci AS (1986). Detection of AIDS virus in macrophages in brain tissue from AIDS patients with encephalopathy. Science 233(4768):1089.
33. Salahuddin SZ, Rose RM, Groopman JE, Markham PD, Gallo RC (1986). Human T lymphotropic virus type III infection of human alveolar macrophages. Blood 68(1):281.

34. Ho DD, Rota TR, Hirsch MS (1986). Infection of monocyte/macrophages by human T lymphotropic virus type III. J Clin Invest 77(5):1712.
35. Hammer SM, Gillis JM, Groopman JE, Rose RM (1986). In vitro modification of human immunodeficiency virus infection by granulocyte-macrophage colony-stimulating factor and gamma interferon. Proc Natl Acad Sci 83(22):8734.
36. Levy JA, Shimabukuro J, McHugh T, Casavant C, Stites D, Oshiro L (1985). AIDS-associated retroviruses (ARV) can productively infect other cells besides human T helper cells. Virology 147(2):441.
37. Nicholson JK, Cross GD, Callaway CS, McDougal JS (1986). In vitro infection of human monocytes with human T lymphotropic virus type III/lymphadenopathy-associated virus (HTLV-III/LAV). J immunol 137(1):323.
38. Cortes E, Koeffler HP, Gaynor R, Mitsuyasu R (1986). Blood 68:123a.
39. Murray HW, Rubin BY, Masur H, Roberts RB (1984). Impaired production of lymphokines and immune (gamma) interferon in the acquired immunodeficiency syndrome. N Engl J Med 310(14):883.
40. Cunningham-Rundles S, Michelis MA, Masur H (1983). Serum supppression of lymphocyte activation in vitro in acquired immunodeficiency disease. J Clin Immunol 3(2):156.
41. Laurence J, Gottlieb AB, Kunkel HG (1983). Soluble suppressor factors in patients with acquired immune deficiency syndrome and its prodrome. Elaboration in vitro T lymphocyte-adherent cell interactions. J Clin Invest 72(6):2072.
42. Donahue RE, Wang EA, Stone DK, Kamen R, Wong GG, Sehgal PK, Nathan DG, Clark SC (1986). Stimulation of haematopoiesis in primates by continuous infusion of recombinant human GM-CSF. Nature 321(6073):872.

Human Retroviruses, Cancer, and AIDS: Approaches to Prevention and Therapy, pages 213–228

EVIDENCE FOR COINFECTION WITH HTLV-I AND HIV IN AIDS RISK GROUP PATIENTS WITH HIGH-GRADE NON-HODGKIN'S LYMPHOMA

Ellen G. Feigal, M.D.[1], Patricia Lekas, M.T.,
Jay H. Beckstead, M.D.[2],
Gregory Reyes, M.D.,Ph.D.[3], Lawrence Kaplan, M.D.[4],
and Michael S. McGrath, M.D.,Ph.D.[1]

AIDS Immunobiology Research Laboratory, Department of Medicine, San Francisco General Hospital, San Francisco, CA 94143

ABSTRACT We examined HTLV-I and human immunodeficiency virus (HIV) seroprevalence by Western blot in 3 patient groups to determine the relationship of these retroviruses to the development of B cell non-Hodgkin's lymphoma. Nineteen patients with high grade non-Hodgkin's lymphoma with AIDS or at risk for AIDS; 20 patients with AIDS, but without lymphoma; and 100 healthy asymptomatic HIV seropositive gay men were studied at San Francisco General Hospital from November of 1985 through July of 1986. Eighteen of 19 high grade non-Hodgkin's lymphoma patients were HIV seropositive, and all 18 were also HTLV-I seropositive (seroprevalence 100%). This result is contrasted to a 5% and 14% HTLV-I seroprevalence rate in patients with AIDS, but without lymphoma and healthy HIV seropositive gay men, respectively ($p<.001$).

[1]This study was supported in part by a grant from the California State AIDS Task Force and the VA Merit Review Grant No.821-103 (MM).

[2]Present address: Department of Pathology, University of California, San Francisco, CA 94143.

[3]Present address: GeneLabs, Inc., Redwood City, CA 94063.

[4]Present address: AIDS Activities, San Francisco General Hospital, San Francisco, CA 94110.

Cytofluorographic analysis revealed a decrease in the number of CD4 lymphocytes in the lymphoma group compared to the other 2 groups (p<0.001). Dot blot analysis detected HTLV-I envelope gene sequences in 5 out of 6 samples of DNA extracted from lymphoma tissue. In a parallel dot blot analysis, only two of these six lymphomas contained significant amounts of Epstein-Barr virus (EBV) DNA. Monoclonal antibodies to the envelope glycoprotein of HTLV-I (gp61/68) identified cells (0.2-1%) within lymphoma tissue sections. These observations suggest that HTLV-I or a similar but cross-reactive retrovirus influences lymphomagenesis associated with HIV infection.

This study also identifies a large subpopulation of gay men in San Francisco (14%) co-seropositive for HTLV-I and HIV; the relative risk for development of high grade lymphoma within this population is currently unknown.

INTRODUCTION

Individuals infected with the human immunodeficiency virus (HIV) are at risk for opportunistic infection and development of neoplasms (1-5). Recently a marked increase in the appearance of high grade B cell lymphomas has been noted in HIV infected individuals (6-9). Little is known of mechanisms by which these lymphomas occur, but a number of hypotheses have been advanced that implicate a role for Epstein-Barr virus (7,10-17), or HIV (6-9,18); however, no etiologic links have been documented. HIV is a lentivirus, and lentiviruses in animal models have not been associated with the development of neoplasms. The role for human leukemia/lymphoma viruses type I and type II (HTLV-I, HTLV-II), have not been thoroughly investigated.

HTLV-I is associated with development of adult T cell leukemia/lymphoma in a subpopulation of HTLV-I infected individuals (19-26). HTLV-I is normally tropic for mature T lymphocytes, especially those expressing the helper-inducer surface antigen CD4 (26). HTLV-I can also infect B lymphocytes, as Longo, et al. (27) reported the isolation of an HTLV-I infected B lymphocyte clone from the peripheral blood of a patient with adult T cell leukemia/lymphoma. The clone was cytogenetically normal and did not express EBV antigens. Co-culture of cells from this B cell clone with cord blood lymphocytes resulted in transmission of HTLV-I and the immortalization of either T or B lymphocytes.

Because HTLV-I has been implicated in B cell transformation (27), the possibility exists that HTLV-I might be involved in the genesis of high grade B cell lymphomas in HIV infected individuals. Evidence for coinfection with HTLV-I and HIV has been reported in selected AIDS risk populations (28-37), but AIDS patients with high grade non-Hodgkin's lymphomas have not been specifically investigated. We present serologic and molecular evidence that HTLV-I or a related retrovirus is present in these patients and may be etiologically linked, in association with HIV, to the development of B cell lymphoma.

METHODS

Patient Population.

Sera were collected from three groups, in accordance with protocols approved by the UCSF Human Subjects Committee. Group 1 consisted of 19 men with recently diagnosed high grade non-Hodgkin's lymphoma who were in a patient population with or at risk for AIDS. Group 2 consisted of 20 patients with AIDS, defined by CDC criteria (38), and excluded patients with lymphoma. Group 3 consisted of 100 healthy, asymptomatic gay men recruited from community clinics for an epidemiologic study of risk factors for HIV seroconversion (A. Moss, personal communication). HIV seropositivity was defined by ELISA (Abbott) and confirmed by Western blot. The first 2 groups of patients were seen at the UCSF or SFGH AIDS clinics, or referred through the UCSF Oncology division for treatment.

Western Blot.

A 1:50 dilution of each serum was incubated with nitrocellulose strips containing either purified HTLV-I, or a lysate from HIV infected H9 ($H9_{HIV}$) cells. Approximately 5 micrograms of purified HTLV-I protein was transferred per HTLV-I strip, and lysate from 5 x 10^5 $H9_{HIV}$ cells, was transferred to each HIV strip after 9% SDS-PAGE. Immunoblot transfer was performed as previously described (38). Antibody reactivity to specific proteins was detected by incubating at room temperature for one hour with ^{125}I-labeled protein A (0.1 uCi per strip, 2-10 uCi/ug specific activity). Western blots were then exposed to X-ray film at -70 degrees C overnight. Sera were considered positive for antibodies to HIV if reactivity to HIV p24, p41, p55, gp120, or gp160 was present. HTLV-I seropositivity was demonstrated by reactivity to HTLV-I envelope glycoproteins gp45 or gp61. Serologic cross-reactivity between HIV antigens and HTLV-I envelope glycoproteins has not been described (32), and in serum samples demonstrating HTLV-I gp61 reactivity, pre-incubation with lysate from 1 x 10^7 $H9_{HIV}$ cells did not inhibit this reactivity.

Source of HIV Infected Cells and HTLV-I.

H9 cells infected with HIV ($HTLV-III_B$) were obtained from Dr. R. C. Gallo, NIH, and grown in vitro in RPMI-1640 supplemented with 10% fetal calf serum (FCS). $H9_{HIV}$ cell lysates for use in Western blots were prepared from pellets of phosphate buffer (PBS) washed cells resuspended at 5 x 10^7 cells/ml in 1% NP-40 containing 1% Trasylol. Insoluble material was removed by centrifugation at 10,000 x g at 4 degrees C for ten minutes. Lysates were kept at -70 degrees C, until use in SDS-PAGE for Western blotting.

HTLV-I was purified from tissue culture supernatants from the HTLV-I producing cell line MT-2. MT-2 cells were grown in RPMI-1640 with 10% FCS. HTLV-I virions were purified by ultrafiltration concentration, followed by Sepharose 4B chromatography, as previously described (40,41). Purified HTLV-I in PBS (2-300 ug/ml) was stored at -70 degrees C until use in SDS-PAGE for Western blotting. Other cell lines used in this study include AL-1, an EBV positive Burkitt's lymphoma, and CEM, a T cell ALL. The cell lines were grown in RPMI-1640/10% FCS.

Preparation of Lymph Node Tissue.

The majority of the non-Hodgkin's lymphoma patients had extranodal involvement. We obtained fresh lymphoma tissue in 6 patients undergoing diagnostic lymph node biopsies. Each tissue sample was divided into sections. One section was snap frozen in dry ice and stored in liquid N_2. The remainder was made into a cell suspension by mincing and passing through a fine wire mesh as previously described (42). Samples were stored in liquid N_2 at 2 x 10^7 cells/ml in RPMI-1640/10% DMSO/20%FCS, until used in dot blot analyses and plastic embedded staining.

Immunologic Phenotyping.

Lymphocyte subset phenotyping was performed as described (43) on peripheral blood from a group of 6 AIDS associated high grade non-Hodgkin's lymphoma patients, 19 AIDS patients, 14 gay men with antibodies to HTLV-I and HIV, and 28 gay men with antibodies to HIV but not to HTLV-I. Mean CD4 and CD8 lymphocyte numbers were calculated by cytofluorographic analysis using an

Ortho Cytofluorograf and fluorescein conjugated OKT4 and OKT8 monoclonal antibodies (Ortho Diagnostics).

Dot Blot Analysis of AIDS Associated Lymphoma DNA.

DNA preparation: 2 to 5 x 10^7 lymphoma cells were lysed in 0.5ml of lysis buffer ((TE: 10mM Tris, 1mM EDTA, 1% SDS, pH 6.5). RNA'se, (100 ug/ml) was added and incubated at 37 degrees C for one hour, with shaking. Proteinase K was then added to a final concentration of 100ug/ml and incubated at 50 degrees C overnight after phenol extraction (25 phenol:24 Chloroform:1 isoamyl alcohol). The DNA containing aqueous phase was collected. Sodium acetate was added to give a final concentration of 0.2M salt prior to adding ice cold ethanol. Ethanol precipitated DNA was then centrifuged, and resuspended in TE. This method was used for all DNA preparations.

Dot blotting. 5 ug of each sample DNA, in 0.17ml of buffer was made up to a final concentration of 0.2M NaOH, and 6.7x SSC (20xSSC = 3 NaCl, 0.3M Na Citrate, pH 7.0). Samples were vortexed, then incubated at 80 degrees C for 10 minutes. The denatured DNA solution was then neutralized with 2 M Tris HCL pH 7.5 (final concentration 0.24 M). The nitrocellulose was wetted with 1x SSC, and samples were loaded into a 96 well dot blot apparatus under suction (Bio-Rad).

Nick translation. Hybridization probes were prepared from the HTLV-I envelope gene (provided by Dr. R. C. Gallo, NCI, NIH) and the large internal BAM HI fragment of EBV (obtained from Dr. Elliot Kieff, University of Chicago). 0.25 ug of each probe, was labeled with ^{32}P dCTP (10 mCi/mM) using a commercially available kit (Amersham). The labeled probe DNA was ethanol precipitated as described above, and added to hybridization buffer for use in dot blot analysis.

DNA hybridization. All blots were pre-hybridized with 50% deionized formamide, 5x Denhardts solution 5x SSC, 0.1% SDS, and 100 ug/ml of denatured salmon sperm DNA, at 43 degrees C, for at least 4 hours. ^{32}P labeled probes were incubated at 100 degrees C for 10 minutes, immediately placed on ice for 10 minutes, and then added to the pre-hybridization mix to give a final concentration of 2 x 10^6 cpm/ml. Blotted nitrocellulose was incubated in Seal-a-Meal bags with labeled probe, at 43 degrees C overnight. After the overnight incubation, blots were washed twice in 2x SSC, 1x Denhardts, shaking at 43 degrees C for thirty minutes per wash. The final two filter washes were with 0.1x SSC, 0.1% SDS, performed at 50 degrees C for thirty minutes each, with agitation. The filters were blotted dry, and exposed to X-ray film at -70 degrees C for 3 to 4 days.

Tissue Staining.

Plastic embedding of lymphoma tissue and immunohistochemical staining with monoclonal antibodies was performed as previously described (44,45). A mouse monoclonal antibody to the HTLV-I envelope glycoproteins (gp61/68) was prepared in our laboratory and immunoprecipitated molecules with the same 2D SDS-PAGE profile as the human 0.5 alpha anti-gp61 (46). Mouse anti-HIV p25 was obtained from Litton-Bionetics (Charleston, South Carolina).

Statistical analysis. The Wilcoxon rank sum test was used to compare the differences between groups for lymphocyte subsets. The Chi Squared test with Yates continuity correction was used to test differences between proportions.

RESULTS

Seroprevalence of HTLV-I.

The seroprevalence of HTLV-I in the three patient groups was investigated by Western blot analysis. Eighteen of the 18 (100%) HIV positive lymphoma patients were seropositive for HTLV-I envelope proteins. In contrast, only one of the 20 (5%) AIDS patients was positive for HTLV-I. Fourteen of the 100 (14%) healthy, asymptomatic HIV seropositive gay men had serum antibody to HTLV-I. Figure 1 shows representative results of the Western blots in the AIDS associated lymphoma group, and Table 1 tabulates the results of the Western blot analysis.

Immunologic Phenotyping.

The results of cytofluorographic analysis of peripheral blood lymphocytes from the three patient groups were divided into 4 separate categories: 1) High grade non-Hodgkin's lymphoma (N=6); 2) AIDS HIV + (N=19); 3) Healthy gay men + for both HTLV-I and HIV (N=14); 4) Healthy gay men + for HIV but not for HTLV-I (N=28). CD4 + cell means and standard error in the 4 categories were 1) 75 $\pm$ SE 15; 2) 335 $\pm$ SE 59; 3) 615 $\pm$ SE 65; and 4) 549 $\pm$ SE 51. The lymphoma group had a significantly lower CD4 mean compared to the other 3 categories with a p value of <0.001.

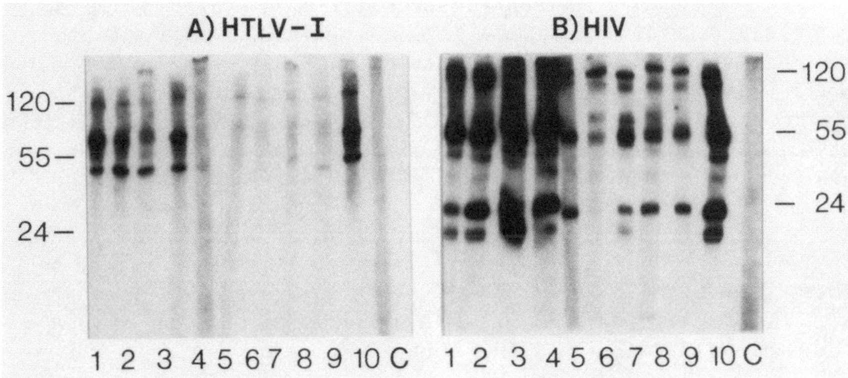

FIGURE 1. Western Blot Analyses of Sera from AIDS Associated High Grade Lymphoma Patients. 1:50 dilutions of patient or control sera were incubated with nitrocellulose strips containing either HTLV-I virus, or a cell lysate from $H9_{HIV}$ cells as described in Methods. Lanes 1-10 represent AIDS associated high grade B cell non-Hodgin's lymphoma patients, with lane C as a negative control.

TABLE 1
HTLV-I SEROPREVALENCE IN AIDS RISK GROUPS

	Sample Size	HTLV-I+ (#)	HTLV-I+ (%)
1) High Grade Non-Hodgkin's Lymphoma	18	18	100[a]
2) AIDS HIV+	20	1	5
3) Healthy HIV+ Gay Men	100	14	14

[a] P value < 0.001.

Molecular Analysis.

To determine whether the presence of HTLV-I reactive antibodies in sera from lymphoma patients would correlate with the presence of HTLV-I genomes, Southern blot analyses were initially performed, but no clonal pattern of HTLV-I hybridizable DNA species were seen. To test whether a nonclonally integrated form of HTLV-I might be present in rare lymph node cells, dot blot analyses were then performed on DNA extracted from lymph node tissue of HTLV-I seropositive and seronegative individuals. Figure 2 demonstrates that DNA which hybridized with the HTLV-I envelope gene probe under stringent washing conditions was present above background in 5 of the 6 lymphoma derived DNA samples (Ia-e). The positive control for HTLV-I consisted of 5 ug of DNA from the MT-2 cell line (IIIa), whereas 5 ug of DNA from the HTLV-I negative cell lines CEM, $H9_{HIV}$ and AL-1 (IIIb-d) did not hybridize above background.

Only two of six lymphoma DNA samples contained significant levels of EBV DNA (Ic,e). This dot blot was deliberately overexposed to determine whether EBV would be present to any degree in these lymphoma tissues. The reactivity of samples b and d represent 1% the level of hybridization noted in samples c and e. The positive control for EBV consisted of 5 ug of DNA from the AL-1 cell line, an EBV positive Burkitt's lymphoma cell line.

Lymphoma Tissue Phenotypic Analysis.

In an attempt to identify cells within lymphoma tissues potentially infected with HTLV-I, plastic embedded sections were stained with a panel of monoclonal antibodies. Figure 3 demonstrates a typical Burkitt's lymphoma lymph node section stained with two monoclonal antibodies. Panel A shows intense HTLV-I gp61/68 reactivity of rare cells within these lymphomas (0.2-1%). Cells staining with the anti HTLV-I gp61/68 antibodies are pleomorphic with some appearing like small lymphocytes and others like macrophages. Panel B demonstrates the complete lack of reactivity using an anti-HIV p25 monoclonal antibody. Plastic embedded cell pellets of MT-2 and $H9_{HIV}$ were positive controls for anti-HTLV-I gp61/68 and HIV p24 respectively. No cross reactivity was noted between antibody reagents.

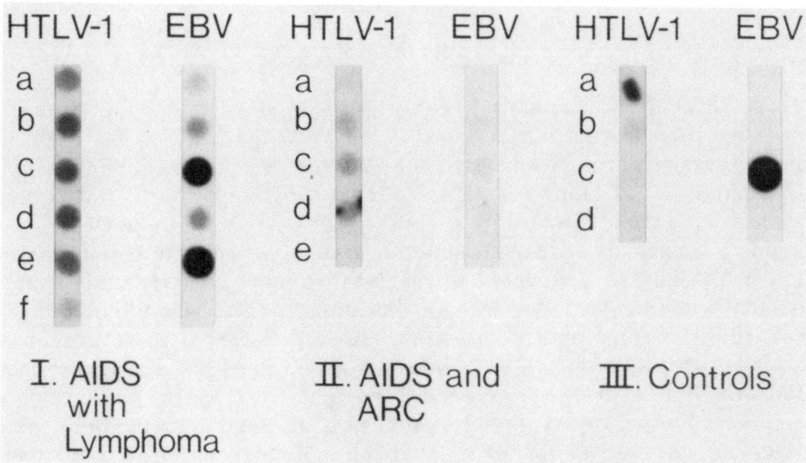

FIGURE 2. Dot Blot Analysis of DNA Derived from AIDS Lymph Nodes with HTLV-I and EBV Gene Probes. In I above the first six DNA samples are from AIDS lymphoma patients. In II: AIDS and ARC lymph node tissues from patients with the following diagnoses were analyzed; a) Kaposi's sarcoma; b) AIDS associated Hodgkin's disease; c) lymphadenopathy syndrome; d) AIDS, with mycobacterium avium intracellulare infection, and e) non-AIDS nodular lymphoma. In III: a) MT-2 cell line (HTLV-I+, EBV-, HIV-); b) CEM-CCRF cell line (HTLV-I-, EBV-, HIV-); c) AL-1 cell line (HTLV-I-, EBV+, HIV-), and d) $H9_{HIV}$ cell line (HTLV-I-, EBV-, HIV+).

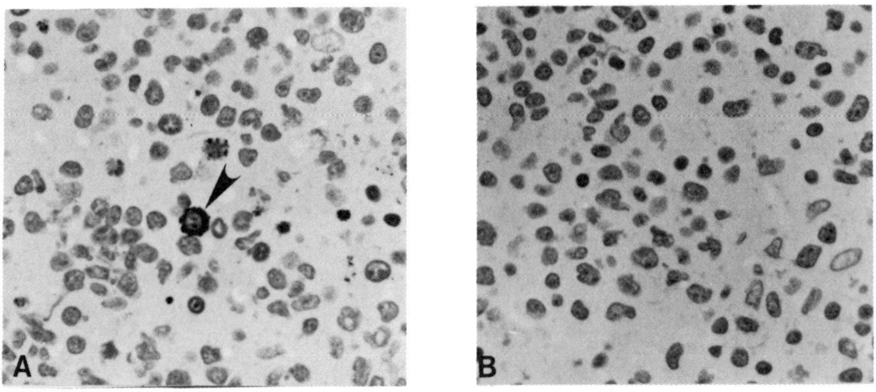

FIGURE 3. Lymphoma Tissue Phenotypic Analysis. Panel A shows intense HTLV-I gp61/68 reactivity. Panel B demonstrates the complete lack of reactivity in any cells using an anti HIV p24 monoclonal antibody.

DISCUSSION

This study shows a greatly increased frequency of serologic reactivity to both HTLV-I and HIV in AIDS patients with high grade lymphoma compared with healthy HIV seropositive gay men or AIDS patients without lymphoma. It is unlikely that HTLV-I represents an opportunistic infecting agent in patients with lymphoma, as only 5 of AIDS patients without lymphoma demonstrated HTLV-I antibodies. Several investigators have documented a coinfection with HTLV-I and HIV in individuals from populations at risk for the development of AIDS (28-37). The highest percentage has been reported in intravenous drug abusers (37). Several explanations of our data come to mind.

First, potential cross-reactivity of serum antibodies to different retroviral antigens must be considered. The lymphoma patient sera evaluated in this study have antibodies to many HIV antigenic determinants, but antibody to the HTLV-I envelope glycoprotein was the most frequently identified HTLV-I seroreactivity. The Western blot reactivity to HTLV-I determinants noted in this study was reproducible using standard radio-immunoprecipitation techniques (not shown). HIV antigens did not inhibit this reactivity, and using an HTLV-I envelope gene probe, nucleotide sequences hybridizing to the HTLV-I envelope gene were identified in DNA extracted from AIDS associated lymphoma tissue. Finally, rare cells within the lymphoma tissue reacted in situ with an HTLV-I specific monoclonal antibody. The reactions we observed could be due to a true HTLV-I infection. Alternatively, another closely related or recombinant retrovirus may account for these observations. Additional studies are in progress in our laboratory investigating several AIDS associated non-Hodgkin's lymphoma cell lines and viral isolates.

HTLV-I may contribute to lymphomagenesis through several mechanisms. It may provide exogenous antigenic stimulation and facilitate transformation in accord with the receptor mediated lymphomagenesis model (40,47). This model predicts that lymphomas would develop from HTLV-I antigen reactive B cell populations either responding to endogenously produced HTLV-I antigens or to HTLV-I antigens produced by macrophages. In the present study, rare macrophages and small mononuclear cells that stained with anti-HTLV-I antibodies would be the likely source of HTLV-I antigens, as the majority of apparent lymphoma cells were negative for HTLV-I antigen expression.

Rare HTLV-I infected T cells and macrophages could contribute to B cell proliferation by the elaboration of various lymphokines such as B cell growth factor (BCGF). Many investigators have documented the production of a spectrum of lymphokines in HTLV-I infected T cell clones and lymphoma cells, including BCGF, B cell differentiation factor (BCDF) and interleukin-2 (48,49). The determination of whether AIDS associated B cell lymphomas may be proliferating in part secondary to lymphokine stimulation by HTLV-I infected cells will require characterization of these cells.

Immunoregulation may be impaired by removal of T lymphocytes. Schwartz (50) has hypothesized that B cell lymphomas arise in part because of impairment of T cell restraint. This could occur because of T cell abnormalities (as were observed in our AIDS cases), or because proliferating B cells became unresponsive to inhibitory signals. The total CD4 mean cell number was very low in the lymphoma group. One may speculate that HTLV-I infects CD4 cells, causes them to proliferate, and this provides more activated target cells for HIV. The determination of whether coinfection accelerates the depletion of CD4 cells in coinfected individuals will need to be studied by prospective analysis.

We also found that only two of six AIDS associated lymphomas contained significant levels of EBV DNA sequences by hybridization. The majority, but not all, of the lymphomas that develop in immunosuppressed patients contain genomic EBV, and a popular hypothesis is that reactivation of EBV due to impaired T cell surveillance leads to B cell proliferation and subsequent polyclonal and monoclonal lymphomas (52). This hypothesis is supported by clear evidence of EBV reactivation of AIDS patients (53). The lack of EBV in some lymphomas may relate to technical problems (52) or to the presence of imcomplete but immortalizing EBV genomes (54). Further work will be needed to clarify the complex relationshiip between HTLV-I and EBV in lymphomagenesis in AIDS.

Finally, this study describes a significant frequency (14%) of gay men in San Francisco co-seropositive for both HTLV-I and HIV. The discovery of a high rate of HTLV-I seroreactivity in a non-endemic area for HTLV-I (but endemic for HIV) suggests that HTLV-I or a related retrovirus has been transmitted sexually and may spread to non HTLV-I endemic areas in a similar manner as HIV. The spectrum of diseases associated with HTLV-I and HIV coinfection is not currently known. The development of high grade lymphomas described in this study, however, appears to be associated with coinfection. The determination of whether the subpopulation of asymptomatic gay men seropositive for both HLTV-I and HIV will predispose them for development of high grade lymphomas will require long term prospective analysis.

ACKNOWLEDGMENTS

We are indebted to Drs. P. Wood and M. Oliver for their technical assistance; to Drs. A. Moss and J. Greenspan for providing the laboratory data on the healthy HIV seropositive gay men; to Dr. D. Feigal for statistical analysis of the data, to Drs. J. Ziegler and J. Lifson for their thoughtful editorial review, and to Sandra Gumpert for her secretarial assistance.

REFERENCES

1. Popovic M, Sarngadharn M, Read E and Gallo RC (1984). Detection, isolation and continuous production of cytopathic retroviruses (HTLV-III) from patients with AIDS and pre-AIDS. Science 225:497.
2. Barre-Sinoussi F, Chermann JC, Rety F, et al (1983). Isolation of a T lymphotropic retrovirus from a patient at risk for acquired immunodeficiency (AIDS). Science 220:868.
3. Levy JA, Hoffman A, Kramer S, Landis J, et al (1984). Isolation of lymphocytopathic retroviruses from San Francisco patients with AIDS. Science 225:840.
4. Reichert CM, O'Leary TJ, Levens DL, Simrell CR, Macher AM (1983). Autopsy pathology in the acquired immune deficiency syndrome. Am J Pathol 112:357.
5. Gottlieb MS, Schroff R, Schanker HM, et al (1981). Pneumocystis carinii pneumonia and mucosal candidiasis in previously healthy homosexual men. Evidence of a new acquired cellular immunodeficiency. N Eng J Med 305:1425.
6. Ziegler JL, Beckstead J, Volberding P, Abrams DI, et al (1984). Non-Hodgkin's lymphoma in 90 homosexual men. Relation to generalized lymphadenopathy and the acquired immunodeficiency syndrome. N Engl J Med 311:565.
7. Ziegler JL, Drew WL, Miner, et al (1982). Outbreak of Burkitt's like lymphomna in homosexual men. Lancet 2:631.
8. Levine AM, Meyer PR, Begandy MK, et al (1984). Development of B cell lymphoma in homosexual men. Clinical and immunologic findings. Ann Int Med 100:7.
9. Levine AM, Gill P, Meyer P, et al (1985). Retrovirus and malignant lymphoma in homosexual men. JAMA 254:1921.
10. Petersen JM, Tubbs RR, Savage RA, et al (1985). Small noncleaved B cell Burkitt-like lymphoma with chromosome (8;14) translocation and Epstein-Barr virus nuclear-associated antigen in a homosexual man with acquired immunodeficiency syndrome. Am J Med 78:141.

11. Magrath IT, Erikson J, Whang-Peng J, et al (1983). Synthesis of kappa light chains by cell lines containing an 8;22 chromosomal translocation derived from a male homosexual with Burkitt's lymphoma. Science 22:1094.
12. Whang-Peng J, Lee EC, Sieverts H, Magrath IT (1984). Burkitt's lympphoma in AIDS: cytogenetic study. Blood 63:818.
13. Chaganti RSK, Jhanwar SC, Koziner B, Arlin Z, Mertelsmann R, Clarkson BD (1983). Specific translocations characterize Burkitt's-like lymphoma of homosexual men with the acquired immunodeficiency syndrome. Blood 61:1265.
14. Lind SE, Gross P, Andiman WA, Stone GC, Schooley RT, Harris NL (1985). Malignant lymphoma presenting as Kaposi's sarcoma in a homosexual man with the acquired immunodeficiency syndrome. Ann Intern Med 102:338.
15. Klein G, Klein E (1985). Evolution of tumours and the impact of molecular oncology. Nature 315:190.
16. de-The G, Geser A, Day NE, et al (1978). Epidemiological evidence for causal relationship between Epstein-Barr virus and Burkitt's lymphoma from Ugandan prospective study. Nature 274:756.
17. Whittle HC, Brown J, Marsh K, et al (1984). T-cell control of Epstein-Barr virus-infected B cells is lost during P. Falciparum malaria. Nature 312:449.
18. Montagnier L, Gruest J, Chamaret S, et al (1984). Adaptation of lymphadenopathy associated virus (LAV) to replication in EBV-transformed B lymphoblastoid cell lines. Science 225:63.
19. Bunn PA Jr, Schechter GP, Jaffe E, et al (1983). Clinical course of retrovirus-associated adult T cell lymphoma in the United States. N Eng J Med 309:257.
20. Hinuma Y, Nagata K, Hanaska M, et al (1981). Adult T-cell leukemia: antigen in an ATL cell line and detection of antribodies to the antigen in human sera. Proc Natl Acad Sci USA 78:6476.
21. Gallo RC, Kalyanaraman VS, Sarngadharan MG, et al (1983). Association of the human type C retrovirus with a subset of adult T-cell cancer. Cancer Res 43:3892-9.
22. Yoshida M, Miyoshi I, Hinuma Y (1982). Isolation and characterization of retrovirus from cell lines of human adult T-cell leukemia and its implication in the disease. Proc Natl Acad Sci USA 79:2031-5.
23. Yoshida M, Seiki M, Yamaguchi K, Takatsuki K (1984). Monoclonal integration of human T-cell leukemia provirus in all primary tumors of adult T-cell leukemia suggests causative role of human T cell leukemia virus in the disease. Proc Natl Acad Sci USA 81:2534.

24. Blattner WA, Kalyanaraman VS, Robert-Guroff M, et al (1982). The human type-C retrovirus, HTLV, in blacks from the Caribbean region, and relationship to adult T-cell leukemia/lymphoma. Int J Cancer 30:257.
25. Blayner DW, Jaffe CS, Blattner WA, et al (1983). The human T-cell leukemia/lymphoma virus associated with American adult T-cell leukemia/lymphoma. Blood 62:401.
26. Poiesz BJ, Ruscetti FW, Reitz MS, Kalyanaraman VS, Gallo RC (1981). Isolation of a new type of C retrovirus (HTLV) in primary uncultured cells of a patient with Sezary T-cell leukemia. Nature 294:268.
27. Longo DL, Gelman E, Cossman J, Young R, Gallo RC, et al (1984). Isolation of HTLV-associated adult T cell leukemia. Nature 310:505.
28. Essex M, McLane MF, Lee TH, Falk L, Howe CWS, Mullins JI (1983). Antibodies to cell membrane antigens associated with human T-cell leukemia virus in patients with AIDS. Science 220:859.
29. Schuback J, Sarngadharan MG, Gallo RC (1984). Antigens on HTLV-infected cells recognized by leukemia and AIDS sera are related to HTLV viral glycoprotein. Science 224:607.
30. Goudsmit J, Miedema F, Wijngaarden-Du Bois RJ, Roos MT, Schellekens PT, et al (1985). Immunoglobulin subclasses of antibodies to human T-cell leukemia/lymphoma virus I-associated antigens in acquired immune deficiency syndrome and lymphadenopahy syndrome. J Virology 1985;53:287.
31. Saxinger W, Blattner WA, Levine PH, Clark J, et al (1984). Human T-cell leukeima virus (HTLV-I) antibodies in Africa. Science 225:1473.
32. Saxinger W, Levine PH, Dean AG, et al (1985). Evidence for exposure to HTLV-III in Uganda before 1973. Science 227:1036.
33. Born M, Von der Helm K, Wernicke D, Deinhardt F (1985). Presence of antibodies to human lymphoma-leukemia virus (HTLV-I) in Germans with symptoms of the acquired immunodeficiency syndrome (AIDS). J Med Virol 15:57.
34. Hunsmann G, Schneider J, Bayer H, et al (1985). Antibodies to adult T-cell leukemia virus (ATLV/HTLV-I) in AIDS patients and people at risk of AIDS in Germany. Med Microbiol Immunol 173:241.
35. Jason JM, McDougal JS, Cabradilla C, Kalyanaraman VS, Evatt BL (1985). Human T-cell leukemia virus (HTLV-I) p24 antibody in New York City blood product recipients. Amer J Hematol 20:129.

36. Robert-Guroff M, Weiss SH, Giron JA, Jennings AM, Ginsburg H, Margolis I (1986). Prevalence of antibodies to HTLV-I, -II, and -III, in intravenous drug abusers from an AIDS endemic region. JAMA 255:3133.
37. Harper ME, Kaplan MIT, Marselle LM, et al (1986). Concomitant infection with HTLV-I and HTLV-II in a patient with T8 lymphoproliferative disease. N Eng J Med 315:1703.
38. Center for Disease Control (1982). Task Force on Kaposi's Sarcoma and Opportunistic Infections. N Eng J Med 306:248.
39. Taang VC, Peralta J, Simons AR (1983). Enzyme-linked immunoelectrotransfer blot techniques (IEBT) for studying the specificities of antigens and antibodies separated by gel electrophoresis. Methods Enzymol 92:377.
40. McGrath MS, Weissman IL (1984). Receptor mediated leukemogenesis: Avian and human leukemia virus interactions with normal and neoplastic B and T lymphocytes. In Gallo R, Essex M, Gross L (eds): "Human T cell leukemia viruses," CSH Press, p.205.
41. McGrath MS, Witte O, Pincus T, Weissman IL (1978). Retrovirus purification: method which conserves envelope glycoprotein and maximizes infectivity. J Virology 25:923.
42. Baird S, Raschke W, Weissman IL (1977). Evidence that MuLV-induced thymic lymphoma cells possess specific cell membrane binding sites for MuLV. Int J Cancer 19:403.
43. Kung PC, Goldstein G, Reinherz EL, Schlossman SF (1979). Monoclonal antibodies defining distinctive human T-cell surface antigens. Science 206:347.
44. Beckstead JH (1983). The evaluation of human lymph nodes using plastic sections and enzyme histochemistry. Am J Clin Pathol 80:131.
45. Beckstead JH (1985). Optimal antigen localization in human tissues using aldehyde-fixed plastic-embedded sections. J Histochem Cytochem 29:577.
46. Matsushita S, Robert-Guroff M, Trepel J, Cossman J, Mitsuya H, Broder S (1986). Human monoclonal antibody directed against an envelope glycoprotein of human T-cell leukemia virus type I. Proc Natl Acad Sci 2673.
47. Wong-Staal F, Gallo RC (1985). The family of human T-lymphotropic leukemia viruses: HTLV-I as the cause of adult T cell leukemia and HTLV-III as the cause of immunodeficiency syndrome. Blood 65:253.
48. Salahuddin SZ, Markham PD, Lindner SG, Gootenberg J. Popovic M, Hemmi H, Sarin P, Gallo RC (1984). Lymphokine production by cultured human T cells transformed by human T cell leukemia-lymphoma virus I. Science 223:703.

49. Volkman DJ, Popovic M, Gallo RC, Fauci AS (1985). Human T cell leukemia/lymphoma virus-infected antigen-specific T cell clones: Indiscriminant helper function and lymphokine production. J Immuno 134:4237.

50. Schwartz RS (1972). Hypothesis. Immunoregulation, oncogenic viruses, and malignant lymphomas. Lancet 1:1266.

51. Masucci G, Mellstedt H, Masucci M, et al (1984). Immunologic characterization of Hodgkin's and non-Hodgkin's lymphoma patients with high antibody titers against Epstein-Barr virus-associated antigens. Can Res 44:1288.

52. Hanto DW, Frizzera G, Kazimiera J, Simmons RL (1985). Epstein-Barr virus, immunodeficiency and B cell lymphoproliferation. Transpl 35:461.

53. Birx DL, Redfield RR, Tosato G (1986). Defective regulation of Epstein-Barr virus infection in patients with acquired immunodeficiency syndrome (AIDS) or AIDS-related disorders. N Eng J Med 314:874.

54. Stevenson M, Volsky B, Hedenskog M, Volsky DJ (1986). Immortalization of human T lymphocytes after transfection of Epstein-Barr virus DNA. Science 233:980.

Human Retroviruses, Cancer, and AIDS:
Approaches to Prevention and Therapy, pages 229–240

HIV GP 120 Serves as a Target for Antibody Dependent Cellular Cytotoxicity

H. Kim Lyerly, Thomas J. Matthews, Alphonse J. Langlois, Dani P. Bolognesi and Kent J. Weinhold

The Department of Surgery, Box 2926, Duke University Medical Center, Durham, North Carolina 27710

Introduction

The human immunodeficiency virus (HIV), the etiological agent for the acquired immunodeficiency syndrome (AIDS), selectively infects cells which bear the CD4 antigen, which includes the helper/inducer subset of T lymphocytes (1,2). In vitro infection of CD4 positive lymphocytes leads to cell death, and the depletion of this population of lymphocytes in vivo by virus induced cytopathology is thought to lead to the profound defects in immune function which renders patients susceptible to life-threatening opportunistic infections and neoplasms (3-8).

The time interval between exposure to HIV and the development of clinical symptoms is quite variable among patients, ranging from months to years, which may be related to the variation in virulence among various HIV strains or to cofactors such as concurrent infection with other immunosuppressive agents (9-11). Variation in the anti-HIV immune response may also be critical to halt or retard the development of symptoms as an effective humoral and/or cellular immune response may prevent spread of virus to susceptible lymphocytes. The nature of this protective immune response is unknown at present. While virus neutralizing antibodies have been shown to exist in seropositive patients, the precise role of these antibodies in relation to disease progression is unclear (12). Furthermore, one must consider control of not only free virus, but also chronically infected cells which may contribute to further spread of infectious virus. An immune response that mediates lysis of infected cells is important because not all HIV infected cells undergo viral-induced cytopathology. In fact, macrophage appear to produce large amounts of infectious virus while remaining resistant to the cytopathic effects of viral infection (13,14).

Cytotoxic immune responses may thus be critical in preventing viral spread and disease progression by eliminating these viral reservoirs. While the role of specific cellular immune responses directed against HIV infected cells is unknown at present, other forms of cytotoxic immune responses may also exist. In animal retroviral infections, protective immunity is thought to be mediated in large part by cooperation between the specific antibody and effector cells in the form of antibody-dependent cellular cytotoxicity (ADCC). ADCC has been demonstrated to be critical in control of feline leukemia virus and AKR virus infections, and antibodies mediating ADCC have crucial roles in not only active immunotherapy but passive immunotherapy as well (15-17). Because of the protective role of antibodies directing ADCC in other retroviral infections, our objective was to determine if antibodies directing ADCC against HIV infected cells were present in serum from individuals infected with HIV and, furthermore, to determine the target antigen for immune attack.

Antibody Binding to Cell Surface Expressed Viral Antigens

As an initial step in examining the ability of patient serum to direct ADCC against HIV infected target cells, we analyzed the ability of patient antibodies to bind to cell surface expressed viral antigens.

CEM.NKR, a transformed T cell line which bears the CD4 antigen and was immunoselected for resistance to natural killer lysis (18), was utilized as a target after infection with the divergent HIV isolates HTLV-III_B, HTLV-III_{MN} and HTLV-III_{RF2} (denoted CEM/III_B, CEM/MN and CEM/RF_2 respectively). Infected cells were analyzed cytofluorometrically following staining with a selected patient serum, monoclonal anti-GP 120 antibody (a generous gift of Dr. Robert Ting, Biotech, Rockville, MD.) and monoclonal OKT4A. As seen in figure 1, patient serum stained all of the infected cells in comparable fashion but did not stain the noninfected cells (denoted CEM).

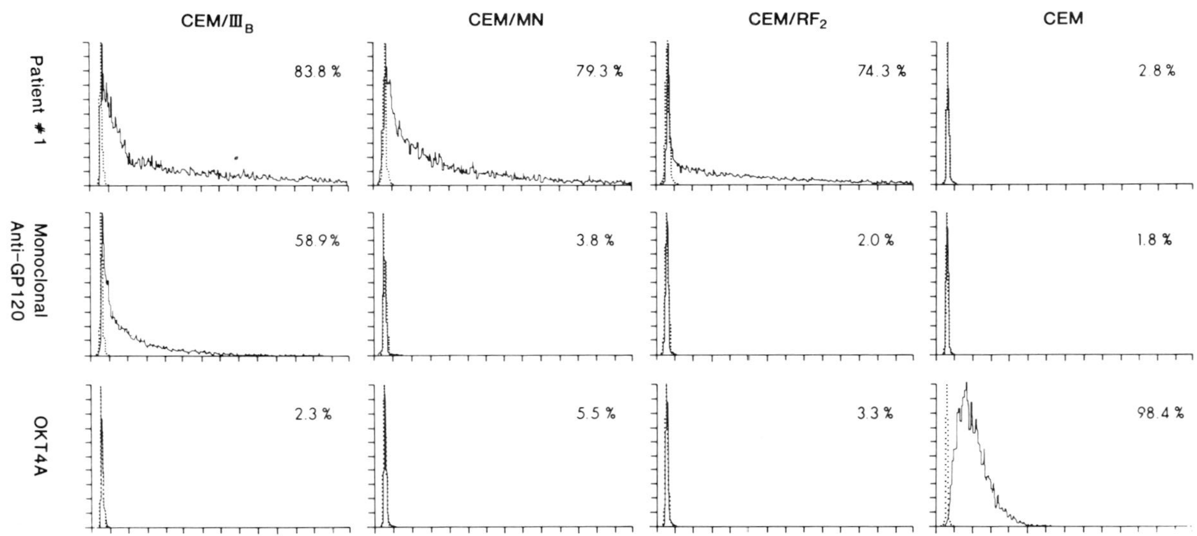

Figure 1 Cytofluorometric analysis of uninfected CEM.NKR and CEM.NKR infected with HTLV-III_B, HTLV-III_{RF2} and HTLV-III_{MN} (CEM, CEM/III_B, CEM/RF_2 and CEM/MN, respectively) using patient serum, monoclonal anti-GP 120 antibody and OKT4A. Linear green fluorescence (x-axis) is plotted versus relative cell number (y-axis).

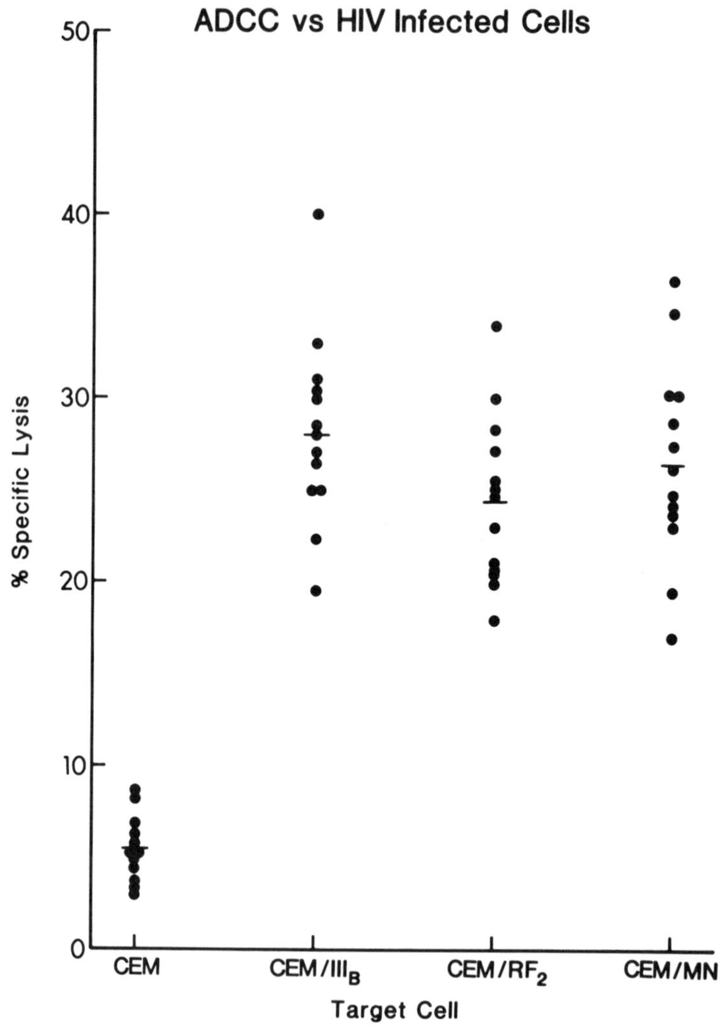

Figure 2 Comparison of antibody-dependent cellular cytotoxicity (ADCC) of CEM.NKR and CEM.NKR chronically infected with HTLV-III$_B$, HTLV-III$_{RF2}$ and HTLV-III$_{MN}$ (CEM/III$_B$, CEM/RF$_2$ and CEM/MN, respectively) with thirteen HIV seropositive sera and normal peripheral blood mononuclear cells. Final serum dilution was 1:1,000 in all experiments. Target cells were plotted versus percent specific lysis (from Lyerly et al, ref. 22).

Monoclonal anti-GP 120 demonstrated only type specific binding, staining only the HTLV-III_B infected cells. Noninfected cells expressed the OKT4A defined epitope, but in contrast the chronically infected cell lines did not. Because other viral antigens, such as P 24, may serve as targets for ADCC and may be expressed on the surface of infected cells, we attempted to stain cells using high titered anti-P 24 antibodies but none of the infected cell lines utilized stained with anti-P 24 antibodies (not shown).

Antibody Dependent Cellular Cytotoxicity

To determine if the broad reactivity of patient serum was reflective of equally broad functional specificity, we tested the ability of patient serum to direct ADCC against a variety of HIV infected cells.

As seen in Figure 2, serum from a wide spectrum of individuals infected with HIV, ranging from asymptomatic to overt AIDS, were found to be effective in directing ADCC not only against cells stably infected with a prototypic strain of HIV (HTLV-III_B), but also against cells infected with widely divergent strains of HIV, including HTLV-III_{MN} and HTLV-III_{RF2}, which differs by about 21% in the amino acid sequence of the viral envelope in comparison to HTLV-III_B (20).

In these studies, we noted that all sera directing ADCC contained anti-GP 120 antibodies. No other correlation appeared to exist between the presence of other anti-HIV antibodies detected by immunoblot analysis, such as anti-P 24 antibodies, to ADCC activity. This, in conjunction with the finding that anti-GP 120 defined epitopes were expressed on the surface of infected cells, suggested that anti-GP antibodies played a major role in ADCC.

Our initial attempts to determine the role of anti-envelope antibodies utilized the well described affinity of HIV GP 120 for specific epitopes of the CD4 molecule. We have recently shown that purified HTLV-III_B GP 120 can readily bind to and saturate all detectable OKT4A defined sites on the surface of normal CD4 positive cells (19). CD4 positive cells coated with HTLV-III_B GP 120 in this manner could be effectively utilized instead of HTLV-III_B infected

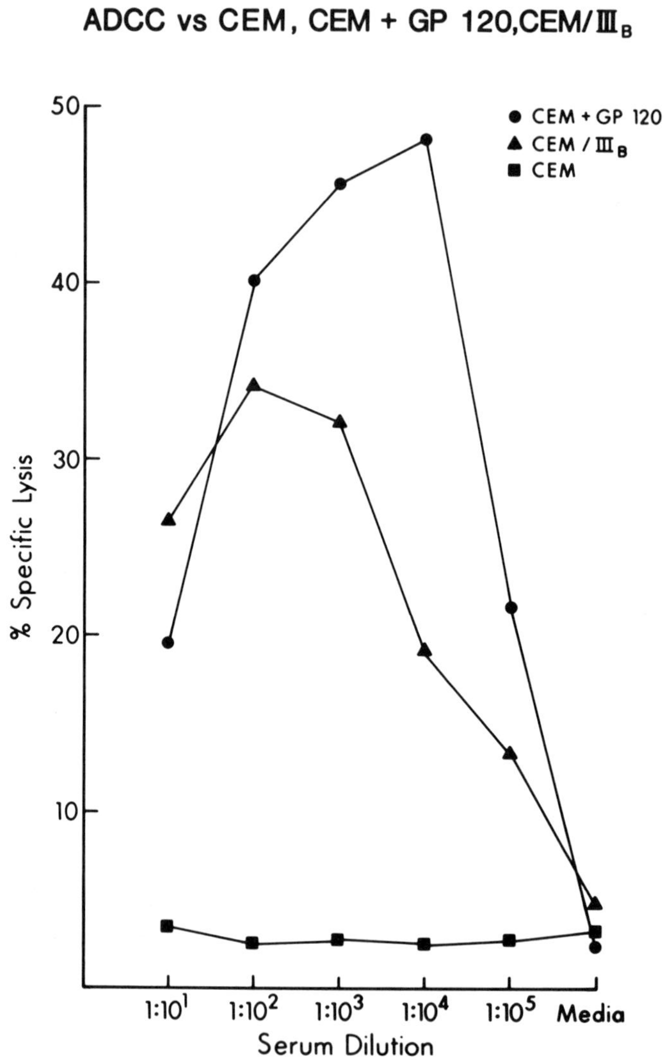

Figure 3 Comparison of ADCC of CEM.NKR, CEM.NKR bearing purified GP 120 and HTLV-III$_B$ infected CEM.NKR (CEM, CEM + GP 120 and CEM/III$_B$, respectively) using seropositive serum and normal donor peripheral blood mononuclear cells at an effector:target ratio of 50:1. Inverse of final serum dilution plotted versus percent specific lysis in 6 hr ^{51}Cr release assay.

cells as target cells in ADCC assays, eliminating all viral antigens but GP 120 as a target for immune attack. Utilizing these GP 120 adsorbed target cells, we were able to detect high titers of anti GP 120 antibodies directing ADCC in patient serum. No patient serum that directed ADCC against HIV infected cells did not direct ADCC against GP 120 coated cells, and conversely no serum which mediated ADCC against GP 120 coated cells failed to direct lysis of HIV infected cells (not shown).

A direct comparison of ADCC activity utilizing a selected patient serum versus GP 120 adsorbed target cells and HIV infected target cells demonstrated a number of features (Fig. 3). GP 120 adsorbed targets always demonstrated a significant "prozone" of suboptimal lysis at low serum dilutions, with maximal lysis achieved at dilutions of 1:100 to 1:10,000. Maximal lysis of GP 120 adsorbed targets was greater than HIV infected cells, which is probably related to the surface expression of GP 120 on infected cells. FACS analysis with monoclonal anti-GP 120 antibody and goat anti-GP 120 serum consistently revealed that GP 120 adsorbed targets consist of a homogenous population with high antigen density. In contrast, surface expression of GP 120 on infected cells was consistently less than on HIV adsorbed targets and the population was much more heterogenous (not shown).

Because of the ability of purified GP 120 adsorbed target cells to define a specific target antigen for ADCC we evaluated the ability of patient serum to mediate lysis of GP 120 from divergent viral isolates. We were able to demonstrate that patient serum directed ADCC equally against cells bearing the envelope glycoprotein from HTLV-III_B or HTLV-III_{RF2} (not shown) (20).

Consistent with these findings was our ability to immuno-affinity purify anti-GP 120 antibodies from seropositive individuals and remove most of the ADCC activity (Fig. 4) (21,22). Utilizing these purified human anti-GP 120 antibodies we again demonstrated broad reactivity to surface expressed envelope glycoprotein on chronically infected cells and ADCC activity against cells infected with widely divergent viral isolates (Fig. 5).

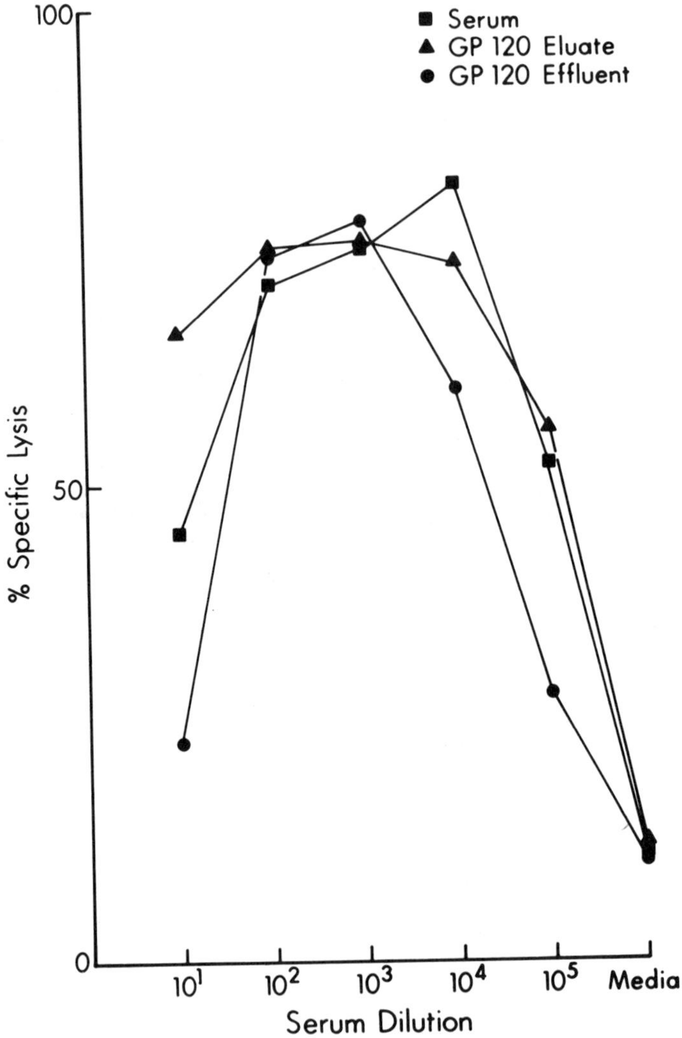

Figure 4 Comparison of antibody-dependent cellular cytotoxicity of CEM.NKR bearing purified GP 120 with seropositive serum, GP 120 column eluate and GP 120 column effluent (■ , ▲ , ● , respectively). Inverse of final serum dilution plotted versus percent specific lysis (from Lyerly, et al, ref. 22).

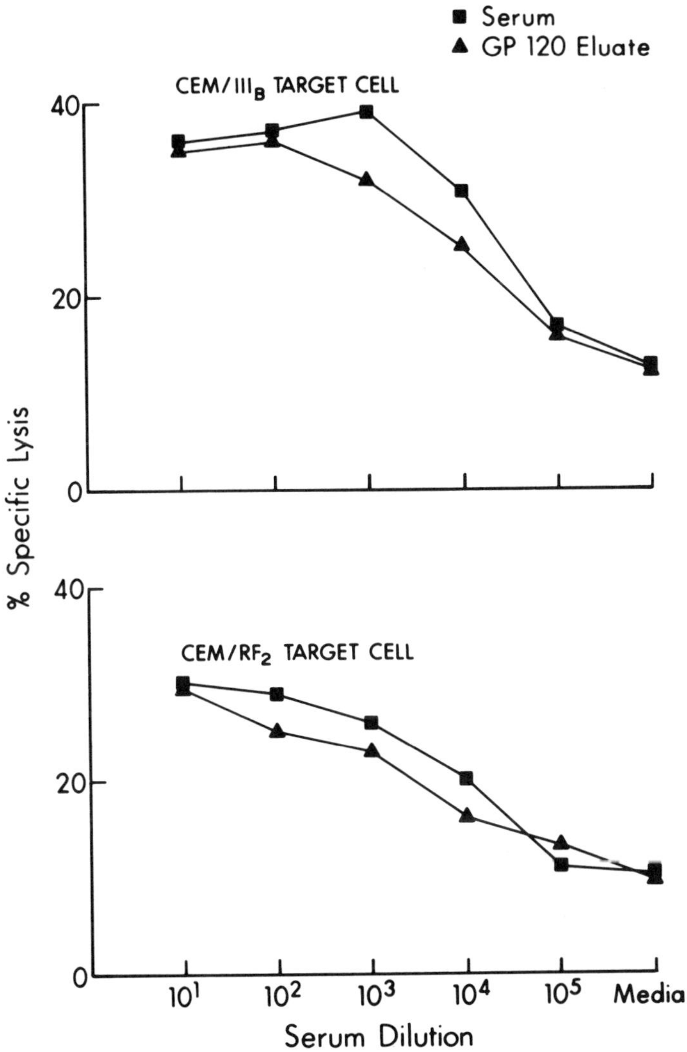

Figure 5 Comparison of antibody-dependent cellular cytotoxicity of CEM.NKR chronically infected with HTLV-III$_B$ or HTLV-III$_{RF2}$ (CEM/III$_B$ or CEM/RF$_2$, respectively) with seropositive serum and GP 120 column eluate (■ , ▲ , respectively). Inverse of final serum dilution plotted versus percent specific lysis (from Lyerly et al, ref. 22).

While the ability of the immune system to generate a protective immune response that is broadly reactive may be critical in preventing or retarding HIV-related disease, it remains to be explained why the high antibody titers present in almost all patients with HIV infection do not appear to protect against disease progression. A plausible explanation is that, in addition to the presence of the appropriate antibody, ADCC requires functioning effector cells which must work in cooperation with specific antibody isotypes. In these studies, normal donor peripheral blood mononuclear cells were utilized as effector cells with patient sera containing anti-GP 120 antibodies. In a separate study, we have also identified a CD16+ population of effector cells in HIV seropositive patients that mediate ADCC (22). Effector cell function appears to decline in advanced stages of disease suggesting that while antibodies may be present the ability to direct ADCC against chronically infected cells may be defective due to a loss of effector cell number or function (unpublished data).

Further studies to define the critical epitopes required to generate broadly reactive antibodies that mediate ADCC and methods to enhance effector cells function in those with preexisting antibodies will be important in developing strategies against HIV related disease.

Acknowledgements

We thank Robert Gallo for HIV isolates, David Durak for patient material, Jean Pratz for excellent technical assistance, Frank Cornew for cytofluorometric analysis and Craig Hughes for manuscript preparation. Supported by the NIH 1-UO1-CA 44082-01.

References

1. Popovic, M., Read-Connole, E., and Gallo, R. C. (1984) Lancet 2 1472-1473.
2. Klatzman, D., Champagne, E., Chamaret, S., Gruest, J., Gretard, D., Hevand, T., Gluckman, J. and Montagnier, L. (1984) Nature (London) 312, 767-768.
3. Barre-Sinoussi, F., Chermann, J. C., Nugeyre, M. T., Chamaret, S., Gruest, J., Dauguet, C., Axler-Blin, C., Brun-Vezinet, F., Rouziuox, C., Rozenbaum, W. and Montagnier, L. (1983) Science 220, 868-871.
4. Popovic, M., Sarngadharan, M. G., Read, E. and Gallo, R. C. (1984) Science 224, 497-500.
5. Levy, J. A., Hoffman, A. D., Kramer, S. A. M., Landis, J.A., Shimabukuro, J. M. and Oshiro, L. S. (1984) Science 225, 840-842.
6. Sarngadharan, M. G., Popovic, M., Brudi, L., Shupbach, J. and Gallo, R. C. (1984) Science 224, 506-508.
7. Brun-Vezinet, F., Rouzioux, C., Montagnier, L., Chamaret, S., Gruest, J., Barre-Sinoussi, F., Geroldi, D., Chermann, J. C., McCormick, J., Mitchell, S., Piot, P., Taelman, H., Mirangu, K. B., Wobin, O., Mazebo, M. N., Kalambayi, K., Bridts, C., Desmyter, J., Fenisod, F. M. and Quinn, T. C. (1984) Lancet 2, 1253-1256.
8. Gallo, R. C., Salahuddin, S. Z., Popovic, M., Shearer, G. M., Kaplan, M., Haynes, B. F., Palker, T. J., Redfield, R., Oleske, J., Safai, B., White, G. and Markham, P. D (1984) Science 224, 500-503.
9. Lui, K.-J., Lawrence, D. N., Morgan, W. M., Peterman, T. A., Haverkos, H. W. and Bregman, D. J. (1986) Proc. Natl. Acad. Sci. USA 83, 3051-3055.
10. May, R. M. and Anderson, R. M. (1987) Nature 326, 137-142.
11. Rees, M. (1987) Nature 326, 343-345.
12. Robey, W. G., Arthur, L. O., Matthews, T. J., Langlois, A. J., Copeland, T. D., Oroszlan, S., Bolognesi, D. P., Gilden, R. V. and Fishinger, P. J. (1986) Proc. Natl. Acad. Sci. USA 83, 7023-7027.
13. Gartner, S., Markovitz, P., Markovitz, D. M., Kaplan, M. H., Gallo, R. C., and Popovic, M. (1986) Science 233, 215-219.
14. Nicholson, J. K. A., Cross, G. D., Calloway, C. O., McDougal, J. S., (1986) J. Immunol. 137(1), 323-329.
15. Weinhold, K. J., Bolognesi, D. P., and Matthews, T. J. (1985) JNCI 75, 717-724.

16. Weinhold, K. J., Huper, G., Matthews, T. J., Fischinger, P. J., Ihle, J. N., Schwarz, H., Thiel, H.-J., Schafer, W., and Bolognesi, D. P. (1984) Virology 135, 105-117.
17. Jarrett, W. (personal communication).
18. Howell, D. N., Andreolti, P. E., Dawson, J. R., and Cresswell, P. (1985) J. Immunol. 134, 971-976.
19. Lyerly, H. K., Matthews, T. J., Langlois, A. J., Bolognesi, D. P., and Weinhold, K. J. (1987) Proc. Natl. Acad. Sci. USA (in press).
20. Starcich, B. R., Hahn, B. H., Shaw, G. M., McNeely, P. D., Modrow, S., Wolf, H., Parks, E. S., Parks, W. P., Josephs, S. F., Gallo, R. C. and Wong-Staal, F. (1986) Cell 45, 637-648.
21. Matthews, T. J., Langlois, A. J., Robey, W. G., Chang, N. T., Gallo, R. C., Fishinger, P. J., and Bolognesi, D. P. (1986) Proc. Natl. Acad. Sci. USA 83, 9709-9714.
22. Lyerly, H. K., Matthews, T. J., Ahearne, P. M., Langlois, A. J., Bolognesi, D. P. and Weinhold, K. J. (1987) Surg. Forum (in press).
23. Lyerly, H. K., Reed, D. L., Matthews, T. J., Langlois, A. J., Ahearne, P. M., Bolognesi, D. P., Weinhold, K. J. (1987) (submitted).

Human Retroviruses, Cancer, and AIDS: Approaches to Prevention and Therapy, pages 241–253

SERUM CAPACITY TO INHIBIT CELL FUSION AND HIV GENE EXPRESSION IN CD4+ CELLS AND THE PRESENCE OF CORE ANTIGENS AND ANTIBODIES: ASSOCIATION WITH CLINICAL DISEASE

Jaap Goudsmit, Livia Giurgia, Lia Smit, Frank de Wolf, Willy Krone, Margreet Bakker, Claudine Bruck, Joep Lange

Human Retrovirus Laboratory
Department of Virology, University of Amsterdam, the Netherlands

Institut Pasteur du Brabant
Brussels, Belgium.

Smith Kline - RIT
Department of Genetics, Rixensart
Belgium

ABSTRACT HIV antigen may be detectable transiently before HIV envelope and core antibody seroconversion. In some cases HIV antigen persists while no HIV core antibodies are detectable. This last serodiagnostic profile is associated with a poor short-term clinical outcome. Similarly in chronic HIV infection low titers of core antibodies, often associated with HIV antigenemia are associated with a high risk of progression to serious HIV-related disease. When HIV-Ab seroconverted men who progressed to AIDS or ARC were compared to men who did not during a follow-up period of 9-21 months, disease progression was associated with low titers of cell fusion inhibiting antibodies (CFI-Ab), low titers of virus neutralizing antibodies (VN-Ab), low titers of core antibodies and high levels of HIV core antigen. These serological difference were already apparent shortly after infection when no clinical distinction between these groups could be made.

INTRODUCTION

The acquired immune deficiency syndrome (AIDS) is caused by a lentivirus, designated human immunodeficiency virus (HIV). In both transsectional (1) and longitudinal (2) studies a grave clinical outcome appeared to be strongly associated with detectable levels of extracellular core antigen in serum. HIV gag gene expression is related to a decline in antibody titer to the major core protein p24 as occurs with impending transition to AIDS (2,3). Enhancement of HIV gene expression appears to lead to clearance of HIV core antibodies in immune complexes (4).

Although individuals without persisting HIV antigen expression in serum appear to have a better clinical prognosis than HIV antigenemic individuals, it has not been clarified why in these men HIV remains dormant. HIV-specific immune responses of the host may limit spread of virus, expression of viral genes in infected cells as well as killing of uninfected CD4 cells. In the present paper we report preliminary data on the relationships between the absence or presence of antibodies inhibiting cell fusion and HIV gene expression in CD4+ cells, core antigens and antibodies, and the progression to ARC or AIDS.

MATERIALS AND METHODS

Cell cultures

A T-cell lymphoma cell line (Sup-T1), established from a pleural effusion in a child with lymphoblastic lymphoma (5) was grown in Iscove's modified medium (Gibco Europe) plus 10% fetal bovine serum. All cells of Sup-T1 express the viral receptor at high density as indicated by the number of cells reactive with the monoclonal antibody (MoAb) OKT4A and the mean fluorescence per cell. A B cell line (B24), kindly provided by T. Tersmette, was obtained by transformation of non-T cells with EBV strain

B95/9 (6). This line was cocultivated with mitomycin-C treated HT9-HTLV-IIIB cells. Five percent of these B cells reacted with MoAbs to HIV gp120 (Dupont) gp41 (Abbott), p24 and p18 (R. Tedder and B. Ferns). These cells produced little virus relative to HT9 -HTLV-III B cells (T. Tersmette, personal communication). The uninfected B24 cells did express CD4 at low levels, since no CD4 expression could be demonstrated by using either the MoAbs OKT4A (Ortho Diagnostic) or leu 3a (Becton Dickinson). These B cells were also grown in Iscove's modified medium supplemented with 10% FBS.

Cell fusion inhibiting antibody (CFI-Ab) assay

Sup-T1 cells (1.5 - 2 x 10^5 cells/well) were attached to 96 well microtiter plates as described before. The medium was removed and B24 cells (5 x 10 cells/well) after washing twice with PBS were added to each well in 100 microliter Iscove's modified medium plus 10% FBS and three dilutions of heat inactivated (30 minutes, 56°C) human serum. Reciprocal dilutions were 20, 60, 180 and 540. After incubation at 37°C for 30 minutes the plates were centrifuged for 10 minutes at 37°C (speed: 1000 rpm). All experiments were done in duplicate and each plate included immune and negative control sera. Syncytia were counted after 24 hrs of incubation at 37°C. Fifty percent reduction of syncytia formation at a certain serum dilution after 24 hrs was taken as the titer of syncytia formation inhibiting Ab of the particular serum.

Virus neutralizing antibody (VN-Ab) assay

Sup-T1 cells were concentrated at 10.10.6/ml in fresh medium. Sera were heat inactivated at 56°C, for 30 minutes and filter-sterilized. For each assay 40 ul of virus purified from HTLV-IIIB producing Molt 3 cells in suspension (1:5 diluted; 1:180 diluted≈25 TCID50) and 40 ul of 1:10, 1:30, 1:90, and 1:180 dilution of serum were mixed and incubated in a microtiter plate for 1 hour at 4°C, and 15 minutes at room temp. 40 ul of Sup-T1 cells were added to each well and incubation continued for 1 hour at 37°C. Aliquots of 60 ul of each mixture were plated into 180 ul medium (containing 5 ugr/ml hydrocortisone) in duplicate wells of another microtiter plate. Infectivity was monitored by 3 criteria: appearance of syncytia; expression of viral proteins in cellular extract by a capture ELISA assay and in cells by immunofluorescence; production of viral particles by RT activity.

Six - 10 days post infection the results in the different assays paralleled each other. As neutralizing titer was considered the inverse of the dilution of serum that induced 50% inhibition of syncytia formation.

Extracellular HIV antigen, HIV core antibody and circulating CD4+ and CD8+ cells.

HIV antigen was detected by enzyme-immunoassay (Abbott Labs) and quantitated using HIV lysate as reference. HIV core antibody was tested by a competitive EIA using recombinant core Ag as target (Abbott Labs). CD4+ cells were identified in the circulation by labeling mononuclear cells with CD4 (CLB-T4/1) and CD8 (CLB-T8) specific MoAbs, subsequent visualization by FITC labelled anti mouse IgG conjugate and quantification using a fluorescence activated cell sorter (EPICS, Coulter, USA).

Human Sera

Sequential serum samples were used of men participating in a Dutch prospective study for the risk to acquire HIV infection and HIV related disease.

Forty-eight men were initially studied, of which 8 developed AIDS or ARC, in order to establish the relationship between HIV antigen in serum and HIV core antibody titers. Subsequently 6 HIV-Ab seroconverted men were selected of which 3 progressed to ARC or AIDS (CDC IV) within the follow-up period for CFI-Ab and VN-Ab studies.

RESULTS

Relationship between clinical disease, HIV core antigenemia and HIV core antibody titers

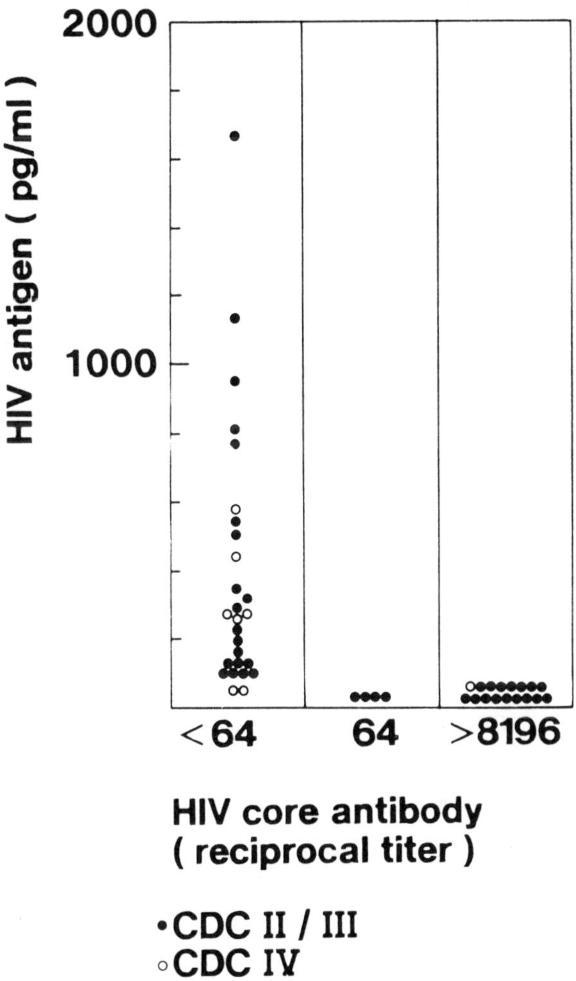

FIGURE 1. Relationship between HIV core antigen levels and HIV core antibody titers in individuals with AIDS or ARC (CDC IV) or without clinical symptoms (CDC II/III).

Sera with HIV core antibody titers over 64 lacked HIV antigen (0/21). Only one individual (1/21) had ARC or AIDS. Twenty-four of twenty-seven sera with HIV core antibody titers below 64 had HIV core antigen. Two ARC or AIDS patients and one asymptomatic individual lacked HIV core antigen in this group. The remaining 5 ARC or AIDS patients had all low titers of HIV core antibody and HIV core antigen.

Serum capacity to inhibit cell fusion and HIV gene expression in CD4+ cells (Fig.2)

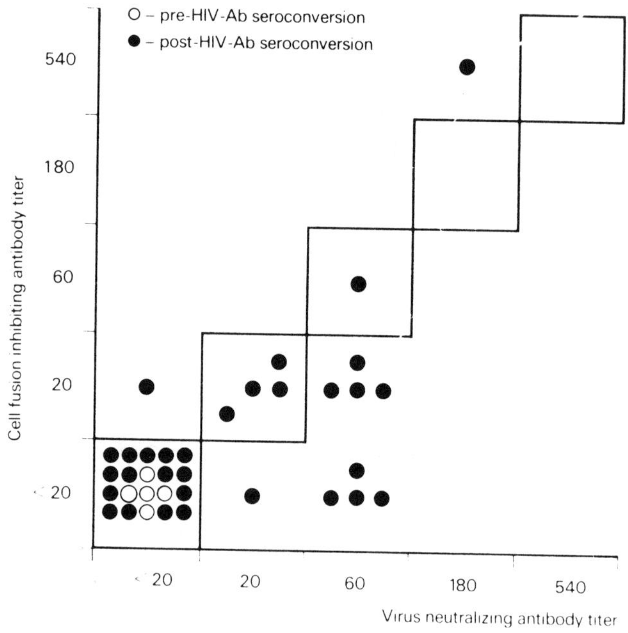

FIGURE 2. Relationship between cell fusion inhibiting antibody (CFI-Ab) titers and virus neutralizing antibody (VN-Ab) titers.

HIV antibody negative sera all lacked both CFI-Ab and VN-Ab (0/5). Of the HIV antibody positive sera 48% (15/31) showed VN-Ab titers of 20 or more and 35% (11/31) had CFI-Ab titers of 20 or more. Fifteen (8%) of 31 HIV-Ab seropositive sera lacked either VN-Ab or CFI-Ab. Among 11 CFI-Ab positive samples (titer over 20) 10 (91%) had VN-Ab titers over 20, and among 20 CFI-Ab negative samples (titer below 20) 5 (25%) were VN-Ab positive. Only one VN-Ab negative sample showed a reciprocal CFI-Ab titer of 20. On the other hand five VN-Ab positive samples had a CFI-Ab titer below 20.

Relationship between clinical immunological status and CFI-Ab, VN-Ab, HIV core Antibodies and Antigen in serum (Table I)

TABLE 1.
CLINICAL AND IMMUNOLOGICAL STATUS RELATED TO CFI-AB AND VN-AB TITERS AS WELL AS HIV CORE ANTIGEN AND ANTIBODY IN 6 HIV-AB SEROCONVERTED MEN.

Clinical category (months after HIV-Ab seroconversion	HIV core Antigen (pg/ml)	HIV core Antibody (titer)	CD4 cell number (10 /l)	CFI-Ab titer	VN-Ab titer
CDC II/III					
Pt 16(21)	-	>8192	0.7	60	60
Pt 172(15)	-	>8192	1.4	>540	180
Pt 666(18)	241	-	0.5	20	20
CDC IV.					
Pt 317(16)	1071	-	0.6	20	<20
Pt 320(9)	350	-	0.2	<20	<20
Pt 1054(12)	226	-	0.1	<20	20

Among three HIV-antibody seroconverted men who did not progress to ARC or AIDS untill the end of the follow-up period two had high titers of HIV core antibodies (Pt16 and 172) and one HIV core antigen (Pt666) CD4 cell numbers were in all three patients within the normal range and all had titers of VN-Ab or CFI-Ab of 20 or more. The lowest titers were observed in the asymptomatic HIV antigen positive man.

Among three HIV-antibody seroconverted men progressing to ARC or AIDS 3 had HIV antigen and lacked detectable levels of antibodies to HIV core antigen. Only one had CFI-Ab titer of 20) at the end of the follow-up period of 16 months after HIV-Ab seroconversion (Pt317) and another (Pt1054) had a VN-Ab titer of 20 at 12 months follow-up.

Longitudinal study of development of CFI-Ab and VN-Ab in HIV Antigen negative asymptomatic individuals. (Fig. 3)

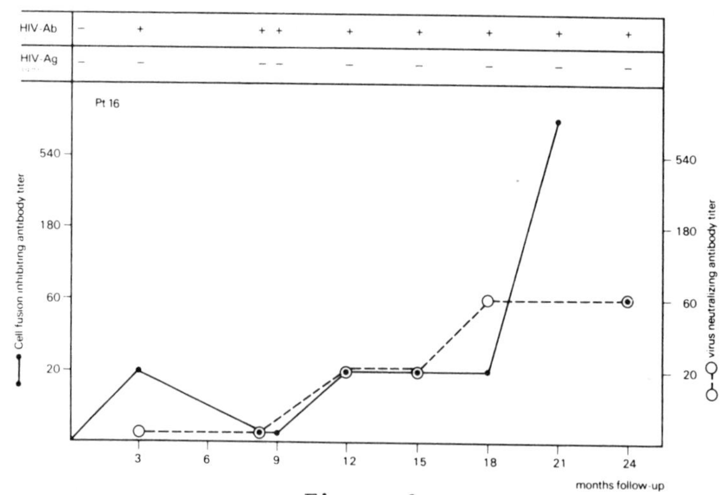

Figure 3

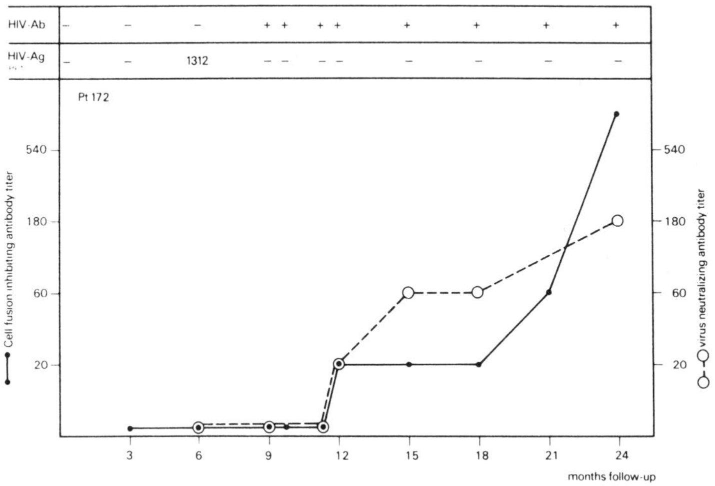

FIGURE 3.Longitudinal study of CFI-Ab and VN-Ab in two asymptomatic and HIV antigen negative men.

In both of these patients the development of CFI-Ab paralleled the development of VN-Ab. In one patient (Pt16) a rise in VN-Ab and CFI-Ab was observed 6 months after HIV-Ab seroconversion, in another (Pt172) three months.

Longitudinal study of development of CFI-Ab and VN-Ab in HIV antigenemic men. (Fig.4)

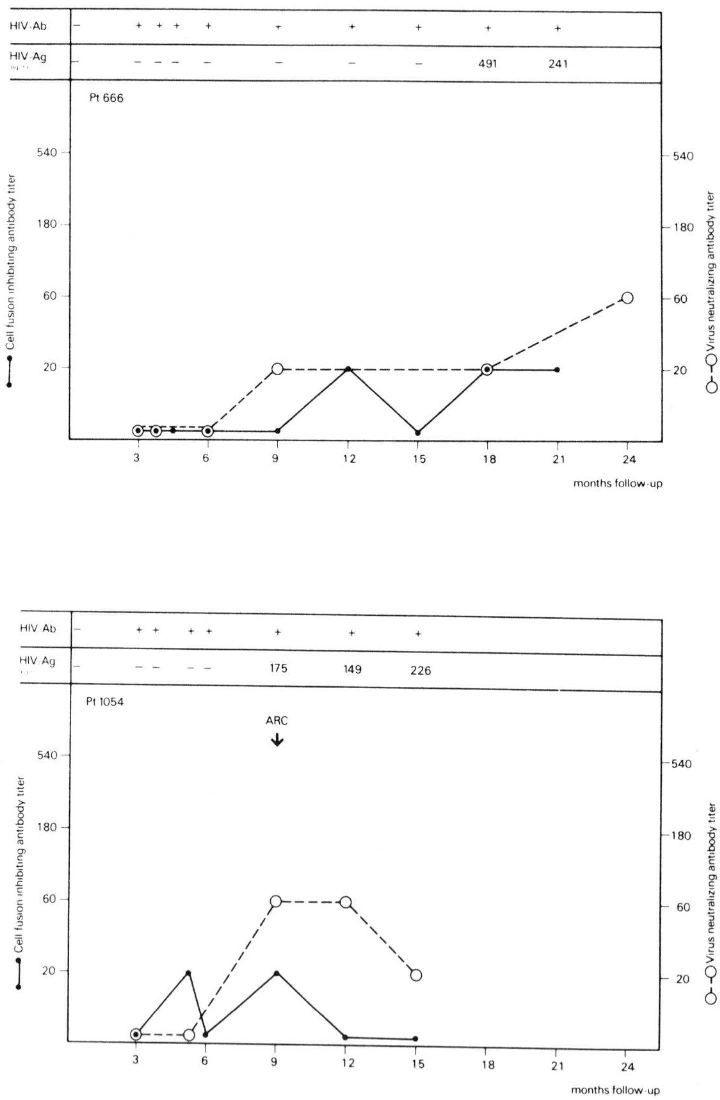

Figure 4

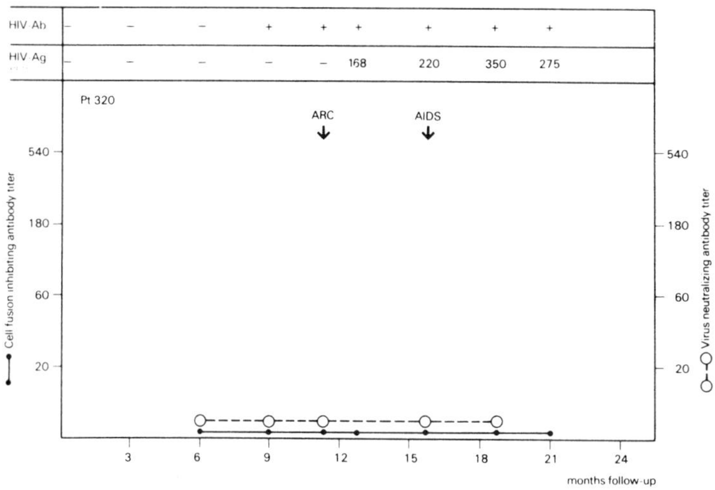

FIGURE 4. Longitudinal development of CFI-Ab and VN-Ab in three HIV-antigenemic men.

Each of these men showed distinct pattern of CFI-Ab and VN-Ab, although CFI-Ab and VN-Ab development paralleled.

The one man (Pt666) who remained asymptomatic 18 months after HIV-Ab seroconversion developed slowly a VN-Ab titer of 60 and CFI-Ab titer of 20, even when HIV antigenemia occurred. One man (Pt1054) developed CFI-Ab as well as VN-Ab titers before he was diagnosed as ARC, however after diagnosis both titers dropped. The man (Pt320) who eventually was diagnosed as AIDS never developed VN-Ab or CFI-Ab titers.

DISCUSSION

The present study confirms our previous reports on the relationship between HIV antigenemia and progression to clinical disease (1,2). However, the data suggest that low titers of HIV core antibodies without detectable levels of HIV antigen may be associated with a poor clinical prognosis as well. We have shown that the present HIV antigen assay detects primarily free uncomplexed HIV antigen (4). The inverse relationship between levels of HIV core antigens and antibodies (Fig. 1) adds evidence to the notion that a dynamic balance exists between HIV antigen expression, antibody production and immune complex formation. Sera inhibiting CD4-dependent cell fusion by HIV glycoprotein have generaly the ability to block HIV infectivity and subsequent HIV gene expression in CD4+ target cells. It remains to be established if this reflects parallel induction or a shared property of the same immunoglbulins.

Progression to ARC and AIDS is associated with low numbers of CD4 cells, low titers of HIV core antibodies and the persisting precence of HIV antigen, although AIDS patients may lack HIV antigen and individuals may have HIV antigen for long time without developing disease. The preliminary data presented indicate that those progressing to ARC or AIDS have low levels of CFI-Ab and VN-Ab. Induction of high titers of CFI-Ab and VN-Ab may limit spread of virus as well as HIV gene expression in already infected cells resulting in low levels of extracellular HIV antigens. Less uninfected CD4 cells may be recruited by HIV glycoprotein bearing cells or virus and escape subsequent cell death.

In those developing AIDS antibodies to core protein may not be produced, trapped in immune complexes by core antigens or both. Although a relationship between CFI-Ab, VN-Ab and titers of antibodies to HIV core proteins is apparent, neutralizing epitopes may be present on several structural proteins of the virus each contributing in part to putative protective immune responses.

REFERENCES

1. Goudsmit J, de Wolf F, Paul DA, et al (1986). Expression of human immunodeficiency virus antigen (HIV-Ag) in serum and cerebrospinal fluid during acute and chronic infection. Lancet ii:177-80.
2. Lange JMA, Paul DA, Huisman HG, et al (1986). Persistent HIV antigenaemia and decline of HIV core antibodies associated with transition to AIDS. Br Med J 293:1459-62.
3. Goudsmit J, Lange JMA, Paul DA, et al (1987). Antigenemia and antibody titers to core and envelope antigens in AIDS, AIDS-related complex and subclinical human immunodeficiency virus infection. J Inf Dis 155:558-60.
4. Lange JMA, Paul DA, de Wolf F, Coutinho RA, Goudsmit J (1987). Viral gene expression, antibody production and immune complex formation in human immunodeficiency virus infection. AIDS 1:15-20.
5. Hecht F, Morgan R, Kaiser-McCaw Hecht B, Smith S (1984). Common region on chromosome 14 in T-cell leukemia and lymphoma. Science 226:1445-6.
6. Tersmette M, Miedema F, Huisman HG, Goudsmit J, Melief CJM (1985). Productive HTLV-III infection of human B cell lines. Lancet ii: 815-6.

V. HIV AND ITS RECEPTOR

Human Retroviruses, Cancer, and AIDS:
Approaches to Prevention and Therapy, pages 257–267

DELINEATION OF A REGION OF THE HUMAN IMMUNODEFICIENCY VIRUS gp120 GLYCOPROTEIN CRITICAL FOR INTERACTION WITH THE CD4 RECEPTOR

Laurence Lasky, Gerald Nakamura, Douglas Smith, Christopher Fennie, Eric Patzer, Craig Shimasaki, Phillip Berman, Timothy Gregory, and Daniel Capon

Department of Molecular Biology and Immunology
Genentech, Inc., 460 Pt San Bruno Blvd.,
South San Francisco, CA 94080

ABSTRACT The primary event in the infection of cells by the Human Immunodeficiency Virus, HIV, is the interaction between the viral envelope glycoprotein, gp120, and its cellular receptor, CD4. A soluble, radiolabeled, recombinant form of gp120 has been found to bind to recombinant CD4 with a high affinity constant (Kd approximately 4×10^{-9}M). We have isolated a murine monoclonal antibody specific for gp120 which blocks the interaction between the viral glycoprotein and the CD4 receptor. The epitope which binds to this monoclonal antibody has been isolated and characterized by amino acid sequence analysis. Using *in vitro* mutagenesis, a small deletion encompassing part of this epitope has been made in the gp120 gene. The resultant mutant gp120 is unable to bind to the CD4 antigen. In addition, we have made a number of point mutants in this region and have found one mutation which alters the ability of gp120 to bind to CD4. These results suggest that sequences within the region which bind to this blocking monoclonal antibody are critical for the interaction between gp120 and CD4.

INTRODUCTION

Human Immunodeficiency Virus (HIV) is the causative agent of the acquired immune deficiency syndrome, AIDS. The virus predominantly attacks the cells of the immune system which bear the CD4 antigen on their surface. Initial evidence using CD4 monoclonal antibodies suggested that CD4 was the receptor for the AIDS virus (1,2). More direct evidence came from studies which demonstrated that a specific complex could be formed between the gp120 surface glycoprotein of HIV and CD4 (3). The most convincing role for CD4 in HIV infection came from recent experiments which demonstrated that non-permissive cell lines could be rendered HIV infectible by transfection and expression of the CD4 gene (4).

While the studies described above suggested that CD4 was the receptor for HIV infection, little is known about the interaction between CD4 and gp120. Amino acid sequence comparisons of various gp120 molecules have shown that there are highly conserved regions interspersed with highly divergent regions in different strains of the virus (5-7). Since all of the HIV strains appear to infect cells via the same receptor, it has been hypothesized that one or more of the constant regions of gp120 are important for interaction with CD4. In order to begin to characterize the gp120-CD4 interaction in greater detail, we have developed a recombinant system for the production of large quantities of gp120 and CD4. In this paper, we report on a conserved region of gp120 which appears to be critical for the interaction between this viral glycoprotein and its receptor, CD4.

Measurement of the gp120-CD4 Affinity Constant

Recombinant gp120 (8) was purified to homogeneity by monoclonal antibody affinity chromatography and radiolabeled by the lactoperoxidase method with I^{125}. As can be seen in Figure 1, the iodinated glycoprotein was predominantly intact after radiolabeling. The interaction of the iodinated gp120 with CD4 was initially analyzed by using coprecipitation of the gp120-CD4 complex. The CD4 used in these experiments was a recombinant form of the antigen expressed in Chinese hamster ovary cells (CHO cells) (D. Smith and

D. Capon, unpublished). As can be seen in Figure 1, the complex could be coprecipitated with the CD4 monoclonal antibodies OKT4 and OKT4b, while no coprecipitation was seen with OKT4a. This agrees with previous results on coprecipitation of the natural gp120-CD4 complex (3) and with previous virus infectivity studies using these CD4 monoclonal antibodies (1,2).

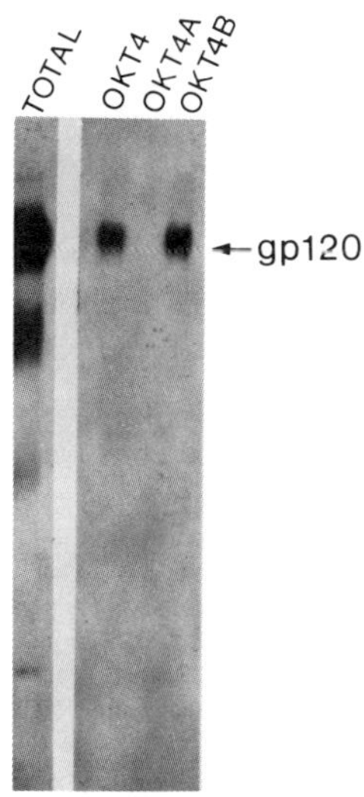

FIGURE 1. Coprecipitation of I^{125} labeled gp120 and CD4 with Various OKT4 Monoclonal antibodies. gp120 was purified by immunoaffinity chromatography and labeled with I^{125} by the lactoperoxidase reaction to a specific activity of 0.53nCi/ng. The isolated, labeled protein was incubated with CHO cells expressing recombinant CD4 at 4°C for 1 hr. The cells were washed, and the complex was solubilized in NP40, immunoprecipitated with a variety of OKT4 monoclonal antibodies, and analyzed by SDS polyacrylamide gel electrophoresis. The first lane shows the purified I^{125} labeled gp120 while the other lanes show coprecipitation of the gp120-CD4 complex with OKT4, OKT4a, and OKT4b monoclonal antibodies.

Figure 2 shows the competitive binding and Scatchard plot analysis of the soluble, recombinant gp120-CD4 interaction. The data reveal a single component binding interaction with a dissociation constant of approximately 4×10^{-9}M. This binding constant is quite high and suggests that the interaction between these recombinant molecules may be representative of the binding of HIV to the CD4 antigen expressed on the cell surface. In addition, these results demonstrate that a soluble form of gp120, ie in the absence of interactions with gp41 or the virus surface, is still able to bind with high affinity to CD4.

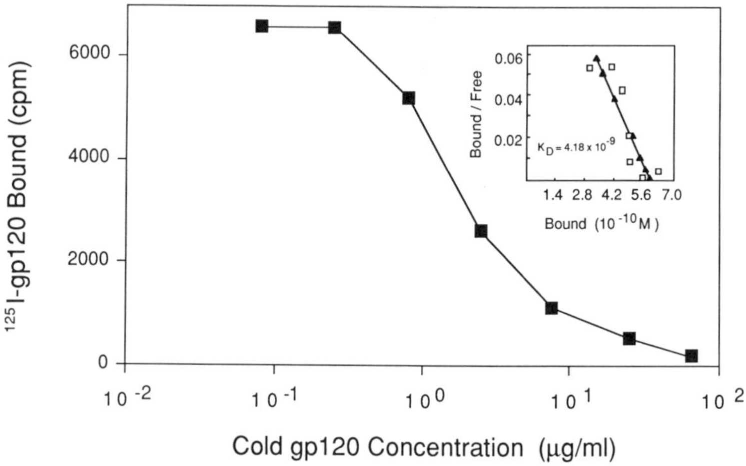

FIGURE 2. Competition Binding and Scatchard Analysis of the gp120-CD4 Interaction. A constant amount of I^{125} labeled gp120 (100,000 cpm) was incubated with CHO cells expressing CD4 and an increasing amount of cold gp120 for 20 hr at 4°C. Unbound counts were washed off, and the specifically bound gp120 was counted in a gamma counter. The resultant data were fitted using the Scatplot program (D. Vandlen, Genentech) and are shown in the inset. Non-specific binding to CHO cells not expressing CD4 was less than 5% of that found for CD4 expressing CHO cells.

Isolation of gp120 Monoclonal Antibodies Which Block the gp120-CD4 Interaction

Several monoclonal antibodies specific for gp120 were analyzed for their ability to block binding in the iodinated gp120-CD4 interaction assay described above. Two monoclonal antibodies, termed 5C2E5 and 7F11, were found to effectively block this interaction. Figure 3 shows an inhibition experiment with one of the blocking gp120 monoclonal antibodies (5C2E5) and a non-blocking gp120 monoclonal antibody (9F6). The figure shows that the blocking of the gp120-CD4 interaction occurs at relatively high 5C2E5 concentrations, possibly due to the high affinity interaction between gp120 and CD4. However, 9F6, is completely ineffective at blocking the interaction. The figure also illustrates that the OKT4a CD4 monoclonal antibody is very effective at blocking the interaction between gp120 and CD4, while the OKT4 monoclonal antibody does not block this binding, a result which agrees with previous studies using either native gp120 binding or virus infectivity (1-3).

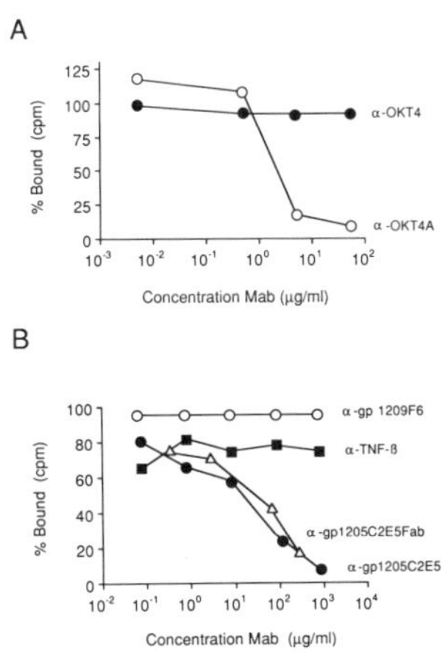

FIGURE 3. Blocking of the gp120-CD4 Interaction by OKT4 and Anti-gp120 Monoclonal antibodies. Panel A shows the results of adding increasing amounts of either the OKT4 or OKT4a CD4 monoclonal antibodies to the I^{125} gp120-CD4 binding assay described in figure legend 2. Panel B shows the results of adding

(continued)

Fig. 3 (continued)
increasing quantities of three other monoclonal antibodies to this assay. As can be seen in this panel, the control monoclonal antibody (anti-TNF beta) as well as a non-blocking gp120 monoclonal antibody (9F6) were both completely ineffective at blocking the gp120-CD4 interaction, while both the intact 5C2E5 monoclonal antibody as well as the Fab fragment of this antibody were both effective at blocking this interaction.

While the blocking of the gp120-CD4 interaction by the 5C2E5 monoclonal antibody may have been due to an antibody-induced conformational change in gp120, it was equally possible that the antibody was recognizing an epitope which was critical for gp120-CD4 interaction. In order to characterize this epitope, an immunoaffinity column using the 5C2E5 monoclonal antibody was produced. Purified gp120 was treated under mild acidic conditions which have been shown to cleave specifically at aspartic acid (D) residues, after which either disulfide-reduced or non-reduced material was passed over the 5C2E5 immunoaffinity column. The resultant bound material was eluted and characterized by N-terminal amino acid sequencing and amino acid analysis. Both techniques unambiguously demonstrated that the 5C2E5 epitope was located within residues 397-439 of the mature, processed gp120 of the 3b strain of HIV. Since both reduced or non-reduced gp120 gave identical results, it appears that the two cysteine residues contained in this region form a disulfide bridge with each other, resulting in a loop in the 5C2E5 binding region. In order to further delineate the 5C2E5 binding epitope, a trypsin-treated gp120 preparation was passed over the column, and the bound material was analyzed as described above. This demonstrated that at least part of the 5C2E5 epitope was within a peptide delineated by the lysine residues at positions 404-415 of gp120. Mapping of both the 5C2E5 and 7F11 blocking monoclonal antibodies by the lambda gt11 epitope mapping system revealed that both monoclonals bound to gp120 in the approximate region described above (D. Dowbenko *et al.*, unpublished data). Finally, the isolated peptide corresponding to residues 397-439 was found to block the 5C2E5 monoclonal antibodies ability to inhibit the gp120-CD4 interaction. In summary, these results suggest that binding of a monoclonal antibody to a region of gp120 located within residues 397–439 appears to disrupt the interaction between this glycoprotein and CD4.

Mutagenesis of the 5C2E5 Binding Epitope

In order to further investigate the role of the 5C2E5 binding epitope in the gp120–CD4 interaction, *in vitro* mutagenesis of this region was done. Figure 4 shows the diversity of amino acid sequences found within this region of gp120. As can be seen in this figure, this region shows an interspersion of relatively divergent sequences with highly conserved residues. In addition, this region contains the last two cysteines of gp120 (residues 402 and 429), one potential N-linked glycosylation site (arginine residue 432), and several potential structure-inducing amino acids such as the two prolines at residues 421 and 422.

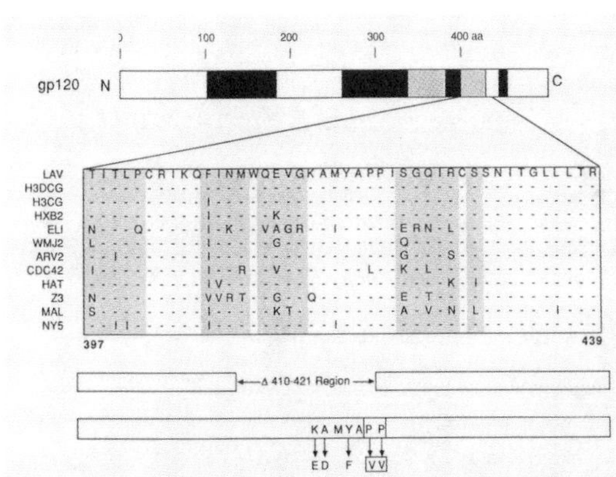

FIGURE 4. Sequence Diversity in the 5C2E5 Binding Region and Location of the gp120 Deletion and Point Mutants. The top of the figure illustrates the highly conserved (clear), moderately conserved (shaded), and non-conserved (dark) regions of gp120 as determined by comparing the protein sequences of all of the published isolates. Also shown is an expanded version of the 5C2E5 binding region illustrating the microheterogeneity in sequence divergence found within this domain. The locations of the $\Delta_{410-421}$, lys$_{416}$-glu, ala$_{417}$-asp, tyr$_{419}$-phe, and pro$_{421,422}$-val mutations are also illustrated at the bottom of the figure.

The first *in vitro* mutant constructed from this region involved the production of a twelve amino acid deletion mutant which was equidistant from the two cysteine residues and which spanned residues 410-421 (Δ410-421) (Figure 4). Mammalian cell lines producing this mutant protein were constructed, and the mutant, secreted antigen was analyzed in coprecipitation experiments with recombinant CD4. Figure 5 shows the coprecipitation experiments using the wild type and mutant proteins produced by mammalian cell lines. As this figure shows, the wild type protein shows apparently quantitative binding to CD4 under the conditions utilized here, while the Δ410-421 mutant shows an apparently complete lack of binding to the CD4 receptor. The mutant glycoprotein appears otherwise identical to the wild type antigen by the criteria of size and immunoreactivity. These results suggest that a small deletion in this region of gp120 has profound effects on the glycoproteins ability to bind to CD4.

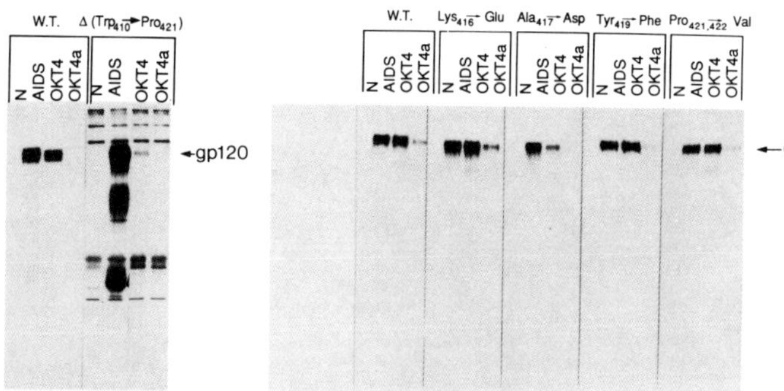

FIGURE 5. Coprecipitations of Wild Type gp120, Δ410-421 gp120, and Various gp120 Point Mutants with Anti-gp120 Polyclonal Sera, OKT4 Monoclonal Antibody, and OKT4a Monoclonal Antibody. Wild type and mutant glycoproteins were expressed transiently in mammalian cells and were labeled with S^{35} methionine. The secreted antigens were mixed with at 4°C with CD4 solubilized from CHO cells expressing the protein, and the complexes were coprecipitated with OKT4 monoclonal antibodies. The total immunoprecipitable material was determined with a high-titre anti-gp120 antiserum from an HIV infected individual.

In order to further analyze the role of conserved amino acids contained within the Δ410-421 region, *in vitro* mutagenesis was done to create various point mutants. Figure 4 shows the amino acid changes which were made within the Δ410-421 region. The resultant mutant glycoproteins were expressed in mammalian cells and the secreted mutant antigens were utilized in the gp120-CD4 binding assay. As Figure 5 shows, many of the point mutants made within this region appeared to have little effect on the overall binding of gp120 to CD4. Thus, the lys_{416}-glu, tyr_{419}-phe, and $pro_{421,422}$-val changes did not appear to grossly effect binding. However, the ala_{417}-asp mutation appeared to profoundly decrease the level of binding of gp120 to CD4 in this experiment. These results strongly suggested that the alanine at position 417, or perhaps the absence of a negatively charged residue at this position, was critical for interaction with CD4.

DISCUSSION

The data reported here represent the initial, detailed characterization of a region of gp120 which appears to be critical for binding of the viral glycoprotein to the CD4 receptor. Although previous expectations led several investigators to assume that the CD4 interaction sites on gp120 would be highly conserved, the region elucidated in this paper shows only partial conservation. The most notable aspect of CD4 interaction site elucidated here is that the regions which are highly conserved are interspersed with relatively divergent regions. This suggests that there is strong selective pressure on the conserved regions to maintain a high degree of sequence preservation. The point mutation studies reported here suggest that complete conservation of amino acids within this region is not necessary for binding to CD4. It should be noted, however, that subtle changes in the affinity which might result from some of the point mutants tested here would probably not be detected. However, the clear decrease in binding with the ala_{417}-asp mutant strongly suggests that a single point mutation in gp120 can have profound effects on the strength of the interaction between this glycoprotein and CD4.

One interesting aspect of the CD4 interaction site elucidated here stems from a recent publication of Maddon et al. (4) which presented potential CD4 binding domains of gp120 predicted from regions of the glycoprotein which bore limited homology with the immunoglobulin superfamily. The second domain presented in this paper encompassed residues 382-422 of gp120 and thus included the region which we have delineated here as critical for CD4 binding. This suggests that the possibility that gp120 interacts with CD4 based upon its distant relationship to the immunoglobulin superfamily may be correct. A second important aspect of the region shown here is found in a comparison of the amino acid sequences of the external envelope proteins of HIV, the Simian T Lymphotrophic Virus Type 3 (STLV3) and a new human retrovirus HIV2 (9,10). STLV3 and HIV2 appear to infect CD4 lymphocytes by utilization of the CD4 receptor in a manner which is similar to that which has been found for HIV (11). Thus, it has been hypothesized that CD4 interaction domain(s) of both viruses may show some sequence homology. A comparison of the gp120 homologues from HIV, STLV3 and HIV2 has revealed very limited homology between the two envelope glycoproteins. However, the region which we have elucidated here shows a relatively high degree of sequence homology between the three viruses. This result lends further support to our contention that the gp120 region elucidated here may be critical for interaction between HIV and its cellular receptor, CD4.

ACKNOWLEDGMENTS

We thank the organic chemistry group at Genentech for the many oligonucleotides utilized in this study as well as Becky Cazares for excellent manuscript preparation.

REFERENCES

1. Dalgleish A, Beverley P, Clapman P, Crawford D, Greaves M, Weiss R (1984). The CD4 (T4) antigen is an essential component of the receptor for the AIDS retrovirus. Nature 312:763.

2. Klatzman D, Champagne E, Chamaret S, Gruest J, Guetard D, Herciend T, Gluckman J, Montaignier L (1984). T lymphocyte T4 molecule behave as the receptor for human retrovirus LAV. Nature 312:767.
3. McDougal J, Kennedy M, Sligh J, Cort S, Mawle A, Nicholson J (1986). Binding of HTLVIII/LAV to $T4^{+}$ T cells by a complex of the 110 K viral protein and the T4 molecule. Science 231:382.
4. Maddon P, Dalgleish A, McDougal J, Clapham P, Weiss R, Axel R (1986). The T4 gene encodes the AIDS virus receptor and is expressed in the immune system and the brain. Cell 47:333.
5. Starcich B, Hahn B, Shaw G, McNeely P, Madrow S, Wolf H, Parks E, Parks W, Josephs J, Gallo R, Wong-Staal F (1986). Identification and characterization of conserved and variable regions in the envelope gene of HTLVIII/LAV, the retrovirus of AIDS. Cell 45:637.
6. Alizon M, Wain-Hobson J, Montaignier L, Sonigo P (1986). Genetic Variability of the AIDS virus: Nucleotide sequence analysis of two isolates from african patients. Cell 46:63.
7. Willey R, Rutledge R, Dias S, Folks T, Theodore T, Buckler C, Martin M (1986). Identification of conserved and divergent domains within the envelope gene of the acquired immunodeficiency retrovirus. Proc. Natl. Acad. Sci. 83:5038.
8. Lasky L, Groopman J, Fennie C, Benz P, Capon D, Dowbenko D, Nakamura G, Nunes W, Renz M, Berman P (1986). Neutralization of the AIDS retrovirus by antibodies to a recombinant envelope glycoprotein. Science 233:209.
9. Hirsch V, Riedel N, Mullins J (1987). The genome organization of STLV3 is similar to that of the AIDS virus except for a truncated transmembrane protein. Cell, in press.
10. Guyader M, Emerman M, Sonigo P, Clavel F, Montaignier L, Alizon M (1987). Genome organization and transactivation of The Human Immune Deficiency virus Type 2. Nature, in press.
11. Kannagi M, Yetz J and Letvin, N (1986). In vitro growth characteristics of simian T-lymphotrophic virus III (STLV III AGM). Proc. Natl. Acad. Sci. 82:7053.

Human Retroviruses, Cancer, and AIDS:
Approaches to Prevention and Therapy, pages 269–281

HIV BINDING TO THE CD4 MOLECULE: CONFORMATION DEPENDENCE AND BINDING INHIBITION STUDIES

J.S. McDougal, J.K.A. Nicholson, W.L. Cosand,
G.D. Cross, S.P. Cort, M.S. Kennedy, and A.C. Mawle

Immunology Branch, Division of Host Factors,
Center for Infectious Diseases,
Centers for Disease Control, Atlanta, GA
and Genetic Systems Corporation, Seattle, WA

ABSTRACT Human immunodeficiency virus (HIV) is cytopathic for CD4 T cells and binds to these cells through a complex of the 110K (or 120K) viral envelope glycoprotein gp110 (or gp120) and the CD4 molecule. We briefly review evidence that the CD4 molecule functions as a receptor for HIV. Various physical, chemical, and enzymic treatments of HIV indicate that there are conformational and structural constraints on the virus with respect to its capacity to bind to CD4. Results from binding inhibition studies using polyclonal and monoclonal antibodies, synthetic peptides, and anti- (anti-CD4) idiotypic reagents and their implications for experimental approaches to defining the binding sites on gp110 and CD4 are presented.

INTRODUCTION

There are now five types of experiments which, when taken together, provide compelling evidence that the CD4 molecule functions as a receptor for HIV--specifically for the envelope glycoprotein gp110. The first, reported by Drs. Popovic, Klatzmann, Dalgleish and their respective colleagues, is the observation that certain α-CD4 monoclonal antibodies (mAb) prevent or limit the infectivity and replication of HIV in T cells (1-3). Inhibition is greatest if CD4 mAb is added to cells before rather than after virus inoculation and maintained in the culture media throughout the culture period; inhibition is not enhanced by combination of α-CD4 mAb with mAbs directed at other cell surface components; nor is the inhibition due to an effect of CD4 mAb on cellular proliferation or activation (4).

The second piece of evidence, also reported by Dr. Dalgleish and coworkers, provided more direct evidence that the CD4 molecule functions early in infection and at the cell membrane. This comes from experiments where CD4 mAb was shown to block penetration of a virus pseudotype formed between vesicular stomatitis virus and HIV and to inhibit fusion (syncytia) between HIV infected and uninfected CD4 cells (3). Syncytia formation is inhibited by treatment of indicator cells with CD4 mAbs and CD4-negative cells do not participate in the fusion process (3,5-6).

The third type of experiment, indirect immunofluorescence, provided evidence that HIV preferentially binds to the surface of CD4 cells but not to CD4 negative cells (4). Binding is saturable, specifically inhibitable by certain α-CD4 mAbs (but not by a reasonably comprehensive panel of mAbs directed against other cell surface components), and reciprocal in that HIV and CD4 mAb each inhibit binding of the other (4). No evidence for qualitative differences in binding avidity was obtained in comparison of direct binding kinetics or inhibition titrations between activated or nonactivated CD4 cells (4). Not all CD4 mAbs inhibit binding equivalently. For instance, figure 1 is a fluorescence histogram of HIV binding to the CD4 cell line, CEM. Virus binding is completely inhibited by pretreating the cells with OKT4A mAb but is not inhibited by OKT4 mAb.

We examined a panel of CD4 mAbs. They titered similarly in direct binding to CD4 but differed substantially in their capacity to inhibit HIV binding. OKT4A, OKT4D, OKT4F, Leu3a mAbs were potent inhibitors of HIV binding whereas binding was not inhibited by OKT4 and OKT4C mAbs and only partially inhibited by OKT4B and OKT4E mAbs (7). Similar results were reported by Sattentau et al. (8) for inhibition of syncytia. The CD4 epitopes detected by these CD4 mAbs map as clusters along the molecule (9), and the pattern of inhibition suggests that HIV interacts with a restricted region in the amino-end of the CD4 molecule.

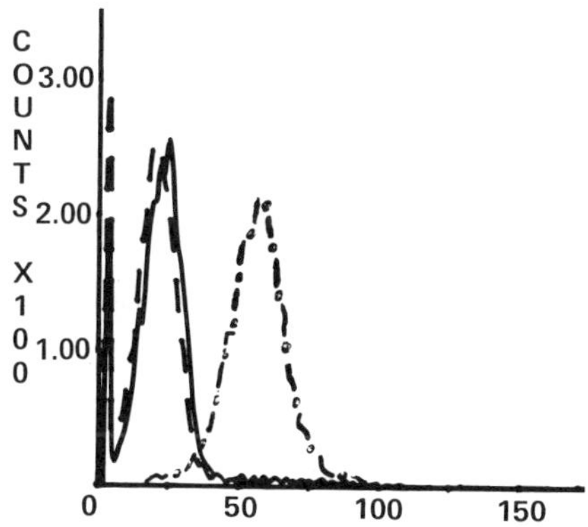

FIGURE 1. Fluorescence histogram (cell number vs. fluorescence intensity) demonstrating inhibition of HIV binding to the CD4 cell line, CEM, by CD4 mAb. Cells were preincubated with OKT4A mAb (— —) or OKT4 mAb (— • —) followed by HIV and washed, and FITC-α-HIV was added. Dashed line is FITC-α-HIV reagent control.

The fourth piece of evidence comes from radioimmunoprecipitation experiments that demonstrate coprecipitation of the CD4 molecule with the gp110 envelope glycoprotein of HIV. If CD4 cells are surface labelled with ^{125}I, exposed to virus, washed, and lysed, immunoprecipitation with anti HIV serum results in coprecipitation of a cell surface protein of 57K which by comigration, blocking, and preabsorption experiments was identified as the CD4 molecule (10). Conversely, if one radiolabels virus and precipitates the CD4 molecule (using an α-CD4 mAb that does not interfere with HIV binding), an HIV protein of 110K coprecipitates with CD4 (10). If CD4 cells that had bound HIV were covalently crosslinked, we could not identify any additional cell surface proteins bound to virus (10).

Further indication that gp110 is the principle viral protein that binds to CD4 has been provided by Bolognesi and colleagues and Lasky and colleagues who demonstrated binding to CD4 using purified native gp110 protein or recombinant-derived gp110 protein, respectively (11,12).

The gp110-CD4 interaction occurs not only at the cell surface but intracellularly as well. Hoxie et al. demonstrated intracellular complexes of CD4 with gp110 (and with the gp160 polyprotein precursor) in CD4 cells productively infected with HIV (13).

The final piece of evidence comes from experiments using cell lines transfected with either the CD4 gene or the HIV envelope gene. If cell lines that ordinarily do not express CD4, do not bind virus, and cannot be infected with native HIV are transfected with the CD4 gene, they express CD4; they bind virus, and in the case of human cell lines, they become permissive for virus replication (14). Murine cell lines transfected with the human CD4 gene express CD4 and bind virus, but virus replication does not occur (14). Since murine cell lines will replicate HIV when HIV is introduced by transfection (15), it is possible the human CD4 protein is not processed, cycled, or internalized appropriately for HIV infection in murine cell lines. To address this possibility, recombinant clones linking the extracellular (HIV binding) domains of human CD4 with the transmembrane and cytoplasmic domains of the murine L3T4 homologue are being constructed.

In the converse type of transfection experiment, Sodroski et al. (6) found that transfection with the gp110 envelope gene rendered cells capable of forming syncytia with CD4 cells. The syncytia model using infected or transfected cells for studying virus-CD4 interactions differs from models using cell-free virus or envelope in one relevant respect. CD4 interaction is readily inhibited in both models by CD4 mAbs, and antibody to HIV inhibits interaction with cell-free virus. However, syncytia formation is not particularly influenced by antibody to HIV (3,6,16). If the syncytia model has in vivo relevance for cell-cell transmission of virus and CD4 cell depletion, immunologic strategies that demonstrably interrupt infection by cell-free virus may or may not be effective against cell-associated virus.

RESULTS AND DISCUSSION

Effect of physical, chemical, and enzymic treatments of HIV on its capacity to bind to CD4 cells. HIV was treated with the regimens listed in Table 1. Specific details of incubation and manipulation are given elsewhere

(7). Treated virus was tested for binding to the CD4 cell line CEM by indirect immunofluorescence and compared to sham-treated virus that had been processed in parallel. The binding protocol included the following. Binding profiles of serially-diluted treated and control virus were compared to detect partial or incomplete effects of treatment. Partial effects on binding were not observed with the regimens listed although partial reduction of infectivity titers were observed with some regimens (e.g. glycolytic enzyme digestions). We tested treated virus for inhibition of binding by OKT4A mAb to ensure that binding occurred by the usual mechanism (the CD4 molecule) rather than having been rendered nonspecifically adsorptive by the treatment. To confirm that treatment regimens that abolished binding were due to effects on the virus rather than on the CD4 cells, we tested 1:1 mixtures of treated and untreated virus and tested untreated virus for binding to CEM cells that had been pretreated with the same reagent or reagent combinations that were present in treated virus preparations at the end of the treatment regimen. Finally, treated virus was tested for antigenicity in immunoblot using polyclonal α-HIV serum and α-gp110 mAb.

Reduction of disulfide bonds followed by alkylation of sulfide groups abolished the capacity of HIV to bind, whereas alkylation alone did not (Table 1). The effect must be due to cleavage of intrachain disulfide bonds since gp110 molecules are not covalently linked to each other or to other virus proteins. If the tertiary covalent structure conferred by disulfide bonding is not disrupted, the proper conformation required for binding appears to be thermodynamically favored. Treatment with urea, SDS, or alcohol followed by removal of the denaturants did not affect binding, nor did heating virus at 56°C or 65°C although irreversible loss of binding occurred at 100°C. The discordance between the effect of certain treatments on the capacity to bind and the capacity to productively infect cells should not be surprising. Disruption of virus particles or inactivation of reverse transcriptase activity by certain treatments may abolish replicative potential but not necessarily prohibit binding of gp110 to the CD4 molecule.

Proteolytic digestion with trypsin abolished binding. We have not observed an effect of glycolytic enzyme digestion or periodate oxidation of carbohydrate groups. However, our digestions may have been incomplete in that

TABLE 1
PHYSICAL, CHEMICAL AND ENZYMIC TREATMENT OF HIV

Treatment regimen[a]	Effect on HIV Binding To CD4 Cells	Effect on HIV Infectivity Titer
1. 100°C x 10 min.	reduce	abolish
2. 65°C x 30 min.	no effect	abolish
3. 56°C x 30 min.	no effect	abolish
4. 8 M urea; dialyse.	no effect	abolish
5. Alcohol (15-20 volumes of 95%), suspend precipitate.	no effect	abolish
6. 0.05% or 1% SDS, 65°C x 30 min; alcohol precipitate as in #5.	no effect	see #5
7. 50 mM dithiotheitol reduction; 55 mM iodoacetamide alkylation; dialyze.	abolish	abolish
8. 55 mM iodoacetamide alkylation; dialyze.	no effect	abolish
9. 10 mM periodate oxidation; 400 µg/ml borohydride reduction; dialyze.	no effect	not done
10. 400 µg/ml borohydride reduction; dialyze.	no effect	not done
11. 50 µg/ml trypsin; 37.5 µg/ml soybean trypsin inhibitor.	abolish	abolish
12. 37.5 µg/ml soybean trypsin inhibitor.	no effect	no effect
13. 5 U/ml neuraminidase.	no effect	reduce
14. 100 mU/ml endoglycosidase H.	no effect	reduce
15. 100 mU/ml endoglycosidase F.	no effect	not done
16. Neuraminidase plus endoglycosidase H.	no effect	not done
17. Neuraminidase plus endoglycosidase F.	no effect	not done

[a]Virus concentration 500 µg/ml.

the apparent molecular weight of gp110 was reduced by digestion to about 85K-92K rather than the 60K predicted from the amino acid composition of gp110. Bolognesi and

TABLE 2

SYNTHETIC PEPTIDES CORRESPONDING TO SEQUENCES OF GP110

Peptide	gp110 Residue #[a]	NH2 leader	Sequence Encoded sequence	COOH tail
24	54-83	Ace-Y	CASDAKAYDTEVHNVWATHACVPTDPNPQE	G-COOH
25	89-108	Ace	VTENFNMWKNDMVEQMHEDI	C-CONH2
26	113-134	NH2-Y	DQSLKPCVKLTPLCVSLKCTDL	CONH2
27	166-190	Ace	ISTSIRGKVQKEYAFFYKLDIIPID	C-CONH2
28	268-280	Ace	GSLAEEEVVIRSA	C-COOH
29	308-328	Ace	TRKSIRIQRGPGRAFVTIGKI	C-CONH2
30	323-336	NH2	VTIGKIGNMRQAHC	CONH2
31	345-360	Ace	ATLKQIASKLREQFGN	C-CONH2
32	362-382	Ace-C	KTIIFKQSSGGDPEIVTHSFN	G-COOH
33	398-423	Ace	STWSTEGSNNTEGSDTITLPC	COOH
34	424-450	NH2	RIKQFINMWQEVGKAMYAPPISGQIRC	CONH2
35	469-493	Ace	GSEIFRPGGGDMRDNWRSELYKYKV	C-CONH2
36	494-517	NH2-C	VKIEPLGVAPTKAKRRVVQREKRA	C-COOH
37	488-499	Ace	LYKYKVVKIEPL	C-CONH2
41	252-266	NH2-K	CTHGIRPVVSTQLLL	CONH2
42	224-233	NH2	APAGFAILKC	K-CONH2
43	210-222	Ace-K	CPKVSFEPIPIHY	CONH2
44	192-201	Ace	DTTSYTLTSC	E-COOH
45	147-162	Ace	SSSGEMMMEKGEIKNC	COOH

[a]Residue number designations from reference 22.

colleagues achieved apparent complete deglycosylation of gp110 and found that this material neither bound to CD4 cells nor inhibited binding of native gp110 (11), and glycosylated but not deglycosylated gp110 blocked syncytia formation (17). However, both glycosylated and deglycosylated gp110 will induce neutralizing antibodies (17). Lifson et al. (18) found that lectins such as conconavalin A (ConA) that bind mannose residues inhibited virus-infected cells from forming syncytia with uninfected CD4 cells whereas lectins that do not bind mannose (e.g. phytohemagglutinin-PHA) did not. We have found that mixing ConA with HIV (1:1 by weight) partially inhibits HIV binding whereas PHA does not. It is premature to ascribe a role for carbohydrate in HIV binding to CD4 cells. The CD4 binding site on gp110 may be a carbohydrate determinant; carbohydrate may form part of the binding site; carbohydrate may be sufficiently close to the binding site such that steric effects of reagents that react with carbohydrate are observed; or carbohydrate may function to maintain protein conformation or protect the molecule from proteolytic attack. The first possibility loses its appeal in view of the results with trypsin and disulfide cleavage and in that it would require that HIV (which has no glycosylation enzymes of its own) acquire its highly specific CD4-binding capacity from host cell glycosylating enzymes.

Effect of synthetic peptides on HIV binding. The above results indicate that the binding site on the gp110 molecule requires a proper protein conformation and not simply the proper primary amino acid sequence making it unlikely that synthetic peptides matching portions of the gp110 molecule would bind to CD4 or inhibit virus binding unless they were formulated in the proper tertiary structure. Nevertheless, receptors that apparently bind to a ligand that is formed from approximation of discontiguous amino acid sequences could conceivably have some affinity for continguous sequences that form part of the bond. The peptides listed in Table 2 were synthesized by Genetic Systems Corp. and tested for inhibition of HIV binding to CD4 cells in the immunofluorescence assay. They were also tested for directed binding to CD4 cells in this assay presuming that direct binding would be detected by the fluorescein-conjugated α-HIV reagent. We preincubated CEM cells with peptide and this was followed (without a wash) by addition of HIV. We used the minimum amount of

TABLE 3

SUMMARY OF α-HIV AND α-(α-CD4) IDIOTYPIC SERA

Reagent	Direct reaction with:[a]					Inhibition of:[b]				
	gp110	OKT4A	OKT4D	OKT4F	Leu3a	virus binding	OKT4A binding	OKT4D binding	OKT4F binding	Leu3a binding
rabbit α-OKT4A idiotype	–	+ (3200)	–	–	–	–	+ (800)	–	–	–
rabbit α-OKT4D idiotype	–	–	+ (3200)	–	–	–	–	+ (800)	–	–
rabbit α-OKT4F idiotype	–	–	–	+ (3200)	–	–	–	–	+ (400)	–
rabbit α-Leu3a idiotype	–	–	–	–	+ (1600)	–	–	–	–	+ (400)
rabbit α-HIV	+ (800)	–	–	–	–	+ (200)	–	–	–	–
human α-HIV serum #1	+ (12800)	–	–	–	–	+ (6400)	–	–	–	–
human α-HIV serum #2	+ (25600)	–	–	–	–	+ (6400)	–	–	–	–
human α-HIV serum #3	+ (25600)	–	–	–	–	+ (6400)	–	–	–	–
human α-HIV serum #4	+ (6400)	–	–	–	–	+ (6400)	–	–	–	–
human α-HIV serum #5	+ (3200)	–	–	–	–	+ (1600)	–	–	–	–
murine α-gp110 mAb	+ (10,000)					+ (10,000)	–	–	–	–

[a]Reactions with gp110 were tested by immunoblot. Reactions with CD4 mAbs were tested by ELISA. Lowest dilution tested was 1:10. Titers are indicated in parentheses.

[b]Lowest dilution tested was 1:10. Endpoint titers resulting in ≥50% inhibition of binding are indicated in parentheses.

HIV required to register binding in the assay (peptide:HIV ratios were ≥10 by weight). Peptides that were covalently coupled to bovine serum albumin (BSA) were also tested for two reasons. First, the relative avidity of low affinity interactions would be enhanced by virtue of the potential for multipoint attachment. Second, some peptides were relatively insoluble in physiologic buffer whereas their BSA conjugates were soluble provided the coupling ratio was not too high. None of the peptides or their conjugates inhibited HIV binding. Antisera to these peptides may be sufficiently reactive with native HIV and provide more informative results. These are currently being produced.

Inhibition of HIV binding by anti-HIV antibodies. We have now tested a total of 11 mAbs directed against various HIV proteins for inhibition of HIV binding: 3 α-p18, 2 α-p24, 5 α-gp41, and 1 α-gp110. Only the α-gp110 mAb inhibited binding. This mAb reacts with a carboxy-terminal epitope of gp110, and although it inhibited binding by 50-80% in high titer, the inhibition was not as complete as with polyclonal sera. For instance, sera from humans exposed to HIV almost inevitably contain antibodies to gp110, and these sera can be potent inhibitors of virus binding. The inhibition results from reaction with virus and is not due to reaction with CD4 cells or to interference with detection of bound virus (7). We tested sera from 107 anti-HIV seropositive homosexual men, and all sera inhibited binding in titers from 1:100 to 1:6400 (titer equals the dilution resulting in ≥50% inhibition of binding). These sera were also titered by Western blot for antibody levels to specific virus proteins. Binding inhibition titers correlated weakly with anti-gp110 titers and not at all with titers to other viral proteins. Of the 107 sera, 25 were from patients with AIDS and 82 were from men who were asymptomatic or had lymphadenopathy at the time of specimen collection. Within the latter group, 25 men have subsequently progressed to AIDS (progressors) and 57 have been followed for an equal or greater period of time and have not developed AIDS (nonprogressors). Progressors had significantly lower binding inhibition titers, CD4 cell levels, and antibody titers to gp110, as well as lower titers to p24, p51, and p65. In multivariate analysis, lower CD4 cell levels were most highly predictive of progression, but lower antibody titers retained a significant association with progression even when the analysis was adjusted for CD4 cell levels (19). These data indicate that lower antibody titers to the envelope protein are at least a marker for disease progression and suggest the possibility that antibody plays a role in limiting the pace at which CD4 cell depletion and progressive disease occurs.

Potential for structural similarity between the CD4 binding site of gp110 and the CD4 binding site of α-CD4 mAbs. If one could find a CD4 mAb that binds to precisely the same epitope of CD4 where gp110 binds, it is conceivable that the two may share sufficient structural homology that antisera raised to one would react with the other and inhibit receptor binding. We selected four CD4 mAbs that were potent inhibitors of virus binding, OKT4A, OKT4D, OKT4F, and Leu3a. Rabbits were immunized with the mAbs and their antisera were absorbed with mouse immunoglobulin. The resultant antisera were idiotype-specific by the criteria that they reacted exclusively with their respective CD4 mAb and inhibited binding of the respective CD4 mAb to CD4 cells. These anti-idiotypic reagents did not react with HIV in ELISA or Western blot nor did they inhibit HIV binding to CD4 cells (Table 3) (7). Conversely, a panel of rabbit and human sera that were reactive with gp110 and that inhibited HIV binding did not react with or inhibit the binding of any of the CD4 mAbs. Two other groups have preliminary indication that antisera raised to the Leu3a mAb in mice inhibits HIV infectivity and/or reacts with gp110 (19,20). This contradicts our data and remains to be resolved. In any event, further examination of the Leu3a and other CD4 mAbs or different strategies may yet yield an idiotype that is an "internal image" of the structure in gp110 that binds to CD4. Considering the conformation dependence of binding, immunogens that maintain structural fidelity with the native binding site of gp110 are particularly attractive.

ACKNOWLEDGMENTS

We are especially grateful to L. Gosting, K. Shriver and L. Goldstein of Genetic Systems Corp. for monoclonal antibodies to HIV proteins and to P. Rao and G. Goldstein of Ortho Pharmaceutical Corp. for monoclonal antibodies to the CD4 molecule. We thank K. Foster for editorial assistance and J. Carter for typing the manuscript.

REFERENCES

1. Popovic M, Gallo RC, Mann DL (1984). OKT4 bearing molecule is a receptor for the human retrovirus HTLV-III. Clin Res 33:560.
2. Klatzmann D, Champagne E, Chamaret S, Gruest J, Guetard D, Hercend T, Gluckman J-C, Montagnier L (1985). T lymphocyte T4 molecule behaves as the receptor for human retrovirus LAV. Nature 312:767.
3. Dalgleish AG, Beverley PCL, Clapham PR, Crawford DH, Greaves MF, Weiss RA (1985). The CD4 (T4) antigen is an essential component of the receptor for the AIDS retrovirus. Nature 312:763.
4. McDougal JS, Mawle A, Cort SP, Nicholson JKA, Cross GD, Scheppler-Campbell JA, Hicks D, Sligh J (1985). Cellular tropism of the human retrovirus HTLV-III/LAV. I. Role of T cell activation and expression of the T4 antigen. J Immunol 135:3151.
5. Lifson JD, Reyes GR, McGrath MS, Stein BS, Engleman EG (1986). AIDS retrovirus induced cytopathology: giant cell formation and involvement of CD4 antigen. Science 232:1123.
6. Sodroski J, Goh WC, Rosen C, Campbell K, Haseltine W (1986). Role of the HTLV-III/LAV envelope in syncytium formation and cytopathicity. Nature 322:470.
7. McDougal JS, Nicholson JKA, Cross GD, Cort SP, Kennedy MS, Mawle AC (1986). Binding of the human retrovirus HTLV-III/LAV/ARV/HIV to the CD4 (T4) molecule: conformation dependence, epitope mapping, antibody inhibition, and potential for idiotypic mimicry. J Immunol 137:2937.
8. Sattentau QJ, Dalgleish AG, Weiss RA, Beverley PCL (1986). Epitopes of the CD4 antigen and HIV infection. Science 234:1120.
9. Fuller TC, Trevithick JE, Fuller AA, Colvin RB, Cosini AB, Kung PC (1984). Antigenic polymorphism of the T4 differentiation antigen expressed on human T helper/inducer lymphocytes. Hum Immunol 9:89.
10. McDougal JS, Kennedy, MS, Sligh JM, Cort SP, Mawle A, Nicholson JKA (1986). Binding of HTLV-III/LAV to $T4^+$ T cells by a complex of the 110K viral protein and the T4 molecule. Science 231:382.
11. Bolognesi DP (1986). Immunobiological properties of the major envelope glycoprotein of HTLV-III_B (HIV). Colloque des "cent gardes." Marnes-la-Coquette, France, Oct. 29-30.
12. Lasky L, Groopman JE, Capon DJ, Berman P (1986). The expression of the HIV envelope in mammalian cell lines: vaccination and biological studies. Colloque

des "cent gardes." Marnes-la-Coquette, France, Oct. 29-30.

13. Hoxie JA, Alpers JD, Rackowski JL, Huebner K, Haggarty BS, Cedarbaum AJ, Reed JC (1986). Alterations in T4 (CD4) protein and mRNA synthesis in cells infected with HIV. Science 234:1123.
14. Maddon PJ, Dalgleish AG, McDougal JS, Clapham PR, Weiss RA, Axel R (1986). The T4 gene encodes the AIDS virus receptor and is expressed in the immune system and the brain. Cell 47:333.
15. Levy JA, Cheng-Mayer C, Dina D, Luciw PA (1986). AIDS retrovirus (ARV-2) clone replicates in transfected human and animal fibroblasts. Science 232:998.
16. Weiss RA, Clapham PR, Cheingsong-Popov R, Dalgleish AG, Carne CA, Weller IVD, Tedder RS (1985). Neutralization of human T-lymphotropic virus type III by sera of AIDS and AIDS-risk patients. Nature 316:69.
17. Putney SD, Matthews TJ, Robey WG, Lynn DL, Robert-Guroff M, Mueller WT, Langlois AJ, Ghrayeb J, Petteway SR, Weinhold KJ, Fischinger PJ, Wong-Staal F, Gallo RC, Bolognesi DP (1986). HTLV-III/LAV-neutralizing antibodies to an E.coli-produced fragment of the virus envelope. Science 234:1392.
18. Lifson J, Coutre S, Huang S, Engleman E (1986). Role of envelope glycoprotein carbohydrate in human immunodeficiency virus (HIV) infectivity and virus-induced cell fusion. J Exp Med 164:2101.
19. McDougal JS, Kennedy MS, Nicholson JKA, Spira TJ, Jaffe HW, Kaplan JE, Fishbein DB, O'Malley P, Aloisio CH, Black CM, Hubbard M, Reimer CB (1987). Antibody response to human immunodeficiency virus in homosexual men. Relation of antibody specificity, titer, and isotype to clinical status, severity of immunodeficiency, and disease progression. J Clin Invest in press.
20. Chanh TC, Dreesman GR, Kennedy RC (1986). A monoclonal anti-idiotype that neutralizes HIV infectivity. Colloque des "cent gardes." Marnes-la-Coquette, France, Oct. 29-30.
21. Weiss RA, Clapham PR, Dalgleish AG, Beverley PCL, Sattentau QJ, Lasky LA, Berman PW, Maddon P, Axel R (1986). HIV-1: neutralizing antibodies and cellular receptors. Colloque des "cent gardes." Marnes-la-Coquette, France, Oct. 29-30.
22. Wain-Hobson S, Sonigo P, Danos O, Cole S, Alizon M (1985). Nucleotide sequence of the AIDS virus, LAV. Cell 40:9.

Human Retroviruses, Cancer, and AIDS:
Approaches to Prevention and Therapy, pages 283–288

THE T4 MOLECULE: ITS POSSIBLE USE IN THERAPEUTIC STRATEGIES AGAINST AIDS

A.G. Dalgleish,[+] R.C. Kennedy,[*] Q. Sattentau,[°] T. Chanh,[*] P. Beverley[°], P. Maddon[▽], R. Axel[▽] and M. Malkovsky[+]

[+] Clinical Research Center, Harrow, UK.
[°] U.C.H.M.S., London, UK.
[*] South West Foundation for Biomedical Research, San Antonio, Texas.
[▽] College of Physicians & Surgeons, Columbia, N.Y.C.

INTRODUCTION

Early studies by us and other authors showed that the human T4 molecule (CD4 antigen) behaved as an essential component of the AIDS virus receptor.[1,2] This has been a consistent feature of all AIDS virus isolates so far tested[3] including members of the HIV-2 family, such as LAV-2 and HTLV-IV (Sattentau *et al.*, unpublished observations). The ability to induce HIV neutralising antibodies appears to be exceptionally poor, considering the strong antibody response mounted against the envelope antigen.[4] Moreover, where neutralising antibodies can be detected in patients' sera they appear to be group specific for various isolates and where antibodies have been made to the envelope region of just one strain, there appears to be poor cross-reactivity with other isolates.[5] These data suggest that a vaccine based on a cloned envelope would be subject to severe limitations in protecting against the many different strains that have now been isolated. However, since all these strains bind and infect via T4 it is conceivable that they have some common structural determinant. This is not readily recognisable by envelope sequence analysis, although conserved regions amongst isolates have been identified. If this is so then an antibody raised against the binding site of the HIV receptor may be used to elicit a further antibody (anti-idiotype) which could mimic the receptor binding site and bind to the constant region on the virus envelope and subsequently neutralise binding and infection. However, for this to be a worthwhile approach, it would be helpful to know that T4 was the only HIV receptor and that HIV could not infect cells when T4 was not available.

We have undertaken studies to determine if this is the case. Firstly, using techniques described in reference 1, we have tried to infect a wide variety of cells which are negative for T4 by immunofluorescence analysis (IF). In the few cases, where this has been possible, (most of these cells have been the B cells which contain the Epstein Barr virus genome), T4 RNA can be detected by Northern blotting using the T4 cDNA probes.[6] However, we have found one HIV-infectable B cell line with very low grade virus production which is T4 negative by IF and Northern blotting. However, using S1 nuclease analysis, these cells are positive for T4 mRNA, whereas B cells which were not infectable were clearly negative using this technique. (M. Malkovsky, Dalgleish A.G., in preparation). We have also tried to determine the presence of another component of the HIV receptor (or an alternative receptor) by using a large number of monoclonal antibodies (MoAbs) to a variety of cellular ligands as well as to class II human leucocyte antigens (HLA). Clinically, cells expressing the T4 molecule become depleted following HIV infection. Furthermore, T4 helper cells can be subdivided by the expression of Leu-8, 4B4 and 4H4, all of which preferentially decrease following HIV infection. Using syncytial induction (SI) inhibition and pseudotype (PT) plaque assays, no inhibition could be detected with these MoAbs with the singular exception of anti-Leu-8 in the SI assay at a dilution of 1 in 10 only.[1] All blocking anti-T4 MoAbs are effective at titres from 1:200 up to greater than 1:3,200. Similarly, weak inhibition of SI is seen with some HLA class II MoAbs, which are rarely effective beyond a titre of 1 in 10. Therefore, it is assumed that these weak inhibitory effects may represent allosteric inhibition. Interestingly, homologies of up to 48% occur between some HLA class II's and T4 molecule.[6]

It is unlikely that HLA class II's have any additional role at all to play with regard to HIV infection as cells which are completely devoid of class II antigens (but T4 positive), e.g. CEM, are as readily infectable *in vitro* as other cell lines expressing abundant HLA class II antigens (e.g. H9). Nevertheless, the level of expression of HLA class II antigens appears to alter following HIV infection in some cells, with both upward and downward regulation of DQ determinants (Sattentau *et al* in preparation)

In order to see whether the expression of the T4 molecule on a cell which does not normally express T4 renders this cell infectable with HIV, the cloned T4 was transfected into a variety of mouse and human cell lines using amphotrophic retrovirus vectors provided by R. Mulligan (M.I.T.). We have shown that the expression of T4 in both lymphoid cells normally devoid of T4 (including B cells) and non-lymphoid T4-negative cells, (e.g. HeLa) rendered these cells infectable with HIV.[6] However, mouse cells which were able to express human T4, were not infectable with HIV. The reasons for this are not clear and they are presently under investigation.[6] It is noteworthy that the AIDS virus has the same affinity to the T4 when it is expressed on human or mouse cells. Furthermore, anti-HIV antibodies co-precipitates the human T4 molecule and no other cellular components.[7]

Using a panel of MoAbs to T4, it has been

Fig. 1. Putative HIV binding site

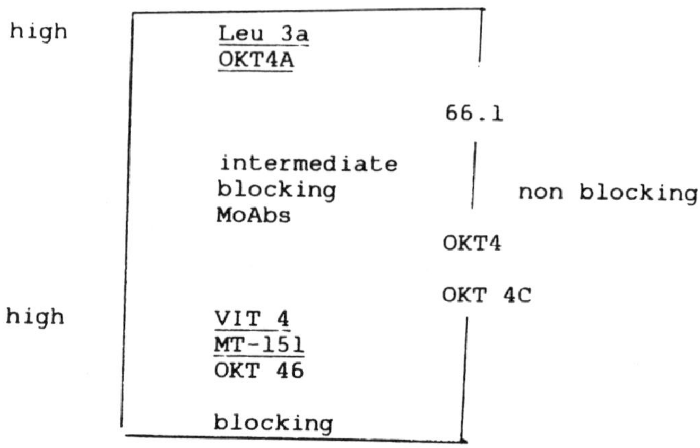

Legend
Putative binding site as determined by competitive inhibition of anti-T4 MoAb's, showing two groups of high titre blocking MoAb's

Table 1
Anti-ID and Anti HIV Reactivity of antisera

Immunising MAB	Mouse No.	RIA anti-ID binding	S.I. by reciprocal dilution of sera			
			Virus isolate			
			H93B	ARV-2	IIIRF	RUT
MT 151	1	2000				
	2	3000				
Leu 3a	1	1740	80	160	40	40
	2	1840	40	80	20	40
			Q. Sattentau, P. Beverley			
Leu 3a	3	>5000	100	100	100	100
	4	> 900	100	100	50	100
	5	>2900	10	10	10	10
Controls	6	126				
	7	300		1/10		

shown that only a few of them efficiently block infectivity (greater than 1:3200), whereas the majority of them block infection only moderately and some of them have no effect on blocking whatsoever, yet clearly bind to the T4 molecule (e.g. OKT4). This strongly suggests that only a particular epitope of T4 is required for HIV infection. We used cross competition assays with radiolabelled anti-T4 antibodies to map the epitopes detected by these antibodies and showed that at least 2 groups of MoAbs against two different epitopes can efficiently block virus antibodies (Fig. 1). Therefore these MoAbs were selected for raising anti-idiotypes that would block virus infection. Initial experiments with MT151 produced strong specific idiotype binding with no neutralising activity. However, mice immunised with anti Leu-3a and OKT 4A produce which neutralise virus infectivity of all tested isolates, in marked contrast, to sera raised against the envelope gene, Q. Sattentau and P. Beverley, A.G. Dalgleish *et al.*, manuscript in preparation (Table 1). Furthermore, MoAbs which recognise the idiotype of anti-Leu-3a and OKT4A have been raised which neutralise HIV, although not as strongly as the polyclonal sera (Kennedy *et al.*, in press, Table 2).

One of these MoAbs (HFI 7) not only binds the immunising antibody (anti Leu-3a) but also the viral envelope as shown by IF and Western blotting. Specific binding to the HIV envelope by polyclonal sera is not as strong as that shown by the MoAb.

Further studies in a variety of animals, using a number of non competing antibodies to T4, with a number of different immunising schedules are now in progress. It may be possible to use an anti T4 to raise neutralising anti-idiotypes in man. Although there are problems which may make this approach difficult, such as the high affinity of the gp110 for the T4 molecule, as well as the more general problems associated with MoAb therapy in humans. Another approach would be

Table 2
Specificity and inhibition of HIV reverse transcriptase (R.T.) by MoAb idiotype HF 1.7

	HF 1.7	GB-2	
AIDS sera			
Binding to HIV ELISA	0.75 ± 0.08	0.05 ± 0.01	1.2 ± 0.11
Reduction in R.T. as compared to control	61% (91%)	2% (13%)	N.T.

Where GB-2 is a negative anti-id control.
The reduction of RT is shown for a virus concentration of TCID$_{50}$ of 1000 and for a TCID$_{50}$ of 100 in parenthesis.

if just the binding domain (when confirmed, see ref. 6), could be administered.

REFERENCES

1. Dalgleish AG *et al.* 1984. Nature 312, 763-766.
2. Klatzmann D *et al.* 1984. Nature 312, 767-768.
3. Dalgleish AG 1986. J Royal Coll Physicians 20, 258-268.
4. Weiss RA *et al.* 1985. Nature 316, 69-72.
5. Weiss RA *et al.* 1986. Nature 324, 572-575.
6. Maddon PJ *et al.*1986. Cell 47, 333-348.
7. McDougal *et al.* 1986. Science 231, 382-385.
8. Sattentau *et al.* 1986. Science 234, 1120-1123.

VI. VACCINE APPROACHES AGAINST HIV

Human Retroviruses, Cancer, and AIDS:
Approaches to Prevention and Therapy, pages 291–311

PERSPECTIVES IN THE QUEST FOR A VACCINE AGAINST AIDS

Maurice R. Hilleman

Merck Institute for Therapeutic Research
Merck Sharp & Dohme Research Laboratories
West Point, Pennsylvania 19486 U.S.A.

ABSTRACT The urgent need for a vaccine against human immunodeficiency virus, HIV, far exceeds the probability for its development in the near future. This review presents an extensive but simplified overview of the technically complex problems involved and the approaches that might lead to their resolution. Brief attention is given to the political, social, ethical, and regulatory restraints that figure into the equation. The best hope is that the AIDS problem can be resolved practically without fully understanding it technically.

The rapid spread of AIDS caused by human immunodeficiency virus, HIV, presents a crisis of potentially phenomenal magnitude that has been likened to the great plagues of history. Spread of the virus to much of the world geography (1), and alarming increases in infection outside the traditional high-risk groups in the U.S.A. (2), has triggered a major thrust toward prevention and control of the disease.

APPROACHES TO CONTROL

The hope to control AIDS (Table 1) rests on epidemiologic, chemotherapeutic and/or vaccine approaches. Traditional case finding and contact tracing is downplayed because of perceptions of

TABLE 1

Approaches to the Control of AIDS

Epidemiologic	
Case finding, screening	Infringes individual rights. There is no cure for infection. Quarantine is impractical.
Education	Breakdown of social and moral traditions. Persuasive alteration of behavior and imposition of mechanical barriers. Fear as a control measure.
Chemotherapy	Viral integration of viral DNA into host DNA. Cure of infection is not feasible. Palliative suppression of clinical disease.
Vaccine	The "Great Hope" but beset with problems and lack of effective precedents.

infringement of individual rights in controlling a disease for which there is no cure and for which quarantine is impractical.

Education, therefore, is the present mainstay for epidemiologic control with the intent to alter human behavior and to introduce mechanical barriers in sexual practice. HIV transmission has been nurtured by a breakdown in the moral codes and social traditions of the past that were created for the purpose of limiting the chance for effective contact between communicable disease agents and their susceptible hosts. There is little doubt that cessation of sexual promiscuity and drug abuse could bring HIV transmission to a halt tomorrow, but that seems unlikely to happen.

In a cartoon that appeared in the February 9, 1987 issue of Current Contents, Cenozoic man thumbed his nose at extinct Mesozoic Monsters. In real life, contemporary man thumbs his nose at living Viral Monsters. Whether explicit language and gentle persuasion will put down the HIV Monster remains to be seen. Old-time Fear is a powerful weapon and might be used propitiously to convey a need for respect for this Modern Leviathan.

Control of viral infections by chemotherapeutic agents is a science that is still too primitive to cope. The chance for cure of infections in which the viral DNA is integrated into that of the host cell is near to impossible, unless one kills the host itself. The best hope for drugs against AIDS is in chemical suppression of viral activity with resultant clinical palliation, using substances that of themselves are not excessively toxic. Past problems with chemical control of viral infections have centered on unsatisfactory toxicity:activity ratios. Newer understanding of the biochemistry of viral replication brings emphasis to the development of drugs against proteins, particularly enzymes and regulatory substances that are produced under the viral genetic code. Such inhibitors offer the best opportunity for specificity of action against the virus while sparing host cell activities, thereby reducing the chance for toxicity and serious side effects.

The great contemporary hope is for prevention of HIV infection by vaccines that have worked so well against other diseases in the past and have provided an easy way out. Funding for the HIV vaccine effort is substantial and the confidence being placed in the virologist-molecular biologist-immunologist is perhaps more flattering than deserved, since the data base for an HIV vaccine is so inadequate and since the problems are so complex.

THE TROUBLE WITH HIV

HIV creates a worst possible scenario of adverse circumstances that is unparalleled for any other known virus (Figure 1). The virus evidently travels both as

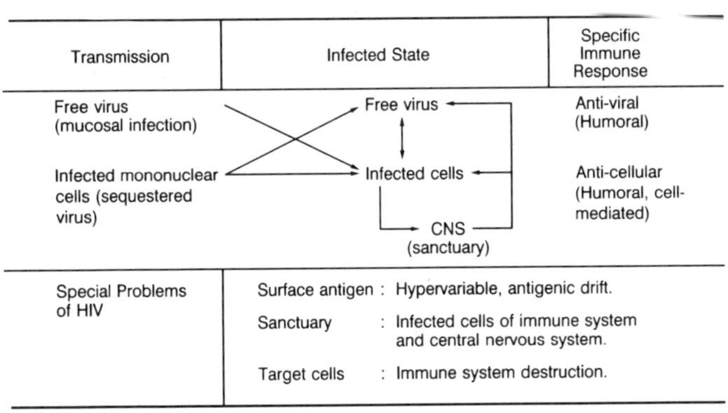

FIGURE 1. Infection, replication, retention, response to HIV.

free particles and within infected mononuclear cells where it is protected from neutralizing antibody and can pass the infection on by cell-to-cell transfer. The virus can also hide in the central nervous system beyond the blood-brain barrier from which it can launch new intrusions into the host at large at any time it chooses to do so. The gene that encodes the surface antigen has hypervariable regions and the virus shows antigenic drift with substantial antigenic differences between isolates (3). Most importantly, the virus destroys the very immune cells in the host that are intended to combat infectious disease agents.

Vaccines are an immunologic tool for prevention and must be given in advance of exposure to infection. They do not cure disease, but may be able to abort some early infections in long incubation diseases such as rabies and hepatitis B. Vaccines against AIDS would properly be given to uninfected persons and would need to be designed to impart an immunity of broad antigenic spectrum against _both_ virus and infected cells.

HIV VIRUS

HIV is a retrovirus (Figure 2) and consists of a lipid bilayer envelope that bears a major envelope

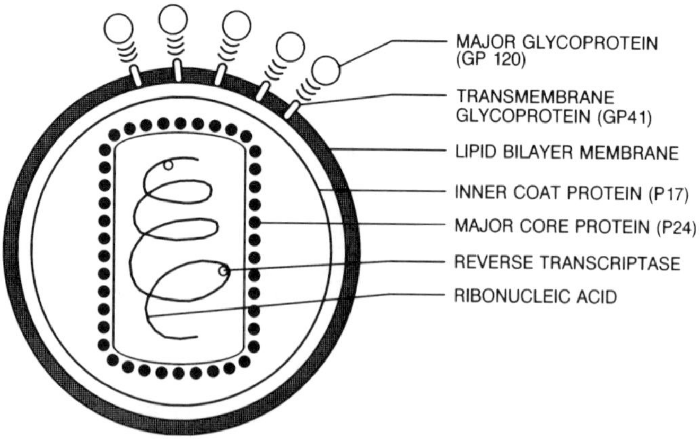

FIGURE 2. Stylized version of HIV (After Gallo, Bolognesi, _et al_.).

glycoprotein, gp120, and a transmembrane segment gp41, that anchors both itself and the gp120 to the particle. Inside the envelope are an inner coat protein and the nucleocapsid or core that bears the viral RNA with its reverse transcriptase. The outer membrane, gp120, carries the acceptor site for the CD4 receptor of susceptible T4 and certain other cells and is responsible for cell fusion by the virus. In most viral infections, the virus travels free and is susceptible to destruction by neutralizing antibody on contact with the immune host. HIV differs in that it may travel within infected cells as provirus or in unassembled form and, in addition, contains at least three regions of hypervariability in its major envelope glycoprotein that may render it insusceptible to neutralization by antibody induced in response to antigenically different strains.

LESSONS FROM COMPARATIVE VIROLOGY (Table 2)

Retroviruses share the attribute of a lipid envelope with both DNA and RNA viruses of the Myxovirus, Herpesvirus, and Hepadnavirus families. Rubeola virus travels as a free agent of constant antigenic structure, and immunity is imparted by neutralizing antibody against the fusion factor on the surface of the virus particle. Influenza virus also travels as a free

TABLE 2
Attributes of Selected Enveloped Viruses

Attribute	Virus				
	Orthomyxo- (Influenza A)	Paramyxo- (Rubeola)	Herpes- (Simplex)	Hepadna- (Hep. B)	Retro- (HIV)
Packaging	RNA	RNA	DNA	DNA (→RNA-DNA)	RNA (→DNA-RNA)
Travel	Virus	Virus	Virus	Virus	Virus and cells
Transmission	Respiratory	Respiratory	Respiratory contact, sex	Sex and blood	Sex and blood
Integration	No	No	Yes	Yes	Yes
Surface antigen variation	Drift-shift	Stable	Stable	Stable	Drift
Immunity	Anti-surface and core	Anti-surface fusion (F)	Anti-surface GP	Anti-surface and core	?
Vaccine	Subunit HA, NA	Live virus	Surface GP	Surface S	?

HA = Hemagglutinin; NA = Neuraminidase; GP = Glycoprotein; S = Surface Antigen.

particle, but must undergo constant antigenic drift and shift in the antigenic specificity of its surface hemagglutinin in order to survive in the experienced human population. There may be some group-specific immunity also since T helper cells (4) recognize a cross-reactive segment of the hemagglutinin that lies in an invariant epitope at the carboxy terminus of the hemagglutinin molecule that is discrete from the binding site of humoral antibody. Additionally, cytotoxic T cells that are active against influenza virus-infected cells appear to be directed against antigen encoded by the virus nucleoprotein gene (4,5). There is no licensed vaccine against herpes simplex virus, but experimental vaccines prepared using outer membrane glycoproteins may impart protective immunity in animals (6). The virus or its genome finds sanctuary in ganglion cells from which it may be activated to cause virus lesions in the skin or mucosa innervated by the corresponding peripheral nerves. This takes place in spite of high a level of neutralizing antibody in the circulation. Hepatitis B virus, like HIV, is blood and sex-transmitted, and goes through RNA-DNA interconversion but, unlike HIV, packages DNA rather than RNA in the virion. Hepatitis B virus DNA integrates into the hepatocyte genomes of some individuals resulting in late sequelae such as cirrhosis or hepatocarcinoma. Prophylactic immunity against hepatitis B is imparted by the invariant a epitopes of the surface antigen of the virus particle. Partial protection against challenge has also been demonstrated in chimpanzees by antibodies against core antigen or its associated e antigen (7,8). It appears that core and e antigens may be present on the surface of cells that are infected with the virus, and it appears also that humoral and/or cell-mediated immune mechanisms may be present in hepatitis B that are functional at the level of the infected hepatocyte (9). Like hepatitis B, viral internal antigens have been identified in the surface membrane of cells infected with murine or feline retroviruses (10-12).

The important takeaway messages from the influenza and hepatitis B examples, I believe, is that invariant conserved antigens may be recognized by the immune system within surface glycoproteins, and invariant gag gene-encoded core antigens may find their way into the membranes of infected cells providing a basis for specific immunologic recognition and removal of cells that are infected with the agent. Findings of this kind provide a weak but valid basis for hope that an effective vaccine against HIV might be developed.

SEARCH FOR EPITOPES

The genome of HIV (Figure 3) is complex and encodes a substantial variety of antigens and immunologic determinants, called epitopes. The virus genome (3) consists of at least seven genes and these encode the envelope (env) glycoproteins; the internal structural (gag) proteins; the polymerase (pol) and other enzymes;

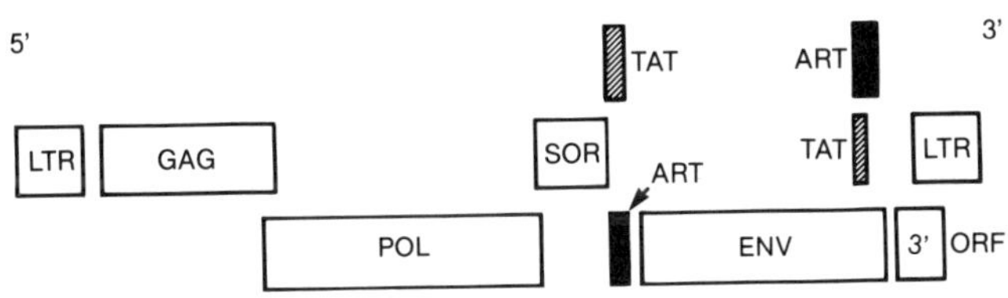

FIGURE 3. Genetic structure of HIV (HTLV-III) virus. (Modified from Reitz & Gallo).

and the tat, art, sor and 3'orf gene products that are regulatory in function or of unknown action.

The quest for vaccine is directed toward broad-spectrum immunologic blocking of infection by both free virus and infected cells. Any and all epitopes encoded by the virus have been fair game, as reviewed recently by Fischinger, et al. (13, see also 14). Constant regions of the envelope glycoproteins will be of interest if they can induce antibody that neutralizes the virus or blocks attachment to CD4 receptor on T4 and other cells. Epitopes encoded by the gag and other internal antigen genes will be of interest if they are broad-spectrum and if they find their way into the surface membranes of infected cells where they may provide a basis for specific immunologic recognition.

Bolognesi (15) has suggested the possibility for preventing attachment of a protruding CD4 receptor on the T4 cells to an acceptor site on gp120. He recognizes that the acceptor on HIV, as for certain Picornaviruses (16), may consist of a highly conserved region that lies protected between the steep walls of a deep cleft ("canyon hypothesis") on gp120. The site may be inaccessible to antibody and a more hopeful approach may lie in blockade of entry to the canyon by antibody against the antigenic constituents of the external rim of the canyon. This effort may be hindered, however, (15) if the rim determinants are encoded by the hypervariable regions of the envelope gene with resulting antigenic diversity.

Concerted efforts are being made to find antigens and epitopes both in whole virus and in segments of viral proteins that are produced by chemical synthesis or by recombinant technology employing vectors bearing gene fragments of HIV. First emphasis in vaccine development has been made in studies of envelope antigens, while the search for internal antigens is following. It is too early either to predict or to evaluate whether important and meaningful progress has already been made.

EPITOPE DELIVERY SYSTEMS

Modern technology has provided a variety of means whereby immunologically important epitopes, once found, can be used (Table 3) to immunize, and these fall into

TABLE 3

Epitope Delivery Systems

Kind	Cautions and Comments
Live Virus	
Natural or genetic attenuation	Mutation, reversion, recombination with or transactivation by indigenous viruses, activation of cellular protooncogenes ("promoter insertion").
Recombinant viral vectors	Virulence, immune response to vector, altered tissue tropism.
Non-living	
Whole killed	Inactivation of double-stranded DNA contaminants, immunosuppression and enhancement.
Subunit	Requirement for appropriate folding, glycosylation (?).
Synthetic	Poor antigenicity and carrier coupling problems; limitation to contiguous polypeptide epitopes.
Recombinant	
Transformed mammalian cells	Residual DNA: Oncogenic transforming virus, oncogenic viral promoters, retroviral contamination.
Yeast	Practical and proved. Scale-up is readily doable. Possible need for appropriate glycosylation.
Antiidiotype	Futuristic. No practical examples.

two broad categories of live or non-living virus vaccines.

Live virus vaccines.

Live virus vaccines against AIDS might consist either of live attenuated HIV or apathogenic live virus vectors into which the genes that express the appropriate HIV antigens and epitopes have been inserted. Live HIV, whether it be an avirulent virus of nature such as HIV-2 (17) that is found in West Africa, or a virus that has been altered genetically in the laboratory, suffers from lack of knowledge of what constitutes attenuation. There are added theoretical and real problems of mutation, reversion to virulence, intracellular genetic recombination with or transactivation by indigenous viruses, activation of cellular protooncogenes by "promoter insertion" and the like (13). Because of these problems, a live attenuated HIV vaccine does not seem a viable possibility.

Attenuated live virus vectors such as herpesviruses, adenoviruses, or particularly vaccinia virus (18,19), carrying an inserted genetic sequence for HIV antigens have been considered for vaccine use, but there are serious concerns. Vaccinia virus, as an example, is not completely avirulent and may cause serious complications, especially when given to persons who are immunocompromised. There will be limitation of viral proliferation and antigen production in previously vaccinated or revaccinated persons due to host immune response to the vector. Additionally, there is the possibility of altering the vector so as to change its tissue tropism or pathogenicity, making it deleterious to the recipient. The most serious limitation of all live virus vaccines is that their safety must be tested for and established in very extensive studies in man that might not be able to be carried out because of ethical and legal liability concerns.

Non-living vaccines.

Non-living virus vaccines are also of two kinds - those consisting of inactivated whole virus and those consisting of viral subunit antigens extracted from the whole virus or produced in the laboratory through application of recombinant technology or by chemical synthesis.

Killed whole retrovirus vaccine, such as the retrovirus D vaccine tested recently in monkeys (20), would not predict success for killed HIV virus unless it were possible to include an appropriate mixture of viral strains that would induce an adequately broad-spectrum immunity against both free virus and infected cells. Killed vaccines impose special issues for safety since the most frequently used inactivating agent, formaldehyde, would not be able to attach to and inactivate contaminating double-stranded DNA (21). Additionally, killed vaccines have been shown in other retroviral systems in mice and cats to cause immunosuppression in the host or enhancement of disease on challenge with live virus (13).

The most likely approach to an AIDS vaccine is that of subunit antigens that fold appropriately to present immunologically meaningful epitopes. Glycosylation of the proteins appears not to be essential, at least for those epitopes studied to date (22,23). Synthetic oligopeptides, that are highly useful in the discovery of epitopes related to immunity, suffer from poor immunizing capability unless satisfactorily coupled to carrier proteins. The synthetic antigen approach is limited also to contiguous epitopes comprised of a linear sequence of amino acids.

The most likely approach to a subunit HIV vaccine is by polypeptide production by application of recombinant technology in appropriate host cells. Antigen production using transformed mammalian cells (21,24,25) is hampered by the need for <u>total</u> removal of contaminating DNA originating from integrated or vector promoter sequences derived initially from oncogenic viruses. Indigenous retroviral contamination may also be present. Transfected yeast cells using yeast gene promoters do not have this safety problem (25), and the process for antigen production has been proved to be practical and doable in the recombinant hepatitis B vaccine example (26). Hepatitis B surface antigen (26) and some identified HIV surface antigens do not require glycosylation for specificity or immunogenicity (13,22,23), since the amino acid backbone alone may present the appropriate epitopes. Antigen glycosylation, if needed for some HIV antigens, might possibly be more appropriate when produced in mammalian than in yeast cells, but there is heterogeneity in the kind of glycosylation among all cell types (27), and there is no example to establish that antigen produced in mammalian cells is superior to any other.

Antiidiotype antibodies, that are produced by immunization against the variable region of specific antibody and that present an image of the original antigen, have been considered for miscellaneous vaccine application (28). In the practical sense, however, there is no present example of a successful antiidiotype vaccine just as there is no example of an adequate synthetic vaccine.

ANTIGEN PRESENTATION AND ADJUVANTATION (Table 4)

Any killed whole virus or subunit vaccine against HIV would probably require, or at least benefit from, immunopotentiation by substances such as alum that is acceptable for routine use in man, or by experimental devices such as incorporation into liposomes or by micellar aggregation as has been applied experimentally to hepatitis B vaccine (29). Immunostimulatory complexes, or ISCOMS (30), are formed by the capture of hydrophobic segments of monomeric polypeptides with Quil A glycoside to form matrices that greatly enhance immune

TABLE 4

Epitope Presentation and Adjuvantation in Non-Living Vaccines

Alum	Used routinely. Permits incorporation of added non-specific immune potentiators.
Experimental	
Liposomes	Presentation of epitopes on surface of lipid. Permits incorporation of enhancers such as MDP.
Micellar Aggregation	Optimizes presentation and enhances immune responses. Hepatitis B example.
ISCOM	Immunostimulatory complexes formed by capture of monomeric polypeptides with Quil A glycoside into a matrix.
Allison's SAF-1	Incorporation of polypeptides with pluronic polymer and muramyl dipeptide-threonine (MDP-T) on spherules of squalene.
Freund's mineral oil adjuvants	Complete with added mycobacteria or incomplete. Safety issues of tissue damage, autoimmune responses, carcinogenicity, non-metabolizability.

responses. Allison's adjuvant (SAF-1) (31) consists of spherules of squalene that incorporate the desired polypeptide with a pluronic polymer and muramyl dipeptide-threonine (MDP-T). This adjuvant shows real promise and deserves special consideration in efforts to prepare a vaccine against HIV, since it promotes both humoral and cell-mediated immune responses. Freund's complete (with added *Mycobacteria*) or incomplete adjuvants are useful tools for animal experimental use, but cannot be considered for routine application to man because of safety issues that include tissue damage, autoimmune responses, carcinogenicity, and non-metabolizability of the mineral oil.

IMMUNOLOGIC SURPRISES IN VACCINATION, A BASIS FOR CAUTION

A frequent though inconstant sequel to vaccination is the development of side-reactions. These may be due to residual virulence of attenuated live viruses that may be necessary to be adequately immunogenic. Adverse reactions to non-living immunogens may result from toxicity or adverse immunoresponsiveness to killed viruses or to their individual components when presented out of context with each other. Because of this, exhaustive pre-clinical testing in animals needs to be carried out and extreme caution must be observed in clinical tests in man.

Retrovirus example.

There are examples of adverse reactions and unexpected responses to vaccines, including those against retroviruses. I feel sure that Jarrett (see 13) must have been surprised when he found that his inactivated feline leukemia virus vaccine, that was poorly immunogenic, actually potentiated the disease on challenge in cats with the same live virus as compared with controls that had not been vaccinated. Likewise, it was probably surprising to learn that transmembrane glycoprotein of animal retroviruses could induce immune suppression, though the very small amount of antigen needed for inclusion in a vaccine would hardly cause any great amount of immunologic impairment. It has been reasonable also to express concern for residual amounts of protoviral DNA in vaccine preparations (21,25) since formaldehyde has no means to inactivate double-stranded DNA and since the insertion of viral LTR's, even though truncated, in proximity to cellular genes could be deleterious (13). This kind of concern has been supported by the classic "promoter-insertion" hypothesis whereby integration of LTR's of avian leukosis virus upstream or downstream from a cellular oncogene may cause lymphoma at a later time (13).

Paramyxovirus example (Figure 4).

Contemporary live attenuated measles virus vaccine is exemplary for its safety and efficacy. The same cannot be said either for killed whole measles virus vaccine or for subunit hemagglutinin vaccine. It was shown in the mid-1960's (32) that children who had received a formalin-killed measles virus vaccine lost their immunity quite rapidly and developed an altered host response on subsequent infection with the virus. Previously vaccinated children, who were exposed to measles virus in nature, developed fever and pain followed by maculopapular rash with petechial vesiculation and urticaria. Peripheral edema and pneumonia, sometimes with pleural effusion, were noted in most patients. Local swelling with maculopapular

First Experience	Antibody Responses		Consequence
	Primary	Viral Exposure* (Proliferation)	
Live Virus Vaccine (or natural infection)			
Fusion antigen (F)	Anti-F →	Boost →	Immunity
Hemagglutinin (HA)	Anti-HA →	Boost	
Formalin-Killed Vaccine (or HA subunit)			
Fusion antigen (F)	Nil →	Viral proliferation →	HA:Anti-HA Complexes causing Generalized Arthus reactions
Hemagglutinin (HA)	Anti-HA →	Boost ↗	

* Natural exposure or revaccination with live virus vaccine.

FIGURE 4. Immunologic surprise: Paramyxovirus (Rubeola).

rash was also seen in killed vaccine recipients who subsequently received live measles virus vaccine. Lennon (see 32) suggested that delayed hypersensitivity might have been induced by the killed vaccine, but Buser (33) suggested that an Arthus reaction was responsible. Analogous reactions have been observed wth respiratory syncytial (RS) virus infections in animals and children who had previously received formalin-killed RS vaccine (34).

It is now known that antibody against the hemagglutinin of measles virus imparts only temporary immunity against measles virus. Antibody against the fusion antigen of the virus, which is critical to induction of immunity, did not appear following use of formalin-killed vaccine since this antigen was destroyed by formaldehyde treatment. Buser's Arthus explanation (33) gains credibility in the light of these observations.

Infection with live measles virus in nature or on vaccination with attenuated live virus induces antibody against both hemagglutinin and fusion antigen, imparting immunity that appears to be lifelong. Immunization with formalin-killed vaccine induces antibody against hemagglutinin alone and protection is of short duration. Exposure to live virus results in unsuppressed measles virus proliferation, while at the same time, inducing a very rapid anamnestic production of antibody against the hemagglutinin. The virus and the anti-hemagglutin antibody, both present in large amount, may form immune complexes that cause an Arthus response.

Hypothetical Hepadnavirus Example (Figure 5).

There is a reported (35) hepatitis B virus example that is probably spurious but that conjures up theoretical concerns for an HIV vaccine that might be aimed at the raising of antibody against the acceptor sequence on the virus which attaches to the CD4 receptor on the host cell referred to above.

Hepatitis B surface antigen is comprised of an S antigen region, that alone stimulates solid and lasting immunity against hepatitis B virus infection, plus a pre-S antigen region that bears the viral acceptor for the host cell receptor whereby attachment of virus to hepatocyte is achieved. In truncated and simplified

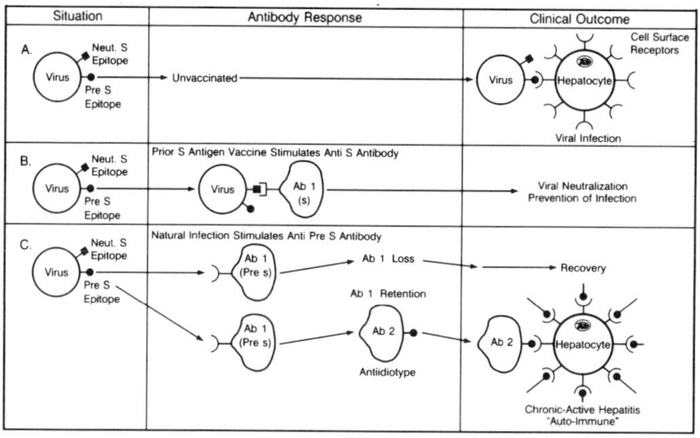

FIGURE 5. Hypothetical immunologic surprise conjured up from hepatitis B.

version, Hellström, et al. (35) reported finding that persons who convalesced satisfactorily from hepatitis B infection quickly lost their antibody against pre-S antigen. By contrast, persons who showed persistence of pre-S antibody went on to develop chronic liver disease. Hellström, et al. explained their findings on the basis of a failure in the down regulation of production of antibody against pre-S antigen. They suggested that antigen in the pre-S region which might be involved in recognition of host self-components should not be considered suitable for vaccines.

Both the basic observations and interpretations of Hellström et al. have been severely attacked (36,37). But the final truth of the matter is unimportant since the Hellström example is being used here to point out a need for caution in developing HIV vaccines that may be directed toward eliciting antibody which will react with the viral acceptor site and block the attachment of virus to host cell receptors.

In the hypothetical hepatitis B example, virus particles in exposed non-immune persons attach to hepatocyte receptors via pre-S acceptor determinants. This leads to viral infection.

Prior immunization of persons with S antigen alone induces antibody that combines with a neutralizing epitope on the virus surface and solid protection is afforded. However, persons who retain their pre-S antibody (Ab1) might reasonably develop antiidiotype antibody (Ab2) that bears the image of the original pre-S acceptor. Such Ab2 might be capable of binding to the hepatocyte receptors bringing about an auto-destructive response of immunologic origin directed against liver cells. Any viral vaccine that is aimed at providing immunity through stimulation of antibodies against the acceptor site might carry this theoretical liability in the event of failure to downgrade antiidiotype (Ab2) responses.

There are no hard data to implicate any adverse response induced by a HIV vaccine since there is no HIV vaccine, at least as of now. The examples given do, however, provide bases for caution and for a need to collect adequate laboratory and animal data on "immunologic safety" before proceeding to clinical trials in man.

The takeaway message from the measles example is that manipulated whole virus antigens or subunit antigens given alone may induce immune responses that are incomplete or are out of context with the natural play of events and may produce immunologic damage rather than protection.

The message from the hypothetical hepatitis B example is that the administration of antigens or monoclonal antibodies (Ab1) that directly or indirectly raise antibodies that attach to host cell receptors may carry large liabilities, even though they might provide a convenient means for preventing viral access to host cells. Importantly, cell receptors must have a purpose in the cell economy, and rendering them non-functional may cause an adverse effect. Additionally, antibodies attached to cell receptors may invite the same kinds of adverse immune response that are believed to be responsible for a variety of autoimmune disorders.

OVERVIEW AND CONCLUSION

Whether and when there might be an effective vaccine against AIDS caused by HIV is clearly open to question. The available data are insufficient to make a meaningful scientific projection either now or in the near future. Even assuming technical resolution of the scientific problems, there still remains the question of incentive for commercial development of a product that may find only a small market and may carry large liability issues for which legislated protection against lawsuits is only a possibility.

Testing of vaccine for protective efficacy in man will be fraught with moral and ethical issues since randomized, double-blind, placebo- controlled trials will need to be conducted. The chimpanzee, which is the only meaningful model for vaccine evaluation at present, is in such short supply as, perhaps, to reverse the traditional concepts for judging the relative worth of man and beast. Chimpanzees, e.g., just might be reserved exclusively for protective efficacy challenge tests and may be committed for this purpose only after adequate pre-chimpanzee testing has been carried out in man. Long-term observations for safety and protective efficacy for any licensed vaccine for use in man will need to be carried out in human beings, and it will be important not to attempt to interfere with the behavior of the volunteers at a time when health education alone might be able to reduce the likelihood of HIV infection in the test subjects - a moral dilemma!

All this brings to mind a recent commentary by Bernard Dixon (38) in his essay on "A Lesson from Louis Pasteur on AIDS Vaccine." Dixon points out that Pasteur, a medically non-qualified person, gave a secretly contrived and untested substance of unknown composition and toxicity to rabies virus-exposed persons with no attempt to solicit informed consent and some of his patients died. Pasteur clearly violated all the then non-existing precepts of the Investigative New Drug Laws (IND) and professional ethics as well. Yet Pasteur, in this brash epoch in medical history, achieved thunderous acclaim for his irresponsible experiments and pushed the science of vaccines by a quantum leap forward. Dixon suggests that Pasteur enjoyed inspirational good fortune but cynics might pass off simply as another adventure of "Lucky Louie".

The parallel is that AIDS, like rabies, is a highly fatal disease in drastic need of prevention. The difference is that rabies vaccine was given to treat already exposed persons while AIDS vaccine would be given to prevent infection in normal individuals. This difference may be equalized by the potentially overwhelming number of HIV infections.

Mitchison (38) raised the question of why even the simplest approaches to a vaccine, such as killed whole virus, are not being given at least small-scale exploratory trials. Some early studies in man using preparations of undisclosed composition have already been initiated in Zaire (39), but, for the most part, elegant laboratory solutions are being sought for a problem of such potential importance that it might not be able to afford the price of elegance. Mitchison questioned whether lawyers and legislators may have too much grip on our society; perhaps the swing toward greater safety in biomedical innovation has gone too far.

No one, I'm sure, would suggest a return to those more relaxed and unregulated days when scientific irresponsibility could be carried to experiments in man. Yet the tremendous potential for harm from AIDS may give cause for rethinking the problem of biomedical regulation, especially if the disease runs rampant in the heterosexual population.

REFERENCES*

1. World Health Organization (1986). Acquired immunodeficiency syndrome (AIDS). Weekly Epidemiological Record 61:361.
2. Committee on a National Strategy for AIDS (1986). "Confronting AIDS: Directions for Public Health, Health Care, and Research." Washington: National Academy Press.
3. Gallo RC (1987). The AIDS Virus (Part II). Scientific American 25:47.
4. Cox JH, Lamb JR (1986). Cellular Immunity to viruses: Antigen recognition and effector function. Eos-Riv Immunol 6:197.
5. Townsend ARM, Gotch FM, Davey J (1985). Cytotoxic T cells recognize fragments of the influenza nucleoprotein. Cell 42:457.
6. Hilleman MR, Larson VM, Lehman ED, Salerno RA, Conard PG, McLean AA (1981). Subunit herpes simplex virus-2 vaccine. In Nahmias AJ, Dowdle WR, Schinazi RF (eds): "The Human Herpesviruses: An

*Where possible, general reviews are cited.

Interdisciplinary Perspective," New York: Elsevier North Holland, p 503.

7. Tabor E, Gerety RJ (1984). Possible role of immune responses to hepatitis B core antigen in protection against hepatitis B infections. The Lancet 1:172.

8. Murray K, Bruce SA, Hinnen A, Wingfield P, van Erd PMCA, de Reus A, Schellekens H (1984). Hepatitis B virus antigens made in microbial cells immunise against viral infection. EMBO J 3:645.

9. Mondelli M, Vergani GM, Alberti A, Vergani D, Portmann B, Eddleston ALWF, Williams R (1982). Specificity of T lympocyte cytotoxicity to autologous hepatocytes in chronic hepatitis B virus infection: Evidence that T cells are directed against HBV core antigen expressed on hepatocytes. J Immunol 129:2773.

10. van der Hoorn FA, Lahaye T, Muller V, Ogle MA, Engers HD (1985). Characterization of $gP85^{gag}$ as an antigen recognized by Moloney leukemia virus-specific cytolytic T cell clones that function in vivo. J Exp Med 162:128.

11. Pillemer EA, Kooistra DA, Witte ON, Weissman IL (1986). Monoclonal antibody to the amino-terminal L sequence of murine leukemia virus glycosylated gag polyproteins demonstrates their unusual orientation in the cell membrane. J Virol 57:413.

12. Holt CA, Osorio K, Lilly F (1986). Friend virus-specific cytotoxic T lymphocytes recognize both gag and env gene-encoded specificities. J Exp Med 164:211.

13. Fischinger PJ, Gallo RC, Bolognesi DP (1986). Toward a vaccine against AIDS: Rationale and current progress. The Mt Sinai J Med 53:639.

14. Frazer IH, Mulhall BP (1986). Second international conference on the acquired immune deficiency syndrome. Med J Australia 145:524.

15. Bolognesi DP. Personal communication. To be published.

16. Luo M, Vriend G, Kamer G, Minor I, Arnold E, Rossmann MG, Boege U, Scraba DG, Duke GM, Palmenberg AC (1987). The atomic structure of Mengo virus at 3.0 A resolution. Science 235:182.

17. Kanki PJ, Barin F, M'Boup S, Allan JS, Romet-Lemonne JL, Marlink R, McLane MF, Lee TH, Arbeille B, Denis F, Essex M (1986). New human T-lymphotropic retrovirus related to simian

T-lymphotropic virus type III ($STLV-III_{AGM}$). Science 232:238.
18. Chakrabarti S, Robert-Guroff M, Wong-Staal F, Gallo RC, Moss B (1986). Expression of the HTLV-III envelope gene by a recombinant vaccinia virus. Nature 320:535.
19. Zarling JM, Morton W, Moran PA, McClure J, Kosowski SG, Hu SL (1986). T-cell responses to human AIDS virus in macaques immunized with recombinant vaccinia viruses. Nature 323:344.
20. Marx PA, Pedersen NC, Lerche NW, Osborn KG, Lowenstine LJ, Lackner AA, Maul DH, Kwang HS, Kluge JD, Zaais CP, Sharpe V, Spinner AP, Allison AC, Gardner MB (1986). Prevention of simian acquired immune deficiency syndrome with a formalin-inactivated type D retrovirus vaccine. J Virol 60:431.
21. Hilleman MR (1979). Line cell saga - An argument in favor of production of biologics in cancer cells. In Petricciani JC, Hopps HE, Chapple PJ (eds): "Cell Substrates," New York: Plenum, p 47.
22. Barnes DM (1986). Strategies for an AIDS vaccine. Science 233:1149.
23. Chanh TC, Dreesman GR, Kanda P, Linette GP, Sparrow JT, Ho DD, Kennedy RC (1986). Induction of anti-HIV neutralizing antibodies by synthetic peptides. EMBO J 5:3065.
24. World Health Organization (1987). WHO meeting on cells for the production of biologicals. Weekly Epidemiological Record 62:13.
25. Hilleman MR, Ellis R (1986). Vaccines made from recombinant yeast cells. Vaccine 4:75.
26. Hilleman MR (1987). Yeast recombinant hepatitis B vaccine. Infection 15:3.
27. Van Brunt J (1986). Glycoprotein remodeling: There's nothing (quite) like the real thing. Bio/Technology 4:835.
28. Koprowski H (1985). Unconventional vaccines: Immunization with anti-idiotype antibody against viral diseases. Cancer Res (suppl) 45:4689s.
29. Skelly J, Howard CR, Zuckerman AJ (1981). Hepatitis B polypeptide vaccine preparation in micelle form. Nature 290:51.
30. Morein B, Simons K (1985). Subunit vaccines against enveloped viruses: virosomes, micelles and other protein complexes. Vaccine 3:83.

31. Allison AC, Byars NE (1986). An adjuvant formulation that selectively elicits the formation of antibodies of protective isotypes and of cell-mediated immunity. J Immunol Meth 95:157.
32. Fulginiti VA, Eller JJ, Downie AW, Kempe CH (1967). Altered reactivity to measles virus: Atypical measles in children previously immunized with inactivated measles virus vaccines. J Am Med Assoc 202:1075.
33. Buser F (1967). Side reaction to measles vaccination suggesting the Arthus phenomenon. N Eng J Med 277:250.
34. Murphy BR, Prince G, Wagner D, Walsh EE, Chanock RM (1986). The immune response of humans and cotton rats to respiratory syncytial virus (RSV) infection or formalin-inactivated vaccine. Abstract in "Modern Approaches to New Vaccines including Prevention of AIDS," Cold Spring Harbor; Cold Spring Harbor Laboratory, p 47.
35. Hellström U, Sylvan S, Kuhns M, Sarin V (1986). Absence of Pre-S2 antibodies in natural hepatitis B virus infection. The Lancet 2:889.
36. Alberti A, Pontisso P, Fraiese A (1986). Pre-S2 antibodies in hepatitis B. The Lancet 2:1457.
37. Aihara S, Ise I, Tsuda F, Takai E, Machida A, Miyakawa Y, Mayumi M (1986). Letter to the Editor. The Lancet 2:1457.
38. Dixon B (1986). A lesson from Louis Pasteur on AIDS vaccine. Bio/Technology 4:753.
39. Newmark P (1987). First human AIDS vaccine trial goes ahead without official OK. Nature 325:290.

Human Retroviruses, Cancer, and AIDS:
Approaches to Prevention and Therapy, pages 313–325

PROSPECTS FOR DEVELOPMENT OF A VACCINE AGAINST HIV

Thomas J. Matthews[1], H. Kim Lyerly[1], Kent J. Weinhold[1], A.J. Langlois[1], James Rusche[2], Scott D. Putney[2], Robert C. Gallo[3] and Dani P. Bolognesi[1*]

Duke University Medical Center, P.O. Box 2926, Durham, North Carolina 27710

Repligen Corporation, One Kendall Square, Cambridge, Massachusetts 02139

Laboratory of Tumor Cell Biology, National Cancer Institute, NIH, Bethesda, Maryland 20892

Introduction

With the etiology and diagnosis of AIDS largely resolved, the challenges for the future clearly lie in its prevention and treatment. Given the alarming projections for the spread of this epidemic within the world population over the next 5 years (1), development of vaccines, anti-viral strategies and immune restorative approaches are imperative. To achieve success in any of these, a better understanding of the virus, the course of infection and the process of disease progression is required. Remarkable progress has been made in defining the genomic structure of the virus as well as the function of its unique genetic elements. Many of the viral genes have been cloned and expressed both in prokaryotic and eukaryotic vectors. The availability of large quantities of these materials in pure form paves the way for both production of vaccines and design of anti-viral agents. Indeed, the life cycle processes of this retrovirus as well as understanding its mechanism of pathogenesis are well within our grasp.

This discussion will be limited to the possibility of developing a vaccine against the human retroviruses associated with AIDS. However, exclusion of all the necessary public health and educational measures should not detract from their critical value toward stemming the tide of infection with this agent in the human population. Likewise, the use of immunoprophylaxis with anti-viral immune elements or chemoprophylaxis mediated by anti-viral compounds could be very effective means of reducing virus load and preventing the onset of disease if applied sufficiently early after exposure. Indeed, it is the combined role of all approaches to prevention which will be necessary to make a significant impact on this disease (1).

Special Consideration for a Vaccine against AIDS

One can sum up the prospects for developing a vaccine as being difficult but achievable. A successful vaccine will have to overcome significant obstacles imposed by HIV and other AIDS-associated retroviruses. The first is the well recognized feature of extensive genomic diversity, particularly in the envelope gene (2), which is highly reminiscent of the situation with lentiviruses (3). An effective vaccine should contain all possible neutralization determinants either in the form of a single universal epitope or as an appropriate cocktail of individual epitopes that span the divergence of the virus in nature. At this point in time, it is not clear how either or both of these alternatives will be pursued.

The second major obstacle is equally foreboding. This is based on the distinct possibility that the disease is transmitted not only by free virus but also via infected cells. This situation, coupled with two unique features of the virus: (1) its ability to exist in latent form and (2) the capacity of infected cells expressing gp120 to fuse with uninfected cells generates mechanisms to disseminate the virus in covert form even in the face of an immune response. One significant hope to overcome these problems is for the vaccine to be able to induce virus specific cell mediated immunity. To accomplish this, not only will the appropriate viral antigens or epitopes need to be identified but also their optimal mode of presentation to the immune system. In addition, or perhaps even in place of cellular immunity, the generation of antibodies able to mediate ADCC (antibody dependent cell cytotoxicity) would be of considerable benefit.

Progress in Characterization of Potential Immunogens for Vaccine Strategies

The structural components associated with the envelope of retroviruses have thus far received the most attention with regard to vaccine strategies. This derives not only from their strategic location on the surface of the virion and the infected cell (4), but because they are responsible for the salient immunobiological properties of the virus such as host tropism, interference and neutralization (5). The envelope glycoproteins associated with HIV are derived from a precursor, gp160, that is proteolytically cleaved to generate the external envelope glycoprotein gp120 and the transmembrane envelope glycoprotein gp41 (Figure 1). Several lines of evidence support the notion that gp120 is involved in important biological processes related to the virus life cycle and that a subunit vaccine based on gp120 may be possible. 1) Antibodies that neutralize HIV infection have been found in sera of people with AIDS, ARC (AIDS related complex), as well as asymptomatic individuals infected with the virus (6,7) and such antibodies bind to affinity resins bearing purified gp120 (8); 2) gp120 elicits production of neutralizing antibodies (9) as does a large segment of gp120 produced in mammalian cells (10); and 3)

FIGURE 1

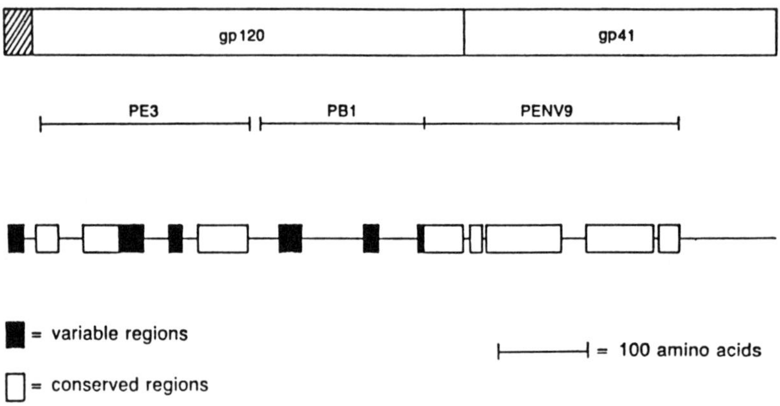

Location of proteins PB1, PE3, and PENV9 in relation to gp120 and gp41. The envelope is synthesized as a precursor, gp160, that is cleaved to give gp120 and gp41. The secretion signal sequence is hatched. The location of the variable and conserved regions are shown as darkened or open boxes, respectively.

direct binding of gp120 to the T4 receptor has been demonstrated and monoclonal antibodies recognizing certain epitopes of the virus receptor prevent viral infection (11,12). Recent studies have also shown that monoclonal antibodies that neutralize HIV are specific for a subregion of gp120 (M. Robert-Guroff, personal communication).

The protein backbone of gp120 represents approximately half of its apparent molecular weight on SDS gels (13) with the remainder consisting of carbohydrate. This extensive degree of glycosylation might be expected to play a role in the determination and accessibility of both binding and neutralizing epitopes. We recently undertook studies to determine the extent of carbohydrate involvement in both the induction of neutralizing antibodies to the virus and in binding of the envelope to CD4 as evidenced by inhibition of HTLV-III mediated cell fusion. To achieve this, antibodies raised against native gp120, gp120 from which the carbohydrate had been enzymatically removed, and selected recombinant fragments of gp120 expressed in *E. coli* were compared in various immunologic and biologic assays (13a also Matthews et al and Putney et al, this symposium).

Immunization with an *E. coli* recombinant segment at the carboxy-terminal half of gp120 (PB1) or with deglycosylated gp120 envelope protein produced antibodies that neutralize HIV infection *in vitro* which were surprisingly superior (10 fold in titer) to those obtained using purified native gp120 as immunogen. Other fragments, including some extending into the gp41 region, were not effective in this regard. Cross-absorption and direct antigen competition studies indeed localize the dominant neutralizing epitopes in PB-1 and document further that the same epitopes elicit antibodies which prevent virus mediated cell fusion (Fig. 2). These results indicate that a segment of the HTLV-III$_B$ envelope produced in *E. coli* may be an important ingredient of a vaccine for AIDS. Studies now in progress are aimed at further definition of the respective biological activities associated with PB-1 as well as other regions of the envelope.

However, in all cases the antibodies produced were specific for the isolate from which the immunogen was derived and did not neutralize divergent HIV viruses (8). This indicates that a variable region of gp120 is a dominant neutralizing epitope in the experimental animal models used

Figure 2

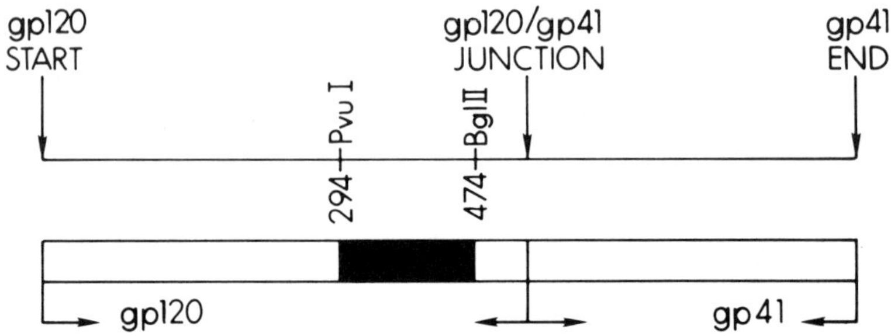

1. A SUBREGION OF GP120 IS RESPONSIBLE FOR INDUCTION OF ANTIBODIES THAT NEUTRALIZE VIRUS INFECTIVITY AND BLOCK CELL FUSION.

2. A BACTERIAL RECOMBINANT FRAGMENT (PB1) REPRESENTING THIS REGION CAN INDUCE HIGH TITERS OF NEUTRALIZING AND FUSION BLOCKING ANTIBODIES.

3. THE REPRESENTATIVE FRAGMENT CAN ITSELF BLOCK THE NEUTRALIZING AND CELL FUSION INHIBITORY ACTIVITIES OF VARIOUS ANTIBODIES RAISED TO LARGER COMPONENTS OF THE *ENV* GENE, INCLUDING GP160 AND GP120.

(goat, chimp); and while conserved regions elicit strong immune responses, the resultant antibodies do not prevent virus infectivity. These findings suggest that "cocktails" of divergent virus envelope components may be required for effective vaccination strategies.

A likely target of opportunity which would represent a conserved region of biologic significance is the binding site on gp120 for the CD4 lymphocyte surface marker. Recent studies demonstrate that binding to CD4 requires the presence of carbohydrate suggesting that a complex rather than a simple linear determinant may be responsible (14). However, this does not exclude the possibility that linear sequences are involved in the binding and that appropriate antibodies or specific peptides could specifically block this interaction. One such site was reported in the symposium by Laskey et al.

Anti-Viral Immune Responses which are Cytotoxic

Various investigative groups are attempting to define both humoral and cell mediated cytotoxic responses against HTLV-III infected cells. Recent studies using gp120 as an immunogen in various animal species, including sub-human primates, indicate that the molecule can induce both T-cell mediated immunity (15) and complement dependent cytotoxic antibodies (16). Similar activities were detected in chimpanzees infected with $HTLV\text{-}III_B$ (16) or with a recombinant vaccina virus containing the virus envelope gene (17). Although no complement fixing cytotoxic antibodies could be demonstrated in humans infected with HIV, virus specific cytotoxic T-cells have recently been identified (see Walker et al., this symposium).

Our recent studies also demonstrate the presence of antibodies in patients which mediate ADCC against virus infected targets (18). This activity was directed against a specific viral antigen, the envelope gp120. Furthermore, using normal CEM cells whose CD4 surface antigens were saturated with exogenously added gp120, virus specific cytotoxic lymphocytes were found in virus exposed individuals (19). The significance of these reactivities, particularly in relation to the stage of infection and disease progression, will be of interest to study and relevant to the vaccine issues discussed here. Definition of the epitopes on the virus envelop which represent targets for the cytotoxic activities is under investigation.

An important aspect with regard to generation of cell mediated immunity is the identity of the virus gene product(s) which are critical in this regard. Based on studies in other virus models (20), it is likely that not only the envelope but also the internal components of the virus may be required. This suggests that unique sequences may be responsible for recognition by T cells during antigen presentation. Two of these have recently been mapped to distinct regions of gp120 with one residing in the PB-1 region (20a). Nevertheless, while the neutralizing and certain T-cell epitopes reside on the virus envelope, a complex vaccine including the internal antigens may be needed to elicit the full immune spectrum necessary for protection against infection.

Animal Models for Pre-Clinical Vaccine Testing

An additional challenge toward developing a successful vaccine is an appropriate animal model where efficacy and safety can be determined. To date the chimpanzee is the only species which can be infected with the human viruses (21,22). Unfortunately, the chimp does not develop the full blown syndrome of AIDS, but a few immunological abnormalities are noted. While imperfect, it is adequate for testing the power of a vaccine preparation to resist challenge by either free virus and/or virus infected cells. At the present time, some promising immunogens are available which, in other animal species, have raised neutralizing antibodies. These are represented by the native gp120 in purified form (23,24), a recombinant gp120 expressed in mammalian cells (25) and recombinant envelope products produced in bacteria (13a) and yeast (26). The major drawbacks for vaccine testing of the chimp model are the scarcity of the animals, their expense and difficulties in handling and, last but not least, the assignation of the chimp as an endangered species. Efforts to find a smaller and more plentiful animal that can be infected with the human isolates would thus represent a major breakthrough in this regard. In this context the close resemblance of STLV-III with HIV indicates that the further development of the experimental models in rhesus macaques and African green monkeys will add a great deal to our knowledge in the meantime. Valuable lessons concerning the nature of immunity required to protect against infection can also be gained by exploiting other animal virus models, particularly those of the ruminant lentiviruses but not excluding either the feline or murine systems which have been so instructive thus far.

Independent of which model is used for testing, the issues of genomic diversity and mode of transmission will have to be seriously considered. Hence, the model must be amenable to challenge with different substrains of HIV including those which exhibit the greatest degree of diversity. In addition, inclusion of infected cells in the challenge will have to be addressed, as will issues such as mode of presentation, routes of inoculation, appropriate adjuvant and intense, immunologic monitoring of the inoculated animals (Figure 3) with particular attention to both neutralizing antibodies and cell-mediated immunity.

However, because any animal model for HIV infection and disease is likely to be imperfect, testing of primary vaccine candidates directly in man must proceed to determine safety, immunogenicity and efficacy.

Concluding Remarks

In summary, while the AIDS epidemic may eventually prove to be one of the most severe devastations by an infectious agent to affect mankind, it remains fortunate that it has occurred during a period when the biomedical community has the opportunity to deal with it. One must find considerable comfort in the vast knowledge that exists about retroviruses in general and their human counterparts in particular and expect that effective countermeasures against these agents will be developed. In the like manner, our rapidly expanding understanding of how the immune system functions will no doubt lead to specific approaches to restore the damage the virus has perpetrated. In both areas, modern biotechnology is likely to provide the methodology and capability of dealing with this problem on a world scale.

As one progresses down the avenues to control this disease, valuable principles will be gained which will apply to other human diseases associated with retroviruses. Because some of these represent malignant neoplasms (27), the opportunity to control a cancer by direct attack on the etiological agent clearly presents itself. The possibility that other widespread diseases such as autoimmune and degenerative syndromes might also involve this group of agents (28) further highlights the valuable byproducts of the intense studies in HIV and AIDS.

Figure 3

HYPOTHETICAL SCHEME FOR EVALUATING CANDIDATE VACCINE ANTIGENS

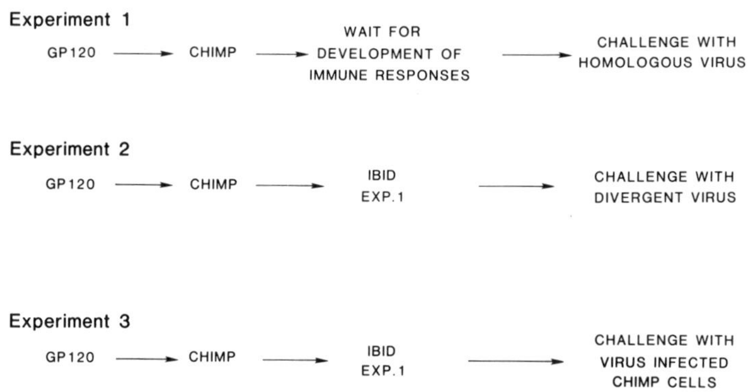

PARALLEL STUDIES SHOULD FOCUS ON:

1) Are other viral antigens necessary (or desirable) to achieve protective response?

2) Approaches to maximize the immunogenicity of viral subunits: role of adjuvants

3) Role of cell mediated immunity in protection

4) Impact of routes of immunization and challenge

5) Role of passively administered antibodies in protection

6) Assessment of immunotoxicity of viral subunit immunogens

REFERENCES

1. Coolfont Report: A PHS plan for prevention and control of AIDS and the AIDS virus. Public Health Reports 101:341, July-August, 1986.

2. Starcich, B.R., Hahn, B.H., Shaw, G.M., et al. Identification and characterization of conserved and variable regions in the envelope gene of HTLV-III/LAV, the retrovirus of AIDS. Cell 45:637-648, 1986.

3. Sonigo, P., Alizon, M., Staskus, K., et al. Nucleotide sequence of the visna lentivirus: Relationship to the AIDS virus. Cell, 42:369-382, 1985.

4. Bolognesi, D.P., Montelaro, R.C., Frank, H., et al. Assembly of type-C oncornaviruses: A model. Science 199:183-186, 1978.

5. Schafer, W. and Bolognesi, D.P. Mammalian C-type oncornaviruses: Relationship between viral, structural and cell surface antigens and their possible significance in immunological defense mechanisms. Contemporary Topics in Immunobiology 6:127-167, 1977.

6. Robert-Guroff, M., Brown, M. and Gallo, R.C. HTLV-III - neutralizing antibodies in patients w/AIDS and AIDS-related complex. Nature 316:72-74, 1985.

7. Weiss, R.A., Clapham, P.R., Cheingsong-Popov, R., et al. Neutralization of human T-lymphotropic virus type III by sera of AIDS and AIDS-risk patients. Nature 316:69-72, 1985.

8. Matthews, T.J., Langlois, A.J., Robey, W.G., et al. Restricted neutralization of divergent HTLV-III/LAV isolates by antibodies to the major envelope glycoprotein. PNAS, in press.

9. Robey, W.G., Arthur, L.O., Matthews, T.J., et al. Prospect for prevention of human immunodeficiency virus infection: Purified 120-kDa envelope glycoprotein induces neutralizing antibody. PNAS 83:7023-7027, 1986.

10. Lasky, L.A., Groopman, J.E., Fennie, C.W., et al. Neutralization of the AIDS retrovirus by antibodies to a recombinant envelope glycoprotein. Science 233:209-212, 1986.

11. Seligman, M., et al. Aids - An immunologic reevaluation. NEJM 311:1286, 1984.

12. McDougal, J.S., et al. Binding of HTLV-III/LAV to T4+ T cells by a complex of the 110K viral protein and the T4 molecule. Science 231:382, 1986.

13. Ratner, Haseltine, W., Patarca, R., et al. Complete nucleotide sequence of the AIDS virus, HTLV-III. Nature 313:277-284, 1985.

13a. Putney, S.D., Matthews, T.J., Robey, W.G., Et al. HTLV-III/LAV neutralizing antibodies to an e. coli produced fragment of the virus envelope. Science 234:1392-1398, 1986.

14. Matthews, T.J., Weinhold, K.J., Lyerly, H.K., et al. Interaction between HTLV-III_B envelope gp120 and CD4: Role of carbohydrate in binding and cell fusion. PNAS, in press.

15. Krohn, K., Robey, W.G., Putney, S.D., et al. Protective immune response towards HIV in animals immunized with HTLV-III_B envelope protein and in HIV-infected individuals. PNAS, in press.

16. Nara, P.L., Robey, W.G., Gonda, M.A., et al. Absence of cytotoxic antibody to HTLV-III - infected cells in man and its induction in animals after infection or immunization with purified gp120. PNAS, in press.

17. Zarling, J.M., Morton, W., Moran, P.A., et al. T-cell responses to human AIDS virus in macaques immunized with recombinant vaccinia viruses. Nature 323:344-346, 1986.

18. Lyerly, H.K., Weinhold, K.J., Matthews, T.J., et al. HTLV-III_B glycoprotein (gp120) bound to CD-4 determinants on normal lymphocytes serves as target for immune attack. PNAS, in press.

19. Weinhold, K.J., Nature, Submitted.

20. Townsend, A.R.M., Gotch, F.M., and Davey, J. Cytotoxic T cells recognize fragments of influenza nucleoprotein. Cell 42:457-467, 1985.

20a. Cease, K.B., Margalit, H., Cornette, J.L., Putney, S.D., Robey, W.G., Ouyang, C., Streicher, H.Z., Fischinger, P.J., Gallo, R.C., DeLisi, C., Berzofsky, J.A. Helper T cell site identification in the AIDS virus gp120 envelope protein and induction of immunity in mice to the mative protein using a 16-residue synthetic peptide. PNAS, in press, 1987.

21. Gajdusek, D.C., Amyx, H.L., Gibbs, Jr. C.J., et al. Infection of chimpanzees by human T-lymphotropic retroviruses in brain and other tissues from AIDS patients. Lancet 1:55-56, 1985.

22. Fultz, P.N., McClure, H.M., Swencon, R.B., et al. Persistent infection of chimpanzees with human T-lymphotropic virus type III/lymphadenopathy-associated virus: A potential model for acquired immunodeficiency syndrome. J. Virology 58:116, 1986.

23. Robey, W.G., Arthur, L.O., Matthews, T.J., et al. Prospect for prevention of human T-cell lymphotropic virus infection: Purified 120,000 dalton envelope glycoprotein induces neutralizing antibody. PNAS, in press.

24. Matthews, T.J., Langlois, A.J., Robey, W.G., et al. Restricted neutralization of divergent HTLV-III/LAV isolates by antibodies to the major envelope glycoprotein. PNAS, in press.

25. Lasky, L.A., Groopman, J.E., Fennie, C.W., et al. Neutralization of the AIDS retrovirus by antibodies to a recombinant envelope glycoprotein. Science 233:209-212, 1986.

26. Levy, J. Personal communication.

27. Sodroski, J., Patarca, R., Rosen, C., et al. Science 229:74-77, 1985.

28. Sodroski, J., Goh, W.C., Rosen, C., et al. A second post-transcriptional trans-activator gene required for HTLV-III replication. Nature 321:412, 1986.

Human Retroviruses, Cancer, and AIDS: Approaches to Prevention and Therapy, pages 327–340

T CELL MEDIATED IMMUNE RESPONSES TO HIV IN IMMUNIZED AND HIV-INFECTED PRIMATES[1]

Joyce M. Zarling,[2] Jorg G. Eichberg,[3] Patricia A. Moran,[2] Jan McClure,[4] William Morton,[5] Harvey Alter,[6] and Shiu-Lok Hu[2]

[2]ONCOGEN, Seattle, Washington 98121
[3]Southwest Foundation for Biomedical Research, San Antonio, Texas 78284
[4]Genetic Systems, Seattle, Washington 98121
[5]Regional Primate Center, University of Washington, Seattle, Washington 98195
[6]Department of Transfusion Medicine, National Institute of Health, Bethesda, Maryland 20892

ABSTRACT T cell-mediated immune responses to HIV were studied in non-human primates immunized with a recombinant vaccinia virus (v-env5) that expresses HIV envelope glycoproteins gp41 and gp110. Peripheral blood lymphocytes, with the phenotype of T cells, from v-env5 immunized macaques and chimpanzees showed strong proliferative responses following stimulation with purified HIV or HIV envelope glycoproteins ('env'). Cytotoxic T cell (CTL) clones directed against 'env' were also isolated from v-env5 immunized chimpanzees thus demonstrating that this immunization primes CTL and that HIV envelope glycoproteins serve as target antigens for CTL. T cells from chimpanzees infected with HIV for three months to three years showed strong proliferative responses to HIV and preliminary results suggest that some HIV infected healthy humans also have T cells that recognize HIV antigens.

[1]Supported in part by PHS grants R01 AI 23249 (to JMZ), RR 0016 (to WM) and NHLBI Contract N01-HB-2-7004 (to JGE).

INTRODUCTION

Human immunodeficiency virus (HIV) causes AIDS, which is a disease that is rapidly increasing in incidence in several developing vaccines against HIV. However, the immune mechanisms that may contribute to the prevention against infection with HIV or against the development of AIDS have not been elucidated and it is not yet clear which HIV antigens may be most important for inducing protective immunity. It is likely that neutralizing antibodies to HIV, which have been demonstrated in certain HIV-infected humans(1,2), may prevent against extracellular spread by the virus, but the virus can also spread from infected to uninfected cells by cell fusion and can thereby escape neutralizing antibodies. Antibodies that can lyse HIV-infected cells by antibody dependent cell-mediated cytotoxicity have recently been detected in healthy HIV seropositive individuals and less frequently, or at lower levels, in patients who have developed AIDS(3).

T cell-mediated immunity, which has been found to be very important in prevention against disease or death caused by a variety of envelope viruses in animals(4-9), may help eradicate HIV-infected cells which can express HIV antigens before spreading virus to uninfected cells. HIV-specific T helper cells may produce lymphokines, such as interleukin-2 (IL-2) to expand HIV-specific cytotoxic T cells or could produce other lymphokines which could activate other effector cells such as natural killer cells or macrophages to lyse HIV-infected cells.

Little has been reported concerning the ability of HIV or potential vaccines against HIV to induce HIV-specific T cell-mediated immunity in animals or man(10,11). Our studies have focused on whether infection with HIV or immunization with a potential AIDS vaccine can induce HIV-specific T cell mediated immunity in primates. Results of these studies, discussed herein, demonstrate that immunization of non-human primates with a recombinant vaccinia virus that expresses HIV envelope glycoproteins induces HIV-specific T helper cells in macaques and chimpanzees and also primes HIV-specific cytotoxic T cells in chimpanzees. In addition, we provide evidence that HIV-infected chimpanzees have strong T-cell mediated immunity to HIV and discuss studies carried out by us and others concerning T-cell mediated immunity to HIV in infected humans.

RESULTS

Induction of HIV-Specific T-Cells in Macaques Immunized with a Recombinant Vaccinia-HIV 'env' Virus

Several macaques (Macaca fascicularis) were immunized with v-env5 which expresses both HIV envelope glycoproteins, gp41 and gp110 and induces HIV-specific antibodies in mice(12). Four weeks following a second intradermal immunization with v-env5 or an unrelated recombinant vaccinia virus (v-HSV-gD1) that expresses herpes simplex virus (HSV) glycoprotein D(12), peripheral blood lymphocytes (PBL) were isolated from the blood of macaques by ficoll-hypaque gradient centrifugation. The PBL were suspended in RPMI 1640 medium containing 10% heat inactivated pooled normal human serum and were stimulated in microwells with sucrose gradient-purified HIV (1 µg/mL) or ultraviolet (UV) light-inactivated v-env5 (1 x 10^6 plaque forming units, PFU/ml prior to UV-light inactivation). Six days later, proliferative response were determined by measuring incorportion of ^{3}H-thymidine (^{3}H-TdR) following a six-hour incubation period. Results shown in Table 1 and previously reported(10) indicate that PBL from all the immunized macaques, but not the non-immunized macaques, responded proliferatively following stimulation with v-env5 due to the immune reponse developed against vaccinia virus. PBL from the v-env5 immunized macaques, but not the v-HSV-gD1 immunized nor non-immunized macaques showed 4 - 15 fold increases in ^{3}H-TdR incorporation following stimulation with purified HIV. This indicates that immunization with v-env5 primes PBL to recognize LAV by proliferating.

In order to determine whether the HIV-stimulated PBL were T cells or B cells, the phenotype of the cells was examined by fluorescence activated cell sorting. Interleukin-2 (IL-2) receptors are expressed on both activated T cells (13) and activated B cells (14) so the percent of IL-2 receptor positive cells expressing T-cell markers CD4 or CD8 or a B-cell marker CD20 (Bp35) was determined using monoclonal antibodies. Results in Table 2 indicate that the majority of the stimulated cells that express IL-2 receptors co-express CD4 or CD8 antigens but not CD20, indicating that the HIV-activated PBLs are, in fact, T cells.

TABLE 1
HIV-INDUCED PROLIFERATIVE RESPONSES OF PBL FROM MACAQUES AFTER IMMUNIZATION WITH A RECOMBINANT VACCINIA VIRUS EXPRESSING HIV ENVELOPE GLYCOPROTEINS[a]

Macaque Number	Immunization	cpm ^{3}H-TdR incorporated (S.I.)[b] No ag	HIV	v-env5
67	v-env5	1,586	7,465 (5)	60,415 (38)
75	v-env5	581	8,645 (15)	47,847 (14)
80	v-env5	1,077	13,922 (13)	24,752 (23)
81	v-env5	965	3,985 (4)	40,572 (42)
73	v-HSV-gD1	612	553 (<1)	56,217 (92)
26	none	2,911	1,822 (<1)	2,532 (<1)
27	none	1,228	1,072 (<1)	2,532 (2)

[a]Modified from Zarling et al., 1986.
[b]S.I. = Stimulation Index =

$$\frac{\text{cpm } ^{3}\text{H-TdR incorporated into stimulated PBL}}{\text{cpm } ^{3}\text{H-TdR incorporated into non-stimulated PBL}}$$

TABLE 2
EXPRESSION OF IL-2 RECEPTORS AND LYMPHOCYTE ANTIGENS ON STIMULATED PBL FROM VACCINATED MACAQUES[a]

Macaque Number	PBL Stimulated With	%IL-2 Receptor^{+} Cells co-expressing CD4	CD8	CD20 (Bp35)
74	v-env5	48.6	52.2	2
80	v-env5	62.4	40	NT
74	HIV	50	59	1.9
80	HIV	50	59	1.9
80	no virus	<0.3	<0.3	<0.3

[a]Modified from Zarling, et al., 1986

TABLE 3
INTERLEUKIN-2 PRODUCTION
BY PBL FROM VACCINATED MACAQUES AFTER STIMULATION[a]

Macaque Number	Immunization	IL-2 (U/mL) in supernatants[b] of PBL stimulated with: No virus	HIV	Recombinant Vaccinia v-env5
67	v-env5	0	28.4	96.0
68	v-env5	0	16.0	124.0
74	v-env5	0	9.0	52.0
73	v-HSVgD1	0	0	108
26	none	0	0	0

[a]Modified from Zarling et al., 1986
[b]IL-2 was measured by testing supernatants for their ability to induce prolipheration of CTLL, an IL-2 dependent cell line.

It is well established that T cells with helper/inducer activity, following antigenic stimulation, can produce IL-2 that can promote proliferation or differentiation of T, B, and natural killer cells(15-18). We therefore asked whether the T cells from v-env5 immune macaques have such HIV-specific helper activity. The results shown in Table 3 indicate that stimulation of PBL from macaques immunized with either of the recombinant vaccinia viruses v-env5 or v-HSV-gD1, produce IL-2 following stimulation with v-env5. However, following stimulation with HIV, IL-2 was detected in culture supernatants only from PBL from the v-env5 immunized macaques. These results thus demonstrate the presence of HIV-specific T-helper cells in v-env5 immunized macaques.

HIV-Specific Proliferative and Cytotoxic T-Cells in v-env5 Immunized Chimpanzees

Chimpanzees are the closest living relatives of man and also the only other species that has been found to be susceptible to infection with HIV (19-21). It was therefore of interest to determine whether immunization with v-env5 would induce T cell-mediated immune response to HIV.

Macaques are small and very limited amounts of blood can be obtained for experimental purposes. In contrast, chimpanzees are large affording us the opportunity to obtain sufficient amounts of blood required to generate and maintain T cell clones to determine whether HIV specific cytotoxic T cells (CTL) are also primed following immunization.

PBL from v-env5 immunized chimpanzees were first tested for their ability to proliferate in response to stimulation with purified UV-inactivated vaccinia virus, purified HIV or with HIV envelope glycoproteins gp41 and gp110 ('env') purified by lentil-lectin sepharose chromatography. As shown in Table 4, PBL from all the chimpanzees immunized with either recombinant vaccinia virus expressing HIV 'env' or HSV-gD1, proliferated following stimulation with UV-inactivated vaccinia virus indicating the presence of vaccinia virus immune PBL in these animals. PBL from the four v-env5 immunized chimpanzees, but not the two V-HSV-gD-1 immunized chimpanzees, showed strong proliferative responses following stimulation with HIV or with purified 'env'. PBL from non-immunized chimpanzees did not respond to vaccinia virus or HIV (data not shown). The amount of ^{3}H-thymidine incorporated into PBL from the v-env5 immunized chimpanzees, after stimulation with HIV or 'env', was 7 to 114 times higher and 17 to 83 times higher, respectively, than without antigen stimulation. The HIV stimulated PBL were concluded to be T cells because the vast majority of the stimulated cells reacted with monoclonal antibodies against CD4 or CD8 antigens.

In order to determine whether CTL that recognize HIV envelope glycoproteins are present in the v-env5 immunized chimpanzees, T cell clones were generated from 'env' stimulated PBL following our previous detailed method (22). Briefly, PBL were stimulated twice at weekly intervals with 'env' (1 μg/ml) and were then cloned by limiting dilution with 'env' and x-irradiated autologous PBL added as antigen presenting cells in medium containing IL-2. After expanding the clones, they were tested for their ability to lyse autologous ^{51}Cr labeled target cells. Results obtained with several clones and with non-cloned 'env' stimulated cells from two different v-env5 immunized chimpanzees are shown in Table 5. Whereas 'env'-stimulated, bulk PBL lysed autologous cells infected with either the recombinant or parental

TABLE 4
PROLIFERATIVE RESPONSES OF PBL FROM v-env5 IMMUNIZED CHIMPANZEES AFTER STIMULATION WITH HIV OR HIV ENVELOPE GLYCOPROTEINS

Chimpanzee	Immunization	Stimulation Index HIV	'env'	Vaccinia
124	v-env5	16.8	18.4	35.5
149	v-env5	7.2	17.1	111.4
72	v-env5	20.4	15.0	48.8
216	v-env5	114.5	83.5	243.6
64	v-HSV-gD1	1.4	1.3	22.8
134	v-HSV-gD1	1.1	1.0	23.4

TABLE 5
LYSIS OF AUTOLOGOUS CELLS EXPRESSING HIV ENVELOPE GLYCOPROTEINS BY T CELL CLONES ISOLATED FROM 'env' STIMULATED PBL FROM v-env5 IMMUNIZED CHIMPANZEES[a]

Chimpanzee	Clone Number	% Specific ^{51}Cr Release From Autologous Target Cells Infected With: v-env5	Parental Vaccinia
149	6	20.0	-0.7
	7	16.3	-0.2
	10	13.8	-1.5
	Bulk (non-cloned)	20.8	14.6
124	1	33.1	-1.4
	4	25.1	-4.8
	5	14.5	1.2
	Bulk (non-cloned)	24.7	23.5

[a]The values shown are the mean values of % specific ^{51}Cr releases from target cells in three replicate wells after six-hour incubation with effector cells at a ratio of 25 effector cells per target cell.

vaccinia virus-infected cells, due to the presence of natural killer-like cells, several clones that specifically recognize HIV envelope glycoproteins were isolated. Clones 6, 7, and 10 from chimpanzee 149 and clones 1,4, and 5 from chimpanzee 124 lysed autologous v-env5 infected cells that express HIV envelope glycoproteins but they did not lyse cells infected with parental vaccinia virus. These results thus demonstrate that v-env5 immunization of chimpanzees results in the generation of CTL that lyse cells expressing HIV envelope glycoproteins. Along these lines, immunization of mice with a recombinant vaccinia virus expressing an influenza viral antigen has been shown to induce influenza virus specific CTL (23).

With many viruses, the antigens that serve as recognition structures for CTL have not been determined. The use of recombinant vaccinia viruses has recently enabled conclusions to be drawn concerning which antigens of influenza virus (23-25) and HSV(22) serve as target antigens for CTL. Because HIV envelope glycoproteins are the only HIV antigens expressed on the v-env5 infected cells, our results showing CTL-mediated lysis of autologous v-env5 infected cells indicate that HIV envelope glycoprotein(s) serve as target antigens for CTL.

T-Cell Responses to HIV in HIV-Infected Chimpanzees

Having demonstrated that immunization of chimpanzees with a recombinant vaccinia virus expressing HIV envelope glycoproteins induces T-cell mediated immunity to HIV, it was of interest to determine whether infection of non-immunized chimpanzees with HIV likewise induces HIV specific T cell immunity. We also asked whether PBL from HIV-infected chimpanzees would respond, as do normal uninfected chimpanzees, to a battery of antigens and mitogens or if they would be impaired in their responses as are PBL from some HIV-infected humans. Chimpanzees 110, 114, 118, 133, and 139 had been infected for approximately three years(19) with HIV and chimpanzees 134 and 64 for less than six months. Results shown in Table 6 indicate that PBL from HIV-infected chimpanzees have normal proliferative responses following stimulation with a B cell mitogen, pokeweed mitogen (PWM), and T cell antigens, including x-irradiated human PBL, and cytomegalovirus (CMV). PBL from HIV-infected chimpanzees also had normal proliferative responses to the T cell mitogen phytohemagglutinin and to other T cell antigens (data not shown).

As shown in Table 6, all HIV-infected chimpanzees studied had stimulation indices greater than eight following stimulation with HIV and greater than four following stimulation with purified HIV envelope glycoproteins ('env'). In contrast, uninfected chimpanzees had stimulation indices of two or less after stimulation with HIV or 'env'. We have also detected significant proliferative responses to HIV gp120 and to the HIV 'gag' protein, p25, in HIV-infected chimpanzees (Eichberg, et al., submitted for publication).

TABLE 6
PROLIFERATIVE RESPONSES OF PBL FROM HIV-INFECTED AND NON-INFECTED CHIMPANZEES[a]

	PWM	Human PBLx	CMV	HIV	'env'
	Stimulation Index				
HIV-Infected Chimps					
110	59*	149	11	14	10
114	37	75	5	8	8
118	8	39	5	NT	10
133	45	150	28	9	19
139	15	41	20	10	8
134	12	35	6	14	5
64	16	65	11	9	5
Uninfected Chimps					
140	15	259	2	1	2
174	53	72	11	2	NT
175	49	53	7	1	2
207	14	53	3	2	1
	Stimulation Index >				
	≥ 8	≥ 35	≥ 3	≥ 8	≥ 4
HIV-Infected Chimps	7/7	7/7	7/7	6/6	7/7
Uninfected Chimps	4/4	4/4	3/4	0/4	0/4

[a]PWM = pokeweed mitogen; PBLx = human x-irradiated PBL; CMV = cytomegolovirus.

It is thus apparent that the chimpanzees which have been infected for a few months to several years with HIV do not have impaired T-cell functions as indicated by their normal responses to a battery of antigens and mitogens. These infected animals also have HIV specific T cells that may play a role in the prevention of AIDS in this species.

Do HIV-Infected Humans Develop T Cell Immune Responses to HIV?

In contrast to chimpanzees that have not, to date, been reported to develop AIDS-related complex (ARC) or frank AIDS, humans can develop either of these conditions. We have begun to carry out experiments with a small number of healthy HIV seropositive individuals to ask whether, like HIV infected chimps, humans develop T cell responses to HIV. One approach we have taken is to compare proliferative responses to parental vaccinia virus with those to the recombinant vaccinia viruses expressing HIV envelope glycoproteins gp110 and gp41 (v-env5) or 'gag' proteins p25 and p18 (v-gag2). The results shown in Table 7 indicate that the HIV-infected humans we have studied have higher proliferative responses to the recombinant vaccinia-HIV viruses than to parental vaccinia virus whereas this difference is not observed in HIV seronegative humans.

TABLE 7
HIGHER PROLIFERATIVE RESPONSE OF PBL FROM HIV-INFECTED HUMANS TO RECOMBINANT VACCINIA-HIV VIRUSES THAN TO PARENTAL VACCINIA VIRUS[a]

HIV	Stimulation Index			HIV	Stimulation Index		
Sero+	Vac	v-env5	v-gag2	Sero-	Vac	v-env5	v-gag2
S1	2	6	34	N1	5	6	6
S2	4	14	48	N2	5	7	6
S3	1	51	79	N3	3	3	3
S4	1	4	5	N4	9	11	11
S5	1	5	10	N5	24	19	15
S6	1	4	4	N6	87	88	52

[a]Vac = parental vaccinia virus; v-env5 expresses gp41 and gp110; v-gag2 expresses p18 and p25 (Hu, et al. in preparation).

These results suggest that PBL from HIV infected humans may recognize HIV 'env' and 'gag' proteins. In some HIV infected individuals, we have detected significant proliferative responses to gp120 and to HIV, but in general the response is lower than what we have observed in HIV infected chimpanzees (Eichberg, et al., submitted). Larger numbers of HIV seropositive and seronegative humans must be studied in terms of T cell responses to HIV and HIV antigens in order to conclude what percentage of healthy HIV infected individuals develop HIV-specific T cell proliferative responses. It is possible that very early after infection humans may generate stronger T cell responses to HIV that may wane during the course of the disease. Prospective studies following early seroconverters would be necessary to test this hypothesis. In addition, it remains to be determined whether HIV-specific CTL clones can be isolated from HIV infected individuals.

DISCUSSION

Our results presented herein demonstrate that immunization of macaques and chimpanzees with a recombinant vaccinia-HIV 'env' virus induces HIV-specific T helper cells and in chimpanzees, also HIV-specific CTL (Zarling et al., submitted for publication). That vaccination with such a recombinant virus may likewise induce strong HIV-specific T cell immunity in humans is supported by recent findings that following a single vaccination with a recombinant vaccinia-HIV 'env' virus, T cells that proliferate in response to HIV were detected in a vaccinee(26).

We have also demonstrated strong HIV-specific T cell immunity in HIV-infected chimpanzees and suggest that this T cell immunity may play a role in the prevention against AIDS in this species. In this regard, it will be interesting and important to determine whether there is an inverse relationship between the level and functional types of HIV-specific T cell responses with the subsequent development of disease in HIV-infected humans. If this is observed, it will add further rationale for developing AIDS vaccines that can induce strong HIV-specific T cell mediated immunity in man and rationale for attempting to augment HIV-specific T cell immunity in humans already infected with the virus, before they develop immunosuppression.

ACKNOWLEDGMENTS

We thank Ms. Phyllis Yoshida for her excellent editorial assistance. This work was supported in part by ONCOGEN and Genetic Systems Corp.

REFERENCES

1. Robert-Guroff M, Brown M, and Gallo RC (1985). HTLV-III-neutralizing antibodies in patients with AIDS and AIDS related complex. Nature 316:72-74.
2. Weiss RA, Clapham PR, Cheingsong-Popov R, Dalgleish AG, Carne AC, Weller IV, Tedder RS (1985). Neutralization of human T-lymphotropic virus type III by sera of AIDS and AIDS-risk patients. Nature 316:69-72.
3. Rook AH, Lane HC, Folks T, McCoy S, Alter S, Fauci AS (1987). Sera from HTLV-III/LAV antibody-positive individuals mediate antibody-dependent cellular cytotoxicity against HTLV-III/LAV-infected T cells. J Immunol 138:1064-1067.
4. Zinkernagel RM and Welsh RM (1976). H-2 compatibility requirement for virus-specific T cell-mediated effector functions in vivo. I. Specificity of T cells conferring antiviral protection against lymphocytic choriomeningitis virus is associated with H-2K and H-2D. J Immunol 117:1495-1502.
5. Starr SE and Allison AC (1977). Role of T lymphocytes in recovery from murine cytomegalovirus infection. Infect Immun 17:458-462.
6. Byrne JA and Oldstone MBA (1984). Biology of cloned cytotoxic T lymphocytes specific for lymphocytic choriomeningitis virus: clearance of virus in vivo. J Virol 51:682-686.
7. Lukacher AE, Braciale VL, and Braciale TJ (1984). In vivo effector function of influenza virus-specific cytotoxic T lymphocyte clones is highly specific. J Exp Med 160:814-826.
8. Larson HL, Feng MF, Horohov DW, Moore RN, and Rouse BT (1984). Role of T-lymphocyte subsets in recovery from herpes simplex virus infection. J Virol 50:56-59.
9. Stohlman SA, Katsushima GK, Casteel N, and Weiner LP (1986). In vivo effects of coronavirus-specific T cell clones: DTH inducer cells prevent a lethal infection but do not inhibit virus replication. J Immunol 136:3052-3056.

10. Zarling JM, Morton W, Moran PA, McClure J, Kosowski SG, and Hu S-L (1986). T-cell responses to human AIDS virus in macaques immunized with recombinant vaccinia viruses. Nature 323:344-346.
11. Wahren B, Morfeldt-Månsson L, Biberfeld G, Moberg L, Ljungman P, Nordlund S, Bredburg-Radén U, Werner A, Lower J, and Kurth R (1986). Impaired specific cellular response to HTLV-III before other immune defects in patients with HTLV-III infection. N Eng J Med 315:393-394.
12. Hu S-L, Kosowski SG, Dalrymple JM (1986). Expression of AIDS virus envelope gene in recombinant vaccinia viruses. Nature 320:537-540.
13. Leonard WJ, Depper JM, Uchiyama T, Smith KA, Waldmann TA, Greene WC (1982). A monoclonal antibody that appears to recognize the receptor for human T-cell growth factor; partial characterization of the receptor. Nature 300:267-269.
14. Anderson KC, Roach JA, Daley JF, Schlossman SF and Nadler LM (1986). Dual fluorochrome analysis of human B lymphocytes: phenotypic examination of resting, anti-immunoglobulin stimulated, and in vivo activated B cells. J Immunol 136:3612-3618.
15. Moretta L, Mingari MC, Moretta A and Fauci AS (1982). Human lymphocyte surface markers. Semin Hematol 19:273-284.
16. Reinherz EL and Schlossman SF (1980). The differentiation and function of human T lymphocytes. Cell 19:821-827.
17. Moretta A (1985). Frequency and surface phenotype of human T lymphocytes producing interleukin 2. Analysis by limiting dilution and cell cloning. Eur J Immunol 15:148-155.
18. Ortaldo JR, Mason AT, Gerard JP, Henderson LE, Farrar W, Hopkins RF 3d, Herberman RB, Rabin H (1984). Effects of natural and recombinant IL 2 on regulation of IFN gamma production and natural killer activity: lack of involvement of the Tac antigen for these immunoregulatory effects. J Immunol 133:779-783.
19. Alter HJ, Eichberg JW, Masur H, Saxinger WC, Gallo R, Macher AM, Lane HC, Fauci AS (1984). Transmission of HTLV-III infection from human plasma to chimpanzees: an animal model for AIDS. Science 226:549-552.

20. Francis DP, Feorino PM, Broderson JR, McClure HM, Getchell JP, McGrath CR, Swenson B, McDougal JS, Palmer EL, Harrison AK, Barre-Sinoussi F, Chermann J-C, Montagnier L, Curran JW, Cabradilla CD, and Kalyanaraman VS (1984). Infection of chimpanzees with lymphadenopathy-associated virus. Lancet 2(8414):1276-1277.
21. Fultz PN, McClure HM, Swenson RB, McGrath CR, Brodie A, Getchell JP, Jensen FC, Anderson DC, Broderson JR, Francis DP (1986). Persistent infection of chimpanzees with human T-lymphotropic virus type III/lymphadenopathy-associated virus: a potential model for acquired immunodeficiency syndrome. J Virol 58:116-124.
22. Zarling JM, Moran PA, Lasky L and Moss B (1986). Herpes simplex virus (HSV)-specific human T-cell clones recognize HSV glycoprotein D expressed by a recombinant vaccinia virus. J Virol 59:506-509.
23. Bennink JR, Yewdell JW, Smith GL, Möller C and Moss B (1984). Recombinant vaccinia virus primes and stimulates influenza haemagglutinin-specific cytotoxic T cells. Nature 311:578-579.
24. Yewdell JW, Bennink JR, Smith GL and Moss B (1985). Influenza A virus nucleoprotein is a major target antigen for cross-reactive anti-influenza A virus cytotoxic T lymphocytes. Proc Nat'l Acad Sci USA 82:1785-1789.
25. McMichael AJ, Michie CA, Gotch FM, Smith GL and Moss B (1986). Recognition of influenza A virus nucleoprotein by human cytotoxic T lymphocytes. J Gen Virol 67:719-726.
26. Zagury D, Leonard R, Fouchard M, Reveil B, Bernard J, Ittele D, Cattaan A, Zirimwabagabo L, Kalumbu M, Justin W, Salaun J-J, Goussard B (1987). Immunization against AIDS in humans. Nature 326:249-250.

Human Retroviruses, Cancer, and AIDS:
Approaches to Prevention and Therapy, pages 341–347

DEFINITION OF HIV DETERMINANTS WITH VACCINE POTENTIAL

Gordon R. Dreesman[1], Tran C. Chanh[1], Jorg W. Eichberg[1], Patrick Kanda[1], Ronald C. Kennedy[1], Jonathan S. Allan[2] and Myron Essex[2]

[1]Department of Virology and Immunology, Southwest Foundation for Biomedical Research, San Antonio, Texas 78284, [2]Department of Cancer Biology, Harvard School of Public Health, Boston, Massachusetts 02115

The complexity of the genetic potential of the human immunodeficiency virus (HIV) (1-3) strongly indicates that methods used to prepare conventional viral vaccines in the past may not be applicable for this virus (4). Thus we have elected to define individual regions or epitopes associated with the HIV envelope glycoproteins (gp120 and gp41) which have potential to induce neutralizing antibody and hopefully protective immunity. Once defined these regions or structures could then be included in the final design of an effective vaccine. I will summarize two studies which are being carried out in our laboratories to accomplish the above goals. These include: 1) characterization of a number of synthetic peptide analogues of gp120 and gp41, and 2) the use of anti-idiotype methodology to define unique viral epitopes.

The first series of studies were designed to identify viral epitopes with vaccine potential by preparing synthetic peptide analogues of several regions of the two major HIV surface glycoprotein subunits, gp41 and gp120. In this presentation, we will summarize the data that has been generated with two given synthetic peptides (5-10). A hydrophilic region with potential turns of gp41 was chosen which encompassed amino acid residues 735-752. The final purified 735-752 peptides conjugated to a carrier protein, keyhole limpet hemocyanin (KLH) via a cysteine residue added to the carboxyl end with a glycine spacer. Peptide 502-532 was assembled on a modified polydimethylacylamide support. After de-protection of amino acid chains, animals were immunized with the resin bound peptide. Both rabbit polyclonal and murine monoclonal antibodies were generated to these conjugates (6-10). Both antibody sources were specific for HIV in that they were positive for viral antigen as determined by a series of different ELISA reactions. In addition, it was demonstrated that the rabbit antibody to 735-752 reacted with gp41 as well as with the envelope precursor glycoprotein gp160, by radioimmunoprecipitation (RIP) and Western blot. In concordance with these observations, rabbit anti-peptide 502-532 reacted with gp120 and gp160 as demonstrated by the above methods.

Gp41 is the major viral transmembrane protein. Therefore, a major question to be addressed with determinants associated with this region, was to demonstrate that antibody specific for the synthetic peptide react with an epitope on the surface of infected cells. Monoclonal anti-peptide (735-752) antibody reacted with the surface of infected H9 cells but not with uninfected cells as shown by flow cytometry. The viral antigen could be detected by 3 days after infection of the H9 cell line with HTLV-IIIB and HTLV-NY5.

The critical question which was addressed with the above reagents was to determine their ability to neutralize viral infectivity _in vitro_. It was shown that rabbit antisera generated to both peptides, 735-752 and 502-532, neutralized two different HIV isolates, HTLV-IIIB and HTLV-NY5 at a sera dilution of 1:32 (8). These observations are of particular importance since these two are known to represent the highest degree of genetic deviation of all North American isolates (M. Martin, personal communication).

Based on these findings, we proceeded to test a potential role of peptide 735-752 for the induction of protective immunity in the chimpanzee animal model (11). Two chimpanzees were injected with the synthetic peptide conjugated to KLH and a third animal was inoculated with an irrelevant peptide of similar length, also conjugated to KLH. A specific anti-HIV response, as determined by ELISA, was noted in both HIV peptide immunized animals after 4 inoculations. One of the two animals produced neutralizing antibody (greater than 70% at a 1:10 dilution). All three animals were challenged after four infectious units of HIV-NY5 (9).

These animals have been followed for a period of 40 weeks post-challenge. Virus has not been isolated from any of the 3 animals during this 40-week period (Fig. 1). However, virus replication has occurred in all three animals as evidenced by the temporal antibody patterns noted in each of the animals. Sera obtained at weekly intervals were analyzed by Western blot and RIP. Both peptide immunized animals produced detectable antibody to gp160 and gp41 prior to challenge. After challenge, the control animal (X-189) and one peptide immunized animal (X-99) produced antibody to p24 by week 7 and antibody to p55 and gp120 by week 10. However, the immune response to gp120 and to the gag proteins was delayed in the second immunized animal (X-183). Antibody to p24 was not detected until week 11 and no antibody was detected to either p55 or gp120 through 12 weeks. It is of interest that chimpanzee X-183 also produced detectable neutralizing antibody prior to challenge. The animals are currently being studied for production of infectious virus.

The second set of studies performed in our studies to define unique HIV epitopes incorporates the use of anti-idiotype methodology. It has been shown that monoclonal antibodies, which have specificity for the CD4 receptor, have the capacity to block infection of T4 lymphocytes with HIV (12-15). These observations clearly show that identification of the chemical structure of the virion which binds to CD4 would be instructive in the engineering of a final vaccine candidate. To accomplish this we prepared a murine monoclonal anti-idiotypic antibody to Leu-3a. Leu-3a monoclonal antibody is a commercial reagent which identifies T4 helper lymphocytes. The monoclonal anti-Id generated in our laboratories (16), referred to as HF1.7, has the following characteristics: The specific reaction with Leu-3a can be inhibited by prior incubation of HF1.7 with CD4 specific monoclonals, namely Leu-3a, OKT-4a and T4, but not by a series of irrelevant murine monoclonal antibodies. It reacted with an HIV antigenic determinant as shown by ELISA. The antibody also reacted with HIV infected H9 but not with uninfected H9 cells by a viable membrane immunofluorescence assay. The antibody preferentially reacted with a viral subunit with an approximate weight of 110,000-120,000 Kd as observed by Western blot analysis. More importantly the monoclonal partially

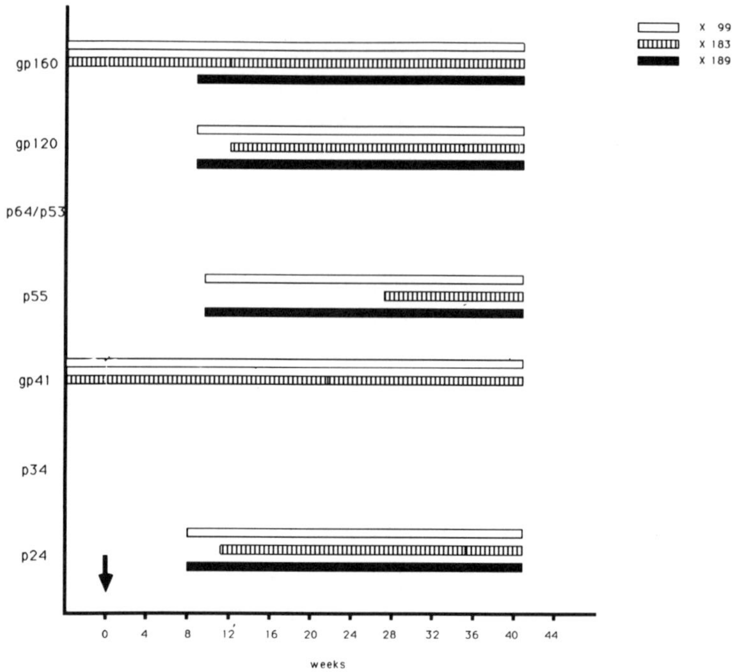

FIGURE 1. Summary of immune response of chimpanzees immunized with gp41 735-752 synthetic peptides (X-99 and X-183) and of control animal immunized with an irrelevant peptide (X-189) observed on day of post-challenge and for 40 weeks post-challenge after IV inoculation with 1000 tissue culture infectious doses of HIV-NY5.

neutralized HIV infectivity *in vitro*. We are presently utilizing this valuable reagent to identify the virion structure (epitope) which reacts with the CD4 receptor of T-helper lymphocytes.

In conclusion, we feel that the two study approaches we have used will be helpful and extremely instructive in the final engineering of an effective vaccine for HIV. Both approaches take into account the extreme variability of the HIV envelope glycoproteins and are consequently directed at epitopes associated with constant regions. It is of interest that the immune response produced by synthetic peptide immunization and by anti-idiotype methodology have resulted in the production of neutralizing antibodies. The chimpanzees inoculated with the single gp41 peptide were not protected when challenged with infectious virus. However, it is noteworthy that infectivity as noted by production of antibody to viral subunits has been delayed in the animal which had detectable neutralizing antibody prior to challenge. Therefore, it appears that peptide 735-752 does present an essential epitope to be included in a final vaccine preparation. The anti-idiotype antibody prepared to a CD4 receptor monoclonal reagent should allow us to identify a second potential epitope. In addition, it is intriguing that a monoclonal anti-receptor antibody, such as Leu-3a, may present yet another potential vaccine candidate.

REFERENCES

1. Shaw, G.M., Hahn, B.H., Arya, S.K., Groopman, J.E., Gallo, R.C. and Wong-Staal, F. (1984). Molecular characterization of human T-cell leukėmia (lymphotropic) virus type III in the acquired immune deficiency syndrome. Science 226:1165-1171.
2. Benn, S., Rutledge, R., Folks, T., Gold, J., Baker, L., McCormick, J., Feorino, P., Piot, P., Quinn, T. and Martin, M. (1985). Genetic heterogeneity of AIDS retroviral isolates from North America and Zaire. Science 230:949-951.
3. Alizon, M., Wain-Hobson, S., Montagnier, L. and Sonigo, P. (1986). Genetic variability of the AIDS virus: nucleotide sequence analysis of two isolates from African patients. Cell 46:63-74.

4. Hilleman, M. (1987). Perspectives in the quest for a vaccine against AIDS. These proceedings
5. Pauletti, D., Simmonds, R., Dreesman, G.R. and Kennedy, R.C. (1985). Application of a modified computer algorithm in determining antigenic determinants associated with the AIDS virus glycoprotein. Anal. Biochem. 151:540-546.
6. Kennedy, R.C., Henkel, R.D., Pauletti, D., Allan, J.S., Lee, T.H., Essex, M. and Dreesman, G.R. (1986). Antiserum to a synthetic peptide recognizes the HTLV-III envelope glycoprotein. Science 231:1556-1559.
7. Chanh, T.C., Kennedy, R.C., Alderete, B.E., Kanda, P., Eichberg, J.W. and Dreesman, G.R. (1986). Human immunodeficiency virus gp120 glycoprotein detected by monoclonal antibody to a synthetic peptide. Eur. J. Immunol. 16:1465-1468.
8. Chanh, T.C., Dreesman, G.R., Kanda, P., Linette, G.P., Sparrow, J.T., Ho, D.D. and Kennedy, R.C. (1986). Induction of anti-HIV neutralizing antibodies by synthetic peptides. The EMBO Journal 5:3065-3071.
9. Kennedy, R.C., Kanda, P., Dreesman, G.R., Eichberg, J.W., Chanh, T.C., Ho, D.D. and Sparrow, J.T. Properties of synthetic peptides that identify neutralizing epitopes on the HIV envelope glycoprotein. In Chanock R, Ginsberg H, Lerner R, Brown F (eds): "Modern Approaches to New Vaccines Including Prevention of AIDS," Cold Spring Harbor Laboratory, Cold Spring Harbor, N.Y.: in press.
10. Kennedy, R.C., Kanda, P., Chanh, T.C., Boswell, R.N., Allan, J.S., Lee, T.H., Essex, M., Sparrow, J.T. and Dreesman, G.R. (1987). Use of a resin bound peptide for identifying a native antigenic determinant associated with the HTLV-III/LAV envelope. J. Biol. Chem. 262:2969-2974.
11. Alter, H.J., Eichberg, J.W., Masur, H., Saxinger, W.C., Gallo, R.C., Macher, A.M., Lane, H.C. and Fauci, A.S. (1984). Transmission of HTLV-III infection from human plasma to chimpanzees: an animal model for AIDS. Science 226:549-552.

12. Dalgleish, A.G., Beverley, P.C.L., Clapham, P.R., Crawford, D.H., Greaves, M.F. and Weiss, R.A. (1984). The CD4 (T4) antigen is an essential component of the receptor for the AIDS retrovirus. Nature 312:763-767.

13. Klatzmann, D., Champagne, E., Chamaret, S., Gruest, J., Guetard, D., Hercend, T., Gluckman, J.-C. and Montagnier, L. (1984). T-lymphocyte T4 molecule behaves as the receptor for human retrovirus LAV. Nature 312:767-768.

14. Nicholson, J.K.A., Cross, G.D., Callaway, C.S. and McDougal, J.S. (1986). In vitro infection of human monocytes with human T-lymphotropic virus type III/lymphadenopathy-associated virus (HTLV-III/LAV). J. Immunol. 137:323-329.

15. McDougal, J.S., Kennedy, M.S., Sligh, J.M., Cort, S.P., Mawle, A. and Nicholson, J.K.A. (1986). Binding of HTLV-III/LAV to T4$^+$ T cells by a complex of the 110K viral protein and the T4 molecule. Science 231:382-385.

16. Chanh, T.C., Dreesman, G.R. and Kennedy, R.C. (1987). Monoclonal anti-idiotypic antibody mimics the CD4 receptor and binds human immunodeficiency virus. Proc. Natl. Acad. Sci. USA, in press.

ACKNOWLEDGEMENTS

This work was supported by grants AI 23619, AI 23472 and HL 32505 from the National Institutes of Health and by contract DAMD 17-86-C-6290 from the U.S. Army Research and Development Command.

**Human Retroviruses, Cancer, and AIDS:
Approaches to Prevention and Therapy, pages 349–361**

RECOMBINANT ADENOVIRUS AS A VEHICLE FOR THE HBV SURFACE ANTIGEN OR HIV ENVELOPE PROTEIN GENES

Paul P. Hung, John E. Morin, Michael D. Lubeck, Joan E. Barton, Katherine L. Molnar-Kimber, Bruce B. Mason, Surendra K.Dheer, Valentina Jarocki-Witek, Beverley Kostek, Gordon Zandle, Anthony J. Conley, and Alan R. Davis

Wyeth Laboratories, Inc., Microbiology Division, P.O. Box 8299, Philadelphia, PA 19101

ABSTRACT Recombinant adenovirus type 5 was made to carry the HBsAg coding sequence in the adenovirus E3 region for the production of HBsAg. This HBsAg was secreted into the medium in tissue culture and has the immunological and biochemical properties of the 22 nm particles found in human serum. Additionally, the recombinant adenoviruses grew normally in all human cells tested. A hamster model was developed to evaluate the immunogenic properties of these recombinant adenoviruses. Upon intranasal inoculation, both wild-type adenovirus and an adenovirus, in which the E3 region was deleted, replicated in the lungs of these animals and induced an antibody response against adenovirus. Hamsters similarly immunized with the live recombinant adenoviruses produced antibody against both adenovirus and hepatitis B virus surface antigen. Recombinant adenovirus type 7 carrying the HIV envelope protein coding sequence was also constructed. Expression of HIV envelope protein was demonstrated using cytoimmunofluorescence and immunoprecipitation.

INTRODUCTION

Live recombinant viral vaccines represent an attractive alternative to the present HBV vaccines. Such vaccines could be derived from the live adenovirus vaccines already in use. The current adenovirus vaccines are safe and efficacious when administered orally as enteric-coated tablets (1,2). They give rise to asymptomatic intestinal adenovirus infections in humans which induce immunity against adenovirus respiratory disease. These characteristics have prompted us to develop recombinant adenoviruses that direct infected cells to produce HBsAg and thus confer immunity against both adenovirus and HBV. Vaccinia virus recombinants, which direct production of HBsAg in animals (3,4), were designed with a similar strategy in mind, however, live recombinant adenovirus vaccines provide the convenience of oral administration. In this study, we describe recombinant adenoviruses which carry the HBsAg coding sequence in the adenovirus E3 region and which direct the production of immunogenic HBsAg as well as a recombinant Ad7 which carries the HIV envelope protein coding sequence and which directs the production of immunoreactive HIV envelope protein.

RESULTS

Construction of Recombinant Adenoviruses.

The HBsAg coding sequence was inserted downstream of the Ad5 E3 promoter at map unit (MU) 78.5 as shown in Figure 1 so that it either immediately precedes, as in the recombinant adenovirus termed Ad5E3HS, or replaces, as in the recombinant adenovirus termed Ad5ΔE3HS, a portion of the E3 region which includes the coding sequence of the viral glycoprotein designated as gp19K. Viruses Ad5E3HS, Ad5ΔE3HS, and Ad5ΔE3 were prepared as shown in Figure 1 by co-transfection of a genomic fragment of Ad5 and a plasmid DNA in a manner such that recombination could occur to form intact viral DNA.

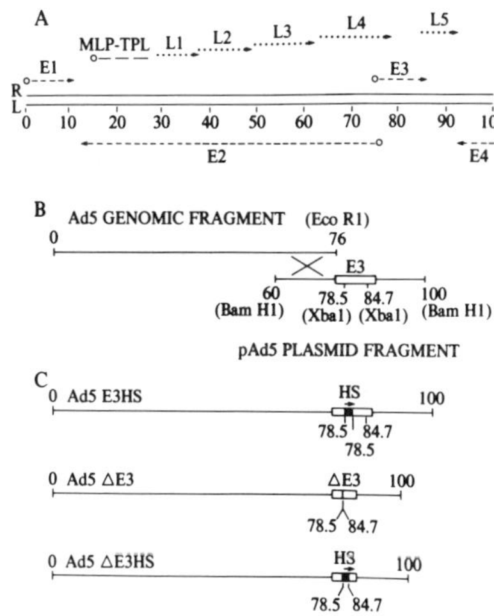

FIGURE 1. Construction of recombinant adenoviruses. (A) Simplified diagram of the transcript map of Ad2, each MU is approximately 360 base pairs. Major late promoter (MLP), tripartite leader (TPL). (B) Recombinant adenoviruses were constructed by transfecting cultured 293 cells with the large Eco R1 fragment of Ad5 genomic DNA together with a partially overlapping fragment of cloned Ad5 DNA from a plasmid (pAd5). (C) Ad5 DNA from MU 60 to MU 100 cloned as described was altered to create new plasmids, pAd5E3HS, pAd5ΔE3 and pAd5ΔE3HS, that were subsequently used to generate the corresponding recombinant adenoviruses Ad5E3HS, Ad5ΔE3 and Ad5ΔE3HS.

Production of HBsAg in Cells Infected With Recombinant Ad5.

Viral stocks of Ad5E3HS (Figure 2A) were used to infect a human cell line, A549, and the synthesis of HBsAg was monitored by RIA. Examination of HBsAg accumulation in the media during the course of infection revealed that cells infected with the virus began to produce HBsAg soon after infection, consistent with the site of insertion of the HBsAg coding sequence downstream of the E3 promoter. Since production of HBsAg by cells infected with Ad5E3HS was unaltered by Ara C, there does not appear to be involvement of the major late promoter.

In contrast, production of HBsAg during the late phase of infection by cells infected with Ad5ΔE3HS (Figure 2B) was abolished by Ara-C, which suggests an involvement of the major late promoter in production of HBsAg using Ad5ΔE3HS. With each virus, the effect of Ara C was reversible by cytidine. The total accumulation of HBsAg in the media at 60 hr post infection in the absence of Ara-C was 1.5 ug per 10^6 cells infected with Ad5E3HS and 2.8 ug per 10^6 cells infected with Ad5ΔE3HS. Human diploid cells, WI-38, produced similar levels of HBsAg when infected with these viruses.

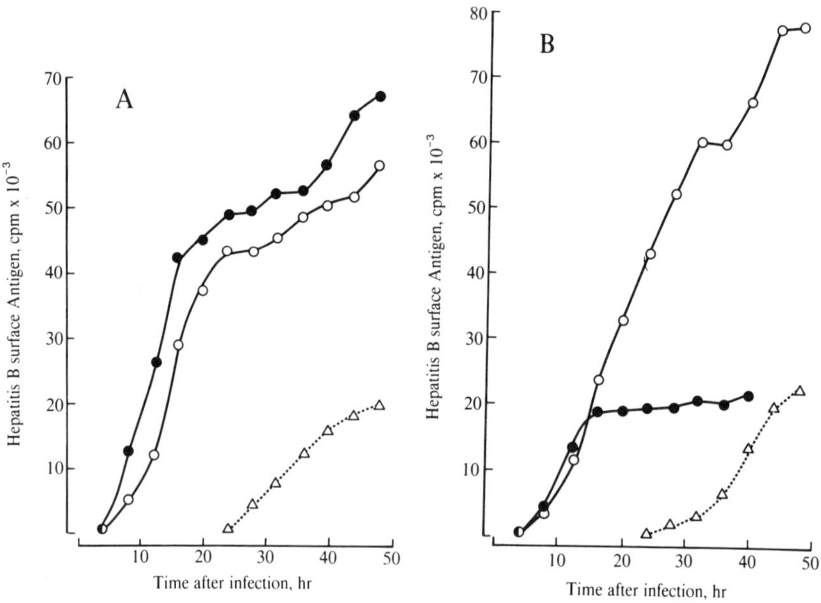

FIGURE 2. Time course of production of HBsAg by A549 cells infected with (A) Ad5E3HS or (B) Ad5ΔE3HS and the effect of Ara-C. Flasks of A549 cells were infected with either Ad5E3HS or Ad5ΔE3HS, (O). Duplicate flasks with 20 ug/ml of Ara-C added were likewise infected with either Ad5E3HS or Ad5ΔE3HS, (●). The media containing Ara-C was removed from one set of duplicate flasks and was replaced with media containing 20 ug/ml of cytidine, (**Δ**). Samples (50 ul) of culture medium were withdrawn at the times indicated and the accumulated HBsAg was estimated by RIA.

Characterization of the HBsAg produced in Cells Infected with Recombinant Ad5.

Electrophoretic analysis of metabolically radiolabeled immunoprecipitates from A549 cells infected with either Ad5E3HS or Ad5ΔE3HS (Figure 3) revealed immunoreactive material with the approximate molecular weights of the unglycosylated (p24) and glycosylated (gp27) forms of HBsAg (5). There was no apparent difference between the molecular weight of HBsAg produced in the early phase of infection and that produced in the late phase. HBsAg immunoprecipitated from lysates of infected cells (Figure 3A) had the same apparent molecular weight as HBsAg secreted into the media (Figure 3B).

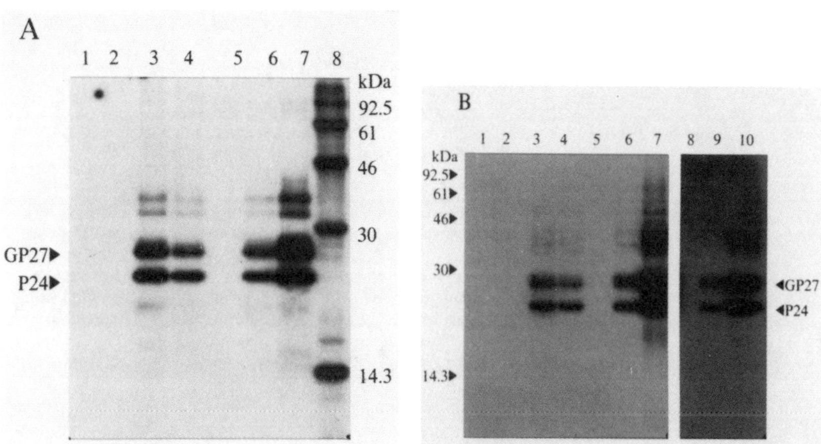

FIGURE 3. Electrophoretic analysis of HBsAg immunoprecipitated from A549 cells infected with recombinant adenoviruses. (A) Immunoprecipitates of lysed cells: lane 1, uninfected; lane 2, Ad5 early phase; lane 3, Ad5E3HS early phase; lane 4, Ad5ΔE3HS early phase; lane 5, Ad5 late phase; lane 6, Ad5E3HS late phase; lane 7, Ad5ΔE3HS late phase. Lane 8, molecular weight markers. (b) Immunoprecipitates of media: lane 1, uninfected; lane 2, Ad5 early phase; lane 3, Ad5E3HS early phase; lane 4, Ad5ΔE3HS early phase; lane 5, Ad5 late phase; lane 6, Ad5E3HS late phase; lane 7, Ad5ΔE3HS late phase. Samples of media (5 ul) were also analyzed without immunoprecipitation: lane 8, uninfected cells; lane 9, Ad5E3HS late phase; lane 10, Ad5ΔE3HS late phase. The size and location of the protein markers are given.

Replication of Ad5 and Ad5ΔE3 in Hamsters.

A small animal model was developed to evaluate the immune response to these recombinant Ad5 viruses. Figure 4 shows the replication of Ad5 and Ad5ΔE3 in hamster lungs after intranasal inoculation. Titers of infectious virus recovered from lungs of animals infected with either Ad5 or Ad5ΔE3 peaked at the same level.

The antibody responses against adenovirus in hamsters inoculated with Ad5 or Ad5ΔE3 are presented as a function of virus dose in Figure 5. Elevated antibody titers were observed in animals receiving a minimum dose of 10^4 PFU of either virus.

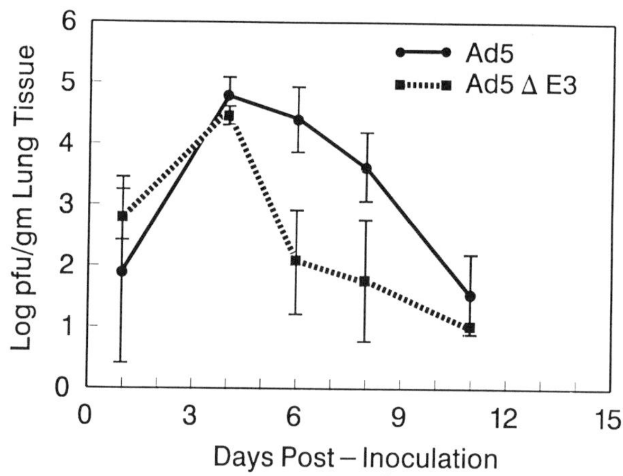

FIGURE 4. Replication of Ad5 and Ad5ΔE3 in hamster lungs. One-month-old hamsters were inoculated intranasally with 10^7 PFU of Ad5 (●) or Ad5ΔE3 (■). Viral titers (PFU/gm lung tissue) were determined for four animals per virus per time point and are expressed as the geometric mean values (± standard deviation).

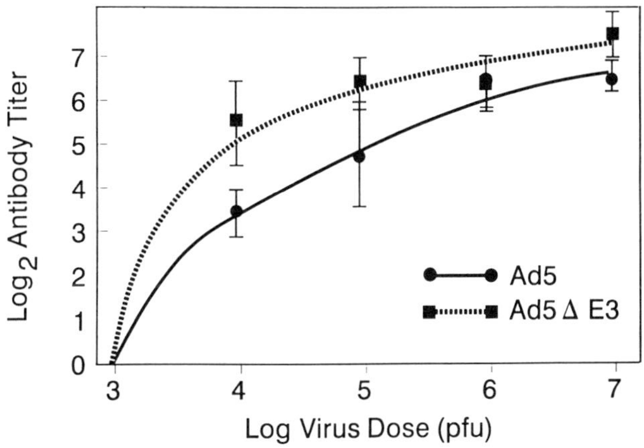

Figure 5. Seroresponses to Ad5 in hamsters inoculated with varying doses of Ad5 and Ad5ΔE3. One-month-old hamsters were inoculated intranasally over a range of doses (10^3 to 10^7 PFU/animal) with Ad5 (●) or Ad5ΔE3 (■) and seroresponses were determined by ELISA analysis 28 days later. Antibody titers represent geometric means (± standard deviation) from 4 animals per dose per virus for all test groups except groups receiving Ad5ΔE3 at doses of 10^7 PFU and 10^5 PFU which consisted of 3 animals per group.

Induction of Antibody to HBsAg in Hamsters.

Hamsters were inoculated with Ad5E3HS or Ad5ΔE3HS and evaluated for production of antibody to HBsAg one month later. Table 1 shows that by 33 days after inoculation with 10^8 PFU of virus, 7 out of 10 hamsters inoculated with Ad5E3HS and 10 out of 10 hamsters inoculated with Ad5ΔE3HS had produced significant levels of antibody to HBsAg. Test animals, inoculated with equivalent dosages of either virus which had been inactivated with ultraviolet light, failed to produce a detectable antibody response to HBsAg.

TABLE 1

SEROCONVERSION OF HAMSTERS TO HBsAg FOLLOWING IMMUNIZATION WITH Ad5E3HS AND Ad5ΔE3HS

Virus[a]	Dose (PFU)	Anti-HBsAg Response #pos./#inoc.	Anti-HBsAg Response mIU[b]
Ad5E3HS	10^8	7/10	126 ± 89
	10^7	4/10	119 ± 121
	10^6	1/10	46
	10^5	0/10	0
	10^4	0/10	0
	U.V.(10^8)[c]	0/10	0
Ad5ΔE3HS	10^8	10/10	75 ± 50
	10^7	5/10	48 ± 39
	10^6	0/10	0
	10^5	1/10	21
	10^4	0/10	0
	U.V.(10^8)[c]	0/10	0
Ad5	10^7	0/10	0

a One-month-old hamsters were challenged intranasally with virus purified by CsCl isopycnic density gradient centrifugation and subsequently shown to be free of HBsAg contamination by RIA.

b mean ± S.D. of positive sera.

c Inocula corresponding to 10^8 PFU/dose were irradiated with ultraviolet radiation to reduce infectivity to approximately 10^2 PFU/dose.

Table 2 shows a detailed analysis of hamster seroresponses to both Ad5 and HBsAg following inoculation with 10^7 PFU of recombinant adenovirus on days 0 and 33. By 33 days after inoculation, 5 out of 8 animals inoculated with Ad5E3HS and 4 out of 8 animals inoculated with Ad5ΔE3HS had seroconverted to HBsAg. By day 33, all animals inoculated with either of the recombinant adenoviruses had produced antibodies against Ad5 as assessed by both ELISA and neutralization analyses.

TABLE 2

ANTI-HBsAg AND ANTI-Ad5 RESPONSES IN HAMSTERS INOCULATED WITH Ad5E3HS AND Ad5ΔE3HS

Virus[a]	Animal Number	Anti-HBsAg[b] (mIU) 33d	65d	Anti-Ad5 (33d) ELISA[c]	Neutralization
Ad5E3HS	1	93*	411*	+	160
	2	59*	502*	+	80
	3	41*	26*	+	80
	4	4	32*	+	160
	5	59*	160*	+	80
	6	2	0	+	80
	7	2	0	+	160
	8	11*	186*	+	80
Ad5ΔE3HS	9	50*	160*	+	160
	10	2	2	+	80
	11	21*	21*	+	80
	12	2	0	+	320
	13	162*	675*	+	80
	14	2	2	+	40
	15	26*	46*	+	20
	16	2	26*	+	80
Neg.Control	17	0	0	-	<20

a One-month-old hamsters were inoculated intranasally on days 0 and 33 with crude viral lysate containing 10^7 PFU recombinant virus per dose.

b Positive sera (≥10 mIU) are highlighted by asterisks (*).

c Positive (+) denotes an ELISA reading of greater than 0.15 absorbancy units at a 1/800 dilution of serum; negative (-) denotes an absorbancy reading of less than 0.15 at a 1/50 serum dilution.

Production of HIV Envelope Protein in Cells Infected With Recombinant Ad7

A recombinant Ad7 was constructed which contains the HIV envelope protein coding sequence within an expression cassette driven by the Ad7 major late promoter. Details of the construction of this recombinant adenovirus, designated Ad7HIVE, will be given elsewhere. A549 cells infected with Ad7HIVE and fixed in acetone 30 hours later showed positive cytoimmunofluorescence when stained with polyclonal human anti-AIDS IgG and fluorescein (Figure 6A). In some cells, the intensity of staining equaled that observed in human lymphocytes infected with HIV (Figure 6B). Staining with a murine monoclonal antibody against HIV envelope protein and fluorescein-conjugated goat anti-mouse IgG yielded similar results.

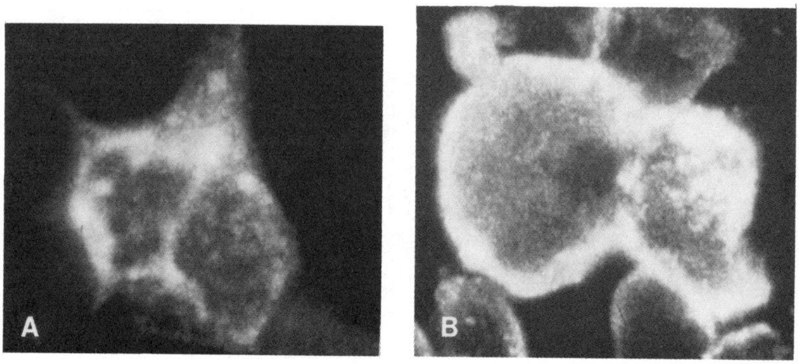

FIGURE 6. Production of HIV envelope protein in A549 cells infected with Ad7HIVE indicated by cytoimmunofluorescence. (A) A549 cells infected with Ad7HIVE. (B) Human lymphocytes infected with HIV. Infected cells were fixed in acetone and stained with polyclonal human anti-AIDS IgG-biotin followed by avidin-fluorescein.

Characterization of the HIV Envelope Protein Produced in Cells Infected With Recombinant Ad7.

Electrophoretic analysis of metabolically radiolabeled immunprecipitates from A549 cells infected with Ad7HIVE revealed immunoreactive material with a molecular weight of approximately 125 kDa (Figure 7A). This material was also immunoprecipitated from the media over A549 cells infected with Ad7HIVE (Figure 7B). The antibody used in these immunoprecipitations was a murine monoclonal IgG directed against the gp120 kDa moiety of HIV envelope protein.

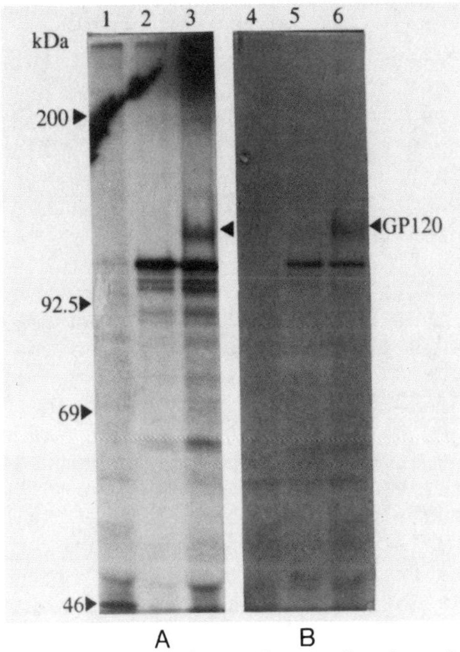

FIGURE 7. Electrophoretic analysis of HIV envelope protein immunoprecipitated from A549 cells infected with recombinant adenovirus. (A) Immunoprecipitates of lysed cells: lane 1, uninfected; lane 2, Ad7; lane 3, Ad7HIVE. (B) Immunoprecipitates of media: lane 4, uninfected; lane 5, Ad7; lane 6, Ad7HIVE. The locations of molecular weight markers are indicated.

DISCUSSION

Our results demonstrate the potential utility of recombinant adenoviruses as live oral vaccines. We describe here recombinant adenoviruses which can replicate in human cells and which direct the production of immunogenic HBsAg or immunoreactive HIV envelope protein. Ad5E3HS, Ad5ΔE3HS and Ad7HIVE were constructed as autonomously replicating adenoviruses in order to enhance antigen production through successive rounds of replication after administration. In addition, the recombinant viruses described here can be propagated as pure isolates in a cell strain appropriate for vaccine production such as WI-38.

Ad5E3HS and Ad5ΔE3HS are not defective because only the nonessential E3 region (6,7,8) is altered. The HBV DNA segment inserted into Ad5 contains only the HBsAg coding sequence and does not include an HBV promoter. The expression of HBsAg in cells infected by Ad5E3HS and Ad5ΔE3HS is therefore dependent on transcription from an Ad5 promoter to produce hybrid Ad5-HBsAg mRNA. The production of HBsAg soon after infection with either Ad5HS or Ad5ΔHS is consistent with the position of insertion downstream of the E3 promoter. The significant difference in the Ara C sensitivity and rate of production of HBsAg during the later phase of infection with Ad5E3HS versus Ad5ΔE3HS may be due to the large E3 deletion in Ad5ΔE3HS, which removes all of the RNA splice sites downstream of the HBsAg coding sequence in the E3 region. It has recently been reported that deletion of a downstream splice acceptor site from the E3 region can increase the relative abundance of mRNAs produced late in infection that contain the portion of the E3 region upstream of the deleted splice acceptor site (9).

Human adenoviruses have a highly restricted host range, which makes development of a useful animal model for adenoviral disease difficult. The best small animal model for human adenoviral disease to date is the recently described cotton rat model (10). This model suffers, however, from the limited commercial availability of these animals. We thus sought a more readily available small animal model to evaluate recombinant human adenoviruses. We demonstrate here that Ad5ΔE3 replicates in hamster lungs to peak titers comparable to those attained by wild-type Ad5. Thus, the Ad5ΔE3 region, which is known to be nonessential for virus replication in tissue culture (6,7,8) is here shown to be nonessential for virus replication _in vivo_.

Both recombinant adenoviruses were equally efficient in seroconverting hamsters to HBsAg and they induced comparable levels of anti-HBsAg antibodies in positive animals. On the whole, these data indicate a good prospect for developing recombinant adenovirus vaccines which will effectively immunize humans against HBV.

The induction of lasting immunity to HIV has not yet been demonstrated with any HIV antigen. Nevertheless, the presentation of immunoreactive HIV envelope protein in the context of an asymptomatic adenovirus infection, _in vivo_, may enhance the immune response. These results illustrate the broad scope of this immunization strategy, which can be readily adapted to deliver essentially pure antigens from a wide variety of pathogenic organisms.

ACKNOWLEDGMENTS

We thank W. Magargle and F. Graupensperger for their excellent assistance.

REFERENCES

1. Couch RB, Chanock RM, Cate TR, Lang DJ, Knight V, Huebner RJ (1963). Immunization with types 4 and 7 adenovirus by selective infection of the intestinal tract. Am Rev Resp Dis 88:394.
2. Top FH, Jr, Buescher EL, Bancroft WH, Russell PK (1971). Immunization with live types 7 and 4 adenovirus vaccines. II. antibody response and protective effect against acute respiratory disease due to adenovirus type 7. J Inf Dis 124:155.
3. Moss B, Smith GL, Gerin JL, Purcell RH (1984). Live recombinant vaccinia virus protects chimpanzees against hepatitis B. Nature 311:67.
4. Paoletti E, Lipinskas BR, Samsonoff C, Mercer S, Panicali D (1984). Construction of live vaccines using genetically engineered poxviruses: biological activity of vaccinia virus recombinants expressing the hepatitis B virus surface antigen and the herpes simplex virus glycoprotein D. Proc Natl Acad Sci USA 81:193.
5. Peterson, DL (1981). Isolation and characterization of the major protein and glycoprotein of hepatitis B surface antigen. J Biol Chem 256:6975.
6. Berkner KL, Sharp PA (1983). Generation of adenovirus by transfection of plasmids. Nucleic Acids Res 11:6003.
7. Kelly TJ, Lewis AM (1973). Use of nondefective adenovirus - simian virus 40 hybrids for mapping the simian virus 40 genome. J Virol 12:643.
8. Jones N, Shenk T (1978). Isolation of deletion and substitution mutants of adenovirus type 5. Cell 13:181.
9. Bhat BM, Wold WSM (1986). Genetic analysis of mRNA synthesis in adenovirus region E3 at different stages of productive infection by RNA-processing mutants. J Virol 60:54.
10. Pacini PL, Dubois EJ, Clyde WA, Jr, (1984). A new animal model for human respiratory tract disease due to adenovirus. J Inf Dis 150:92.

VII. TREATMENT APPROACHES AGAINST HIV

Human Retroviruses, Cancer, and AIDS: Approaches to Prevention and Therapy, pages 365–380

STRATEGIES FOR ANTI-VIRAL THERAPY IN AIDS

Samuel Broder

Clinical Oncology Program, Division of Cancer Treatment, National Cancer Institute, Bethesda, MD 20892

ABSTRACT An analysis of the life cycle of retroviruses suggests a number of targets for therapeutic intervention. The reverse transcriptase is a particularly promising target, and one member of the dideoxynucleoside family (AZT) has already been shown to confer some clinical benefits in certain patients.

Acquired immunodeficiency syndrome (AIDS) was initially defined as the development of either an opportunistic infection or Kaposi's sarcoma (an unusual neoplasm that had previously been recognized to be associated with certain immunosuppressed states) in a person without a known cause for immunodeficiency (1, 2). Shortly thereafter it became apparent that these patients had a cellular immunodeficiency characterized by an inexorable depletion of helper/inducer ($T4^+$ or $CD4^+$) T cells, and within 3 years it had been proven that a retrovirus which has the capacity to replicate within cells of the immune system, leading to a profound destruction of $T4^+$ T cells, is the cause of AIDS (3, 4). The retrovirus is the third known human T-lymphotropic virus (HTLV-III). The virus has also been called lymphadenopathy-associated virus (LAV)(5) or AIDS-associated retrovirus (ARV) (6).* This virus poses one of the most

*Recently, the human retrovirus subcommittee of the International Committee on the Taxonomy of Viruses has proposed that the retrovirus which causes AIDS be designated as human immunodeficiency virus, HIV (7), and in the near future HIV may be the general designation for this virus.

serious threats to modern medicine, and even if education and a future vaccine prove effective, physicians will still need new therapeutic options for patients who are already infected.

The immunodeficiency of AIDS is manifested as a loss of delayed-type cutaneous hypersensitivity reactions, a loss of certain *in vitro* T-cell proliferative responses, excessive immunoglobulin production by B cells, perhaps due to abnormal regulation coupled with a T-cell dependent mitogenic effect mediated by the virus, and a loss of *in vitro* cytotoxic T cell responses. In addition, the opportunistic agents which most characteristically cause illness in this patient population (*Pneumocystis carinii*, *Mycobacterium avium* and *Candida albicans*) are normally controlled by cell-mediated (T-cell) immune responses. Once established, the immunodeficiency state is generally progressive and leads to death. The hope is that this progression can be handled and even reversed by anti-viral agents that prevent replication of the virus and its cytopathogenicity in cells of the immune system. Some recent clinical studies provide support for this idea.

In addition to its effects on the immune system, there is a growing recognition that serious neurological diseases, ranging from peripheral neuropathy to fulminant dementia, can be caused by HTLV-III with or without a clinically evident immunodeficiency (8-10). Perhaps infected macrophages play a role in the traffic of virus across the blood-brain-barrier (11, 12). While it is still not known for sure how the virus enters the brain and how it brings about neurologic damage, it is a virtual certainty that successful therapeutic strategies must address the consequences of and probably prevent, viral replication within the central nervous system. Fortunately, the prevailing assumption that AIDS-virus dementias were irreversible may not be valid with the advent of anti-retroviral chemotherapy.

As with any virus, the different stages in the life cycle of HTLV-III present a variety of distinct potential targets for anti-viral agents. In this article, we will focus on the reverse transcriptase inhibitors since there has already been some success in this area, notably with 3'-azido-2',3'-dideoxythymidine (AZT)(13, 14). The testing of new anti-retroviral agents has been facilitated by the availability of rapid and sensitive *in vitro* screening systems that determine whether a putative drug can inhibit the replication and T-cell killing activity of HTLV-III

(15). At the outset, it is worth stressing that effective therapy of HTLV-III infections may well depend on a combination of strategies that attack multiple steps in viral replication and cytopathogenicity, in part because the emergence of drug-resistant strains might be less likely.

HTLV-III as a Retrovirus

In the era before the etiology of AIDS was recognized, one of the most notable features of retroviruses was the capacity to induce neoplastic transformation in infected target cells; hence the expression "RNA tumor virus" or "leukemia virus" appeared in the literature to denote this category of virus (16). But the virus that causes AIDS has not been shown to have a transforming capacity.

By definition, retroviruses replicate through a DNA intermediate (that is, at one step of their cycle of replication, genetic information flows from RNA to DNA, a reverse or "retro" direction) (17, 18). Reverse transcriptase (the viral DNA polymerase) that catalyzes this step, is encoded by the *pol* gene of the virus, a gene that is conserved to a considerable extent in its amino acid and nucleotide sequences among retroviruses (19). The reverse transcriptase gene of the AIDS virus is one component of the *pol* region and in general this region is expressed as a polyprotein containing a protease, reverse transcriptase and an endonuclease (integrase). Subsequent cleavage yields the reverse transcriptase. These viruses have as their major structural components a core of genomic RNA; group-specific antigen (*gag*) proteins, which play a role both in the structure of the core and assembly of the virion; a lipid bilayer; and an outside envelope glycoprotein. HTLV-III is the most complex retrovirus yet characterized (20, 21) in that it contains at least five genes that are not found in previously defined retroviruses. The functions of three of these five genes are not known. The functions of two other genes, *tat-III* (22, 23) and *art* (24) or *trs* (25), will be discussed later.

Cell Binding and Entry

The first step in the infection of a cell by HTLV-III is its binding to the target cell receptor. In the case of helper/inducer T cells, this receptor seems to be linked to the cell-surface protein that is recognized by T4 or CD-4 antibodies (26, 27). The process of specific binding between the T4 antigen and parts of the viral envelope glycoprotein may be vulnerable to attack by antibodies either to the virus or to the receptor, and theoretically certain chemicals or small peptides (28) could be designed to occupy the receptor and accomplish the same thing.

It might be worthwhile deviating from the chronology of the retroviral life cycle briefly to address the cytopathogenicity of the virus which causes AIDS. There is as yet no consensus on how the virus kills T cells. From one perspective, the T4 molecule and the envelope glycoprotein of the virus determine events both at the beginning and end of the life cycle of HTLV-III within susceptible T cells. In addition to a role in the receptor mediated entry of the virus into target T cells, the T4 receptor plays a part in the susceptibility of a target T cell, once it begins to produce virus, to be killed by that virus. Precisely how HTLV-III destroys T cells *in vivo* is not known. The cytopathic effect is thought to be mediated in part by an interaction between the T4 molecule and the HTLV-III envelope protein that brings about lethal cell-to-cell fusions (syncytia) or a surface autofusion phenomenon that destroys the integrity of the cell membrane (29, 30). But other factors are also thought to play a role in the cytopathic effects of the virus. Recent results raise the possibility that the carboxyl terminus of the envelope protein, a region different from the portion that directly binds to the T4 molecule, is important in the destruction of T-cells by the virus (31).

Conceivably therapeutic agents could be designed to alter the properties (for example, the lipid composition) of the viral surface or target cell surface to reduce viral infectivity or cytopathic effects. An alternative target is the envelope protein itself. Although there is considerable variation in the protein from one viral isolate to another, the range of alterations in the binding site is most likely constrained by the need to bind to T4, which is relatively constant in structure. An antibody directed against this site might bind to (and neutralize) most strains of HTLV-III and perhaps kill infected cells as they begin to express envelope antigens so that spread of virus to uninfected cells can be reduced.

Thus, monoclonal antibodies to the envelope protein could have a therapeutic role in patients with AIDS or related diseases. We have recently been able to produce a complement-fixing human IgG_k monoclonal antibody against the major envelope glycoprotein of the first known pathogenic human T-lymphotropic retrovirus (HTLV-I) (32), and similar approaches could be used to develop human monoclonal antibodies against HTLV-III. A potential difficulty of this approach, however, is that virally infected cells could make infectious cell-to-cell contacts. Antibodies might not gain access to relevant epitopes and the envelope protein under such circumstances. Also, it has been shown that AIDS can occur in the face of what *in vitro* appears to be neutralizing antibodies to HTLV-III. Whether this occurs because the titers of such antibodies are low or because such antibodies do not block epitopes that mediate *in vivo* cytopathogenicity is under investigation. One must at least consider that humoral immunity *per se* does not protect the host, and what protection is possible is mediated by cellular immunity.

After binding to a cell, HTLV-III enters the target cell by an incompletely defined mechanism, most likely by a fusion process. It is conceivable that drugs could be developed to block this step just as calmodulin antagonists block the entry of Epstein-Barr virus into B cells. Another theoretical target is the stage of 'uncoating' of the virus after it enters a target cell. In this stage, the virus loses its envelope-coat and RNA is released into the cytoplasm (each virion is thought to convey a dimer of two identical genomic RNA subunits into the cell). Pharmacologic agents which block viral uncoating might eventually be developed in the treatment of AIDS.

Uncoated viral RNA is used as a template for the production of DNA by reverse transcriptase. As already mentioned, this enzyme has become a prime target for antiretroviral agents both because it should be possible to find inhibitors that will discriminate between this enzyme and the DNA polymerases of the host cell, thus avoiding side effects, and because a great deal is already known about reverse transcriptase. It is likely that the reverse transcriptase gene will yield important information when studied by site-directed mutagenesis. HTLV-III reverse transcriptase uses a lysine transfer RNA primer to make a minus strand DNA copy of the viral RNA as an RNA-DNA hybrid (21).

The production of reverse transcriptase in an infected cell depends on a translational frame-shift between *GAG* and *pol* and drugs that perturb this frame shift could conceivably be found to inhibit viral replication. Retroviral DNA polymerase possesses an inherent RNase H activity that specifically degrades the RNA of the RNA-DNA hybrid. The

C-terminal region of the reverse transcription protein may be a domain with RNase H activity. Theoretically, inhibition of this process would suppress viral replication. The reverse transcriptase then catalyzes the production of a positive strand DNA, and eventually, a double-stranded viral DNA is formed. In some cells, the double-stranded viral DNA can migrate to the nucleus by a poorly characterized mechanism.

The reverse transcriptase of HTLV-III has been purified and seems to exist as a p51 and a p66 molecule (33). Large quantities of the HTLV-III reverse transcriptase should become readily available because the enzyme has been expressed in bacteria (34) and yeast (P.J. Barr and P.A. Luciw, unpublished) using recombinant DNA technology. This should aid the testing of potential reverse transcriptase inhibitors. The use of such agents in patients with AIDS is predicated on the assumption that there is continuing viral replication in the disease and that its inhibition would permit some regeneration, or at least prevent further deterioration of the immune system. Two drugs (suramin and HPA-23), which early on were chosen for clinical trials because they inhibit reverse transcriptase (and were already being given to human beings for other purposes), have not appeared to confer clinical benefits to patients (35-37). Nevertheless, agents which inhibit reverse transcriptase have the most likelihood of achieving an immediate clinical impact on the virus. Several promising agents that inhibit this enzyme are either already available, having been developed for the therapy of conventional viral diseases (for example, phosphonoformate (38)) or are being developed specifically for AIDS on the basis of *in vitro* screening systems for activity against HTLV-III (13, 15). We will return to one class of such inhibitors, the dideoxynucleosides later. One member of this class of nucleosides (AZT), has already been shown to prolong survival in patients with AIDS and to confer certain other clinical benefits as well.

Integration, Latency and Reactivation

The DNA copy of HTLV-III may be circularized during or soon after its formation, and apparently can either remain in an unintegrated form or can become integrated into the genome of the host cell. It is possible that chemicals could be developed to interfere with the viral endonuclease or "integrase" (thought to be a function of one of the *pol* gene products) which mediates this integration step. Later, perhaps after activation of the infected cell, the DNA is transcribed to mRNA and viral genomic RNA using host cell RNA polymerases, and this RNA is then translated to form viral proteins, again using the biochemical apparatus of the host cell.

It has recently been shown that HTLV-III has a gene (tat-III) coding for a diffusible protein that markedly enhances the expression of other viral genes and viral replication. The tat-III gene, like the tat genes of the other two known human pathogenic retroviruses, is so called because it was originally thought to mediate a trans-activation of transcription, that is, it worked through a mechanism that affected the transcription of genes not in direct proximity to itself (22, 23). But ideas about the tat-III gene are still evolving (39, 40). The tat-III protein seems to cause an increase of viral products at a transcriptional level. However, the protein may also increase viral expression by acting beyond transcription of DNA to RNA by either enhancing mRNA stability and/or translational efficiency. Whatever the mechanisms are, the tat-III protein is thought to provide the virus with a positive feedback loop by which a viral product can amplify the production of new virions. The protein is small (86 amino acids) with a cluster of positively charged amino acids, and is thought to affect the synthesis of other proteins by binding to critical regulatory sequences at the 5' end of viral mRNA. It may be possible to find drugs that inhibit the tat-III product itself, a crucial nucleic acid binding site for this protein, or both.

Employing the same mRNA which codes for tat-III, but using a different reading frame, the art or trs gene of HTLV-III produces a different small (116 amino acids) positively charged protein, which is thought to function as a second essential trans-acting factor in viral replication (24, 25). Again, drugs which bind or inactivate this protein would be expected to inhibit viral replication. In the absence of this second regulatory factor, gag and env encoded protein synthesis is severely diminished. While there is no doubt about the existence of this new regulatory gene, its mechanism of action is still a matter for study. The suggested mechanism of action of the gene was first described as an abrogation of negative regulatory effects on translation of viral mRNA encoding HTLV-III structural proteins (hence the name art for anti-repression trans-activator)(24). It is possible that tat-III controls art, which in turn regulates the activity of gag-pol and env. A more recent report by Feinberg et al. (25) suggests that the gene product balances the amount of spliced and unspliced viral RNA to permit the preservation of gag-pol and env mRNA (hence the alternative name, trs for trans-acting regulator of splicing).

Thus, although the precise mechanisms are matters of future study, it is clear that this retrovirus has evolved an astonishingly complex system of genetic regulation. Perhaps this is because of the race between viral replication within a cell and the destruction of the cell that the virus has commandeered, leaving no tolerance for inefficiency or improper timing in the synthesis of viral components. We can hope that the very complexity of the virus will contribute to its defeat.

Protein Production and Assembly

It is conceivable that drugs that interfere with the structure and function of retroviral mRNA transcribed from integrated DNA in infected cells could be of therapeutic value in AIDS. One drug, ribavirin, is believed to act as a guanosine analogue that interferes with the 5'-capping of viral mRNA in other viral systems, and perhaps could be useful in retrovirally-induced disorders (41).

Another approach would be the use of "anti-sense" oligodeoxynucleotides, already tested in vitro (42). Basically, this approach employs short sequences of DNA (or DNA which is chemically modified to enable better cell penetration and resistance to enzymatic degradation) whose base-pairs are complementary to a vital segment of the viral genome. In theory such anti-sense oligodeoxynucleotides could block expression of the viral genome through a kind of hybridization arrest of translation or possibly interfere with the binding of a regulatory protein such as tat-III. Indeed, since the tat-III gene and the art/trs genes are expressed on the same mRNA transcript, it is possible that one anti-sense oligodeoxynucleotide could interrupt two functions that are vital for HTLV-III replication. Elsewhere in this symposium, Matsakura et al. discuss the use of phosphorothioate analogs of various oligodeoxynucleotides, some of these analogs are exceedingly potent inhibitors of the AIDS virus (and other lentiviruses) in vitro. However, there may be an unexpected level of non-specificity in terms of the oligonucleotide sequence and the precise anti-viral mechanism is not known. Whether these phosphorothyioate analogues work through a process of hybridization arrest or affect earlier stages of viral replication such as primer binding to reverse transcriptase is now under study.

The final stages in the replicative cycle of HTLV-III involve crucial secondary processing of certain viral proteins by a protease (a function of one of the pol gene products) and myristylating and glycosylating enzymes (provided by the host) as a prelude to assembly of infectious virions. Therefore, additional strategies for the treatment of AIDS might conceivably involve certain kinds of protease inhibitors or drugs which dampen or alter myristylation and glycosylation steps in the synthesis of viral components (43, 44). Finally, retroviruses are released by a process of viral budding, which may be inhibited by interferons (45).

While we have focused the discussion on how to suppress HTLV-III, it might be worth noting that the virus could set off a chain of secondary events in vivo (autoimmune reaction, toxic lymphokine production, etc.) necessary for the expression of clinical disease. It is also intriguing to speculate that a combination of anti-retroviral therapy coupled with bone marrow or lymphocyte replacement therapies might be successful in certain subsets of patients with HTLV-III infections.

Dideoxynucleosides

We would now like to turn to a discussion of a broad family of 2', 3'-dideoxynucleoside analogues that can be metabolized to become potent chain-terminating inhibitors of HTLV-III reverse transcriptase. Even at large viral doses, these analogues can completely inhibit in vitro HTLV-III replication and its capacity to destroy T-cell cultures at concentrations that are 10-20 fold lower than those that impair the proliferation and survival of target cells (46). In several cases studies of these compounds have been done over the past twenty years or so (47-53), and in triphosphate form, they are familiar to every molecular biologist as reagents for the Sanger DNA-sequencing procedure (53). But their application to human anti-retroviral therapy demands a new perspective. The dideoxynucleoside analogues are of special interest because they prove that a simple chemical modification of the sugar moiety can predictably convert a normal substrate for nucleic acid synthesis into a compound with a potent capacity to inhibit the replication and cytopathic effect of HTLV-III, at least *in vitro* (46).

We are currently developing 2',3'-dideoxycytidine as a possible agent for treating patients infected with HTLV-III. On a molar basis, dideoxycytidine is the most potent anti-viral nucleoside that we have tested, but, of course, *in vitro* potency need not necessarily be linked to a therapeutic effect. Under certain *in vitro* conditions, the drug can suppress HTLV-III at concentrations $\leq$ 10 nanomolar. This dideoxynucleoside analogue was selected for clinical development because of its *in vitro* potency against HTLV-III (46), relative resistance to cytidine deaminase (a major catabolic enzyme for cytidine analogues) (54), good oral bioavailability, straight-forward pharmacokinetic clearance by the kidney, failure to reduce normal intracellular pyrimidine pools, and comparative lack of toxicity when administered to animals. We have recently begun to administer this drug to patients. In the near future, it is expected that dideoxyadenosine will similarly be available. The adenosine analogue is interesting in terms of its low relative toxicity for human bone marrow cells *in vitro*.

While there are many issues related to the anti-retroviral effects of 2',3'-dideoxynucleosides which are as yet not resolved, it would appear that as they are successively phosphorylated in the cytoplasm of a target cell to yield 2',3'-dideoxynucleoside-5'-triphosphates, they become analogues of the 2'-deoxynucleoside-5'-triphosphates that are the natural substrates for cellular DNA polymerases and reverse transcriptase. (It is generally thought that nucleoside-5'-triphosphates do not cross cell membranes and are not active as drugs because of their ionic character and comparatively low lipophilicity.) Such analogues could compete with the binding of normal nucleotides to DNA polymerases, or could be incorporated into DNA and bring about DNA chain termination because normal 5'->3 phosphodiester linkages cannot be completed. We know that, at concentrations that are achievable in human cells, dideoxynucleotide analogues can serve as substrates for the HTLV-III reverse transcriptase to elongate a DNA chain by one residue, after which the chain is terminated (55).

Pyrimidine and purine dideoxynucleoside analogues can inhibit the *in vitro* replication and pathogenic effects of a range of animal and human retroviruses, even when the pathogenic effect being monitored (transformation) requires only a single round of replication; moreover, with certain lentiviruses (a family of animal retroviruses related to HTLV-III (56)), these drugs can reduce the *in vitro* viral infectivity by more than five orders of magnitude (57). We have found that two dideoxynucleosides, 2',3'-dideoxycytidine and 3'-azido-2',3'-dideoxythymidine (vide infra) can block the infectivity of another human retrovirus, HTLV-I, against helper/inducer T-cells *in vitro* (S. Matsushita, H. Mitsuya, M.S. Reitz, and S. Broder, unpublished). Indeed, we have not as yet observed any type or strain of retrovirus that is resistant to 2',3'-dideoxynucleoside analogues in appropriate target cells; however, the emergence of drug-resistant mutants must always be considered possible. One might speculate by analogy to herpes simplex that *pol* mutations might lead to attenuation in pathogenicity of the mutant virus. It is important to stress that the phosphorylation reactions crucial to the activation of the nucleoside analogues are catalyzed by host cell kinases, and therefore, extreme caution must be used in extrapolating from cells of one type (or species) to another. If these kinases are lacking in the host cell, the retrovirus will appear resistant to the nucleoside analogues, but if the retrovirus is permitted to replicate in a different target cell which has the appropriate enzymes for anabolic phosphorylation, it will appear sensitive again. Similarly, we have observed that one dideoxynucleoside (2',3'-dideoxythymidine) behaves as a relatively poor substrate inhibitor for human thymidine kinase. The substitution of an azido group at the 3'-carbon of this analogue, yielding 3'-azido-2',3'-dideoxythymidine (AZT), produces a compound that is an excellent substrate for thymidine kinase (Km= 3 uM) and is a very potent inhibitor of HTLV-III replication. In this context, the lack of activity against HTLV-III that we have observed using 2',3',5'-trideoxyadenosine probably relates to the unavailability of the 5'-site to undergo phosphorylation. To re-emphasize, the retrovirus does not provide its own enzymes for phosphorylation, and therefore, unlike *Herpes* viruses, cannot adopt a strategy of mutating a kinase gene to develop drug resistance.

There are data to suggest that the HTLV-III reverse transcriptase is much more susceptible to the inhibitory effects of these drugs as triphosphates than is mammalian DNA polymerase alpha (H. Mitsuya, Z. Spigelman, R.P. McCaffrey, and S. Broder, unpublished), an enzyme which has key DNA synthetic and repair functions in the life of a cell. Indeed, the reverse transcriptase has a higher affinity for dideoxynucleotides than normal substrates. This parallels what had been learned in animal retroviral systems (see discussion in references 46 and 58). Although 2',3'-dideoxynucleoside-5'-triphosphates can inhibit mammalian DNA polymerase beta (a repair enzyme), and DNA polymerase gamma (a mitochondrial enzyme) (58), we have observed that dideoxynucleosides can suppress HTLV-III replication and protect sensitive helper/inducer T cell target cells *in vitro* for long periods without interfering with the function and survival of target T cells (55). As discussed above, our working explanation for the activity of these drugs against pathogenic retroviruses is that following anabolism to nucleoside-5'-triphosphates, they bind to the viral DNA polymerase and/or bring about a selective chain termination as the RNA form of the virus attempts to make DNA copies of itself. The inherent RNase H activity of the viral DNA polymerase or cellular enzymes might be expected to degrade the viral RNA, giving the virus no second chance.

AZT

Synthesized over twenty years ago by Horwitz et al. (48) and shown to inhibit C-type murine retrovirus replication *in vitro* by Ostertag et al. more than 12 years ago (59), no medical application of 3'-azido-2',3'-dideoxythymidine (AZT) had emerged prior to our studies. We found that AZT is a very potent *in vitro* inhibitor of HTLV-III replication and its cytopathic effect in susceptible target T cells, and that it has an anti-retroviral effect against widely divergent strains of HTLV-III (13). The drug undergoes anabolic phosphorylation in human T cells to a nucleoside-5'-triphosphate (60), which can compete with thymidine-5'-triphosphate (TTP) and serve as a chain-terminating inhibitor of HTLV-III reverse transcriptase.

In that sense, AZT parallels the other dideoxynucleosides. But it can also bring about severe alterations of nucleoside metabolism within host cells, which may be of clinical significance. For example, thymidine kinase catalyzes the formation of a monophosphate derivative of AZT, which then serves as a competitive inhibitor, with very low V_{max}, of thymidylate kinase (an enzyme that catalyzes the second phosphorylation step to thymidine diphosphate), leading to the reduced formation of the third phosphorylation product, TTP (60). From this perspective,

AZT has an interesting capacity to lower the level of its natural substrate competitor (TTP) for viral and cellular DNA polymerases. AZT can also reduce 2'-deoxycytidine triphosphate (dCTP) levels (60), but the mechanism of this effect is unknown. How these reductions of normal pyrimidine pools might affect the balance between anti-retroviral activity and drug-induced cytotoxicity remains unknown. Nevertheless, a form of pyrimidine starvation is likely to contribute to bone marrow suppression, one of the key side-effects of the drug. This feature of the drug might lend itself to regimens that combine AZT with an agent that does not appear to deplete intracellular pyrimidine pools, such as dideoxycytidine. There are also other features which might have substantial clinical relevance, but remain unexplained at this time, including the capacity of acyclovir (a guanosine analogue with potent activity against *Herpes* viruses but rather weak anti-retroviral activity *per se*) to potentiate the anti-retroviral effect of AZT *in vitro*.

We began administering AZT to patients with AIDS and related conditions in a phase I (feasibility and toxicity-testing) trial in July of 1985, about 4 months after we showed that the drug suppressed the AIDS virus *in vitro*. In that study, it was found that the drug had good oral bioavailabilty and excellent penetration across the blood-brain-barrier. Our conclusion from the phase I study (14) and extensions of that study (R. Yarchoan and S. Broder, unpublished) is that during short courses of administration, AZT can bring about partial restoration of immune function and improve certain other clinical abnormalities associated with AIDS. The limiting toxicity observed was bone marrow suppression, predominantly in the form of anemia and leukopenia. In some patients with HTLV-III-mediated dementia, we observed at least some neurologic improvement, often quite prompt and dramatic; however, the durability of the improvement is still not known (61).

AZT was recently tested in a randomized study of patients with fulminant AIDS and poor prognostic AIDS-related complex under double-blind, placebo-controlled conditions at several centers under the coordination of the Burroughs-Wellcome Co. The study was begun in February 1986, and approximately 140 patients were accrued to each arm shortly thereafter. By September 1986 there were 19 deaths in the placebo arm and only one death in the AZT arm ($p<0.001$). At the same time, patients in the drug arm showed other evidence of clinical and immunological improvements. At that point, an independent data-monitoring board recommended that the placebo group begin to receive the drug. The study is still underway (with both arms now receiving drug) and at this time the long-term safety and efficacy are being assessed. Nevertheless, the results at hand warrant the initiation of appropriate controlled studies to see if therapy with AZT at an early point of retroviral infection can block the onset of AIDS in individuals who are at risk, but who are otherwise free of symptoms, at the time of treatment. It is worth noting that the Food and Drug administration recently approved AZT as a prescription drug in the USA for certain patients with AIDS and its related syndromes.

Thus, AZT, a drug chosen on the basis of its selective *in vitro* antiviral effect against HTLV-III, has been shown as a single agent to confer a clinical benefit in patients with advanced disease. In this respect, it represents a first step in developing practical chemotherapy against pathogenic human retroviruses. While the clinical results might be important in their own right, they are also important because they appear to validate the idea that therapy for established retroviral infections is a feasible goal. This was not a foregone conclusion at the beginning of these studies.

REFERENCES

1. Gottlieb, M.S. et al. *N. Engl. J. Med.* 305, 1425-1431 (1981).
2. Broder, S. & Gallo, R.C. *New Engl. J. Med.* 311, 1292-1297 (1984).
3. Gallo, R.C., et al. *Science*, 224, 500-503 (1984).
4. Popovic, M., Sarngadharan, M.G., Read, E., & Gallo, R.C. *Science*, 224, 497-500 (1984).
5. Barre-Sinoussi et al. *Science*, 220, 868-871 (1983).
6. Levi, J.A. et al. *Science*, 225, 840-842 (1984).
7. Coffin, J. et al. *Nature*, 321, 10 (1986).
8. Shaw, G.M. et al. *Nature*, 227, 177-182 (1985).
9. Ho, D.D. et al. *New Engl. J. Med.* 313, 1493-1497 (1985).
10. Resnick, L. et al. *New Engl. J. Med.* 313. 1498-1504 (1985).
11. Gartner, S. et al. *Science*, 233, 215-219 (1986).
12. Koenig, S. et al. *Science*, 233, 1089-1093 (1986).

13. Mitsuya, H. et al. Proc. Natl. Acad. Sci. USA. 82, 7096-7100 (1985).
14. Yarchoan, R. et al. Lancet, i, 575-580 (1986).
15. Mitsuya, H., Matsukura, M. & Broder, S. in AIDS: Modern Concepts and Therapeutic Challenges (ed. Broder, S.) 303-333, (Marcel Dekker, Inc., New York, 1987).
16. Gross, L. Oncogenic Viruses, 3rd edition (Pergamon, Oxford, 1983).
17. Baltimore, D. Nature, 226, 1209-1211 (1970).
18. Temin, H. & Mizutani, S. Nature, 226, 1211-1213 (1970).
19. Toh, H., Hayashida, H., & Miyata, T. Nature, 305, 827-829 (1983).
20. Ratner, L. et al. Nature, 313, 277-284 (1985).
21. Wain-Hobson, S., Sonigo, P., Danos, O., Cole, S., Alizon, M. Cell, 40, 9-17 (1985).
22. Sodroski, J. et al. Science, 227, 171-173 (1985).
23. Sodroski, J. et al. Nature, 319, 555-559 (1986).
24. Sodroski, J. et al. Nature, 321, 412-417 (1986).
25. Feinberg, M.B., Jarrett, R.F., Aldovini, A., Gallo, R.C., & Wong-Staal, F. Cell, 46, 807-817 (1986).
26. Dalgleish, A.G. et al. Nature, 312, 763-767 (1984).
27. Klatzmann, D. et al. Nature, 312, 767-768 (1984).
28. Pert, C.B. et al. Proc. Natl. Acad. Sci. USA. 83, 9254-9258 (1986).
29. Sodroski, J., Goh, W.C., Rosen, C., Campbell, K., Haseltine, W.A. Nature, 322, 470-474 (1986).
30. Lifson, J.D. et al. Nature, 323, 725-728, (1986).
31. Fisher, A.G. et al. Science, 233, 655-659 (1986).
32. Matsushita, S. et al. Proc. Natl. Acad. Sci. USA. 83, 2672-2676 (1986).
33. Veronese, F.D. et al. Science, 231, 1289-1291 (1986).
34. Tanese, N., Sodroski, J., Haseltine, W.A., & Goff, S.P. J. Virol. 59, 743-745 (1986).
35. Mitsuya, H. et al. Science, 226, 172-174 (1984).
36. Broder, S. et al. Lancet, ii, 627-630 (1985).
37. Rosenbaum, W. et al. Lancet, i, 450-451 (1985).
38. Sandstrom, E.G., Kaplan, J.C., Byington, R.E., Hirsch, M.S. Lancet, i, 1480-1482 (1985).
39. Cullen, B.R. Cell, 46, 973-982 (1986)
40. Okamoto, T. & Wong-Staal, R. Cell, 47, 29-35 (1986).
41. McCormick, J.B., Getchell, J.P., Mitchell, S.W., Hicks, D.R. Lancet, ii, 1367-1369 (1984).
42. Zamecnik, P.C., Goodchild, J., Taguchi, Y., & Sarin, P. Proc. Natl. Acad. Sci. USA, 83, 4143-4146 (1986).

43. Henderson, L.E., Krutzsch, H.C., & Oroszlan, S. *Proc. Natl. Acad. Sci. USA.* 80, 339-343 (1983).
44. Schultz, A.M. & Oroszlan, S. *J. Virol.* 46, 355-361 (1983).
45. Ho, D.D. et al. *Lancet*, i, 602-604 (1985).
46. Mitsuya, H. & Broder, S. *Proc. Natl. Acad. Sci. U.S.A.* 83, 1911-1915 (1986).
47. Robins, M.J. & Robins, R.K. *J. Am. Chem. Soc.* 86, 3585-3586 (1964).
48. Horwitz, J.P., Chua, J. & Noel, M. *J. Org. Chem.* 29, 2076-2078 (1964).
49. Doering, A.M., Janse, M. & Cohen, S.S. *J. Bact.* 92, 565-574 (1966).
50. Horwitz, J.P., Chua, J., Noel, M., & Donatti, J.T. *J. Org. Chem.* 32, 817-818 (1967).
51. Atkinson, M.R., Deutscher, M.P., Kornberg, A., Ruseel, A.F., Moffat, J.G. *Biochemistry*, 8, 4897-4904 (1969).
52. Toji, L. & Cohen, S.S. *J. Bacteriol.* 103, 323-328 (1970).
53. Sanger, F., Nicklen, S. & Coulson, A.R. *Proc. Natl. Acad. Sci. USA.* 74, 5463-5467 (1977).
54. Cooney, D.A. et al. *Biochem. Pharmacol.* 35, 2065-2068 (1986).
55. Mitsuya, H. et al. *Proc. Natl. Acad. Sci. USA.* (in the press).
56. Chi, I.-M. et al. *Nature*, 317, 366-368 (1985).
57. Dahlberg, J.E. Mitsuya, H., Broder, S., Aaronson, S.A. *Proc. Natl. Acad. Sci. USA.* (in the press).
58. Waqar, M.A., Evans, M.J., Manly, K.F., Hughs, R.G., Huberman, J.A. *J. Cell. Physiol.* 121, 402-408 (1984).
59. Ostertag, W. et al. *Proc. Natl. Acad. Sci. USA.* 71, 4980-4985 (1974).
60. Furman, P.A. et al. *Proc. Natl. Acad. Sci. USA* 83, 8333-8337 (1986).
61. Yarchoan, R. et al. *Lancet* i:132-135, 1987.

Human Retroviruses, Cancer, and AIDS:
Approaches to Prevention and Therapy, pages 381-392

ISSUES IN THE DEVELOPMENT OF ANTIVIRAL TREATMENT OF HIV INFECTION [1]

Paul A. Volberding, M.D. [2]

Medical Oncology
AIDS Activities Division
San Francisco General Hospital
San Francisco, California 94110

ABSTRACT The development of antiviral agents against the human immunodeficiency virus (HIV) has three goals: to prevent viral transmission; to prevent progression to disease manifestations in infected individuals; and to reverse established disease. Issues to be resolved in achieving these goals are discussed and knowledge gained from the clinical testing of antiviral drugs in AIDS and ARC patients is reviewed.

INTRODUCTION

The acquired immune deficiency syndrome (AIDS) is defined for surveillance purposes as the presence of unusual opportunistic infections and rare malignancies in individuals who are otherwise healthy and have no other reason for immune system compromise (1). The lifethreatening diseases associated with AIDS are endstage manifestations of infection with the human immunodeficiency virus (HIV), a retrovirus independently identified in 1983-84 by researchers in France (2) and the United States (3,4).

[1] This work was supported by a grant from the University of California AIDS Task Force.
[2] Present address: San Francisco General Hospital, Ward 84, 995 Potrero Avenue, San Francisco, California 94110

HIV infection produces a spectrum of clinical manifestations ranging from no symptoms in some individuals to rapid disease progression and death in others. Within this spectrum, several syndromes have been identified, including the persistent lymphadenopathy syndrome (PGL) (5,6,7) the AIDS-related complex (ARC) (8,9) and the acquired immunodeficiency syndrome (10,11,12). At first thought to represent discrete manifestations of response to the virus, these syndromes are now considered to be clinical stages on a continuum of retroviral destruction of the immune system. Strong evidence is accumulating that a majority of people with HIV infection will eventually manifest some symptoms of disease (7,13) and more than half will progress to ARC or AIDS (G. Rutherford, personal communication, 1987). Given the possibility that 1 to 2 million people may currently be infected in the United States and millions more worldwide, the full impact of HIV infection in terms of morbidity, mortality, and socioeconomic costs is only beginning to be felt.

In the United States, more than 35,000 cases of AIDS and more than 20,000 deaths have been reported [14]. By the early 1990s, 270,000 AIDS cases and 179,000 deaths are projected 15. Mortality from AIDS is extremely high. Two-year mortality in patients with an opportunistic infection or Kaposi's sarcoma approaches 90% and the ultimate mortality may be 100% (16). In patients with ARC, two-year mortality is low, but as many of these patients will progress to AIDS, the ultimate mortality may be very high.

In cities where the majority of AIDS cases have been diagnosed, the health care systems are already being overwhelmed by the complex medical, psychological, and social needs of AIDS patients. Estimates of the average lifetime costs per AIDS patient range from $50,000 to $150,000 (17-19). At San Francisco General Hospital, which developed a model system of comprehensive AIDS patient care, costs have been kept relatively low through the emphasis on outpatient services, coordination of inpatient and outpatient care, and the contribution of voluntary agencies in providing home care and psychosocial and educational services (20). Lifetime hospital charges for AIDS patients at San Francisco General Hospital are about $30,000 (21). If out-of-hospital costs are included, however, an estimate of $50,000 to $70,000 per AIDS patient is more realistic.

As the AIDS epidemic continues to expand, medical strategies to control this disease focus increasingly on the development of antiviral drugs to treat the underlying infection with the human immunodeficiency virus (HIV). No matter how successful treatments become for the opportunistic infections and malignancies of AIDS, so long as the retroviral infection persists and the immune deficiency worsens, mortality will remain extremely high.

Antiviral therapy for HIV infection has three goals: 1) to prevent further transmission of the virus, either by treating currently infected individuals to reduce their contagious risk to others or by drug prophylaxis in uninfected individuals to prevent establishment of infection; 2) to prevent progression of disease in those already infected; and 3) to reverse established disease and restore immune system function. To achieve these goals, we need to know more about the mechanisms of HIV transmission, the natural history of the virus, and the pathogenesis of immune deficiency. In addition, many practical and economic issues need to be resolved if antiviral drugs are to be used on millions of people worldwide. Although much has been learned about HIV since it was first discovered, many basic questions with important clinical implications remain unanswered.

PREVENTING HIV TRANSMISSION

HIV may be found in essentially any body fluid, but only blood, semen, and vaginal and cervical secretions are believed to be important in viral transmission (22). Although HIV has been detected in saliva and tears, there is no evidence that the virus is commonly transmitted through these fluids. It is well established that HIV is transmitted through contact with infected blood and blood products and through sexual intercourse with an infected partner. Sexual transmission of the virus can occur through vaginal, anal, and possibly oral intercourse. Infected males can transmit the virus sexually to homosexual or heterosexual partners, and infected females can transmit the virus sexually to males and perinatally to their unborn infants. Since the HIV antibody test has been used to screen donated blood, the risk of viral transmission through blood transfusion is greatly reduced. The primary blood-borne route of transmission is through contaminated hypodermic syringes shared by intravenous drug users. As evidenced by studies of health care workers (23-25) and household contacts of AIDS patients (26-28), HIV is not casually transmitted.

Retroviral infection occurs when HIV attaches to the T4 antigen on the surface of a cell. Many cells appear to carry the antigen, including T-helper lymphocytes, macrophages, and possibly glial cells in the central nervous system (29). It is not yet known whether infection requires exposure to the naked virus or to cells infected with the virus. If infection occurs through exposure to infected cells, it is less likely that a vaccine will prevent that form of transmission.

Within 8 weeks following infection, antibodies to HIV may be detected by the ELISA antibody test in 50% of people (30). Almost all infected individuals seroconvert within 6 months following infection. Unlike antibodies to other viruses, the HIV antibody implies neither immunity nor that a person is no longer contagious to others. The HIV antigen and antibody appear almost simultaneously and both imply that an individual is actively infected, probably for life, and represents a continuing contagious risk to others through sexual, parenteral, or perinatal routes of viral transmission. There is no credible evidence that a person infected with HIV may spontaneously clear the virus or become immune.

Antiviral drugs designed to prevent HIV transmission would have to reduce either the infectiousness of someone who already carries the virus or susceptibility to infection in someone who might be exposed to the virus. To reduce infectiousness, the ideal drug would have to markedly decrease viral replication and viral titre in semen, blood, and vaginal secretions. To reduce susceptibility to infection, the drug would have to block attachment of the virus to the T4 antigen or neutralize the effects of possible co-factors involved in promoting susceptibility to infection.

We do not yet know what determines the infectious risk of an infected person or what factors are most important in determining susceptibility to infection. Are all infected people capable of transmitting the virus at all times? How much virus needs to be inhibited to reduce the likelihood of transmission? Are all people equally susceptible to HIV infection, if exposed? Do factors such as nutrition or recreational drug use affect susceptiblity to HIV infection? Does the presence of a coincident venereal disease, such as herpes or gonorrhea, facilitate viral transmission or infection? Answers to these questions will assist the development of effective antiviral treatments or prophylactics to prevent HIV transmission.

PREVENTING PROGRESSION OF DISEASE

People with AIDS and ARC have both qualitative and quantitative loss of immune function. The absolute number of T-helper cells is probably the best index of immune competence. At various lengths of time following HIV infection, the virus begins to destroy the T-helper cell population. It is not known whether the virus simply kills helper-T cells so that fewer cells are in circulation or whether it disrupts hormones responsible for normal cell proliferation and functioning. As the immune system is destroyed, people gradually begin to manifest the various symptoms collectively referred to as ARC, and with further immune damage, the clinical manifestations of AIDS.

HIV may penetrate the central nervous system very early in the disease process. Evidence for this comes from clinical observations of aseptic meningitis in patients who experience the acute retroviral syndrome within a few weeks following infection (31). Viral culture of cerebral spinal fluid in these patients confirms the presence of HIV. To prevent the neurologic damage and dementias associated with AIDS, therefore, an antiviral drug must be capable of crossing the blood-brain barrier.

An antiviral drug that prevents disease progression must block viral replication without compromising the restoration of normal immune function. Treatment probably should start as soon as possible following infection and probably must continue for at least for 10 years and perhaps for life. Experience with other chronic and potentially life-threatening diseases, such as hypertension, suggests that longterm compliance with drug treatment regimens is extremely difficult to maintain. Any effective antiviral drug for HIV, therefore, will have to be convenient to take, orally administered, have minimal toxicity and essentially no subjective side effects. Moreover, if millions of people might be required to take it for the rest of their lives, the drug must be inexpensive. This is especially important for use in Third World countries with few health care resources.

REVERSING ESTABLISHED DISEASE

By the time an individual has AIDS or ARC, damage to the immune system may be irreversible by using antiviral drugs alone. Among the questions to be answered is whether the virus has infected the stem cells needed to repopulate the immune system. If these cells are destroyed early in the viral infectious process, inhibiting the virus will be insufficient to reverse the disease and bone marrow transplants may be required to restore the immune system.

More knowledge is needed about the mechanisms of neuronal destruction that produce the dementias and neurologic syndromes associated with AIDS. If viral infection of brain cells is the primary mechanism, the chance of reversing this process is small. However, the neurologic dysfunction may result from the action of lymphokines or other secreted factors in the brain. If so, inhibiting the virus might result in some improvement.

Combining antiviral drug therapy with drugs that stimulate the immune system might be effective in restoring immune function. Experiments using interferon (32) and recombinant interleukin-2 alone to stimulate the immune system have been unsuccessful. Among the possible explanations for this failure is that immune system stimulation simply creates new target cells for the virus to infect, or that these drugs cause cells infected with HIV to proliferate and produce more virus. Unless antiviral drugs are used first to inhibit the virus, immune system stimulators will be ineffective in restoring normal function.

CLINICAL TESTING OF ANTIVIRAL AGENTS

Clinical testing of anti-HIV drugs is fraught with problems. Testing in patients with fully established AIDS may not be useful because even if a drug were effective against HIV, disease might be so far advanced that this would be difficult to prove. On the other hand, testing an experimental drug in a completely healthy person raises serious ethical problems. Is it appropriate to test a drug that might be toxic in someone who might not really need therapy for another 10 years? Although the first clinical drug trials were in AIDS patients, today researchers are more interested in testing drugs in asymptomatic seropositive people in order to prevent progression to disease.

Suramin and HPA23 were the first antiviral drugs clinically tested in the United States (33-37). When suramin testing began, people clamored for access to the drug and a black market for it developed. Unfortunately, suramin proved to have no efficacy and considerable toxicity, resulting in the death of some patients who had not yet developed AIDS. Two patients became adrenal insufficient during the clinical trial and still have no detectable adrenal function. Moreover, four of five patients who became viral culture negative had progression of disease even in the absence of the virus.

Tests of HPA23, a French drug, had a similar outcome. HPA23 had no real effect against HIV or in slowing disease progression, and even when the virus was inhibited, the clinical outcome was unaffected.

These experiences taught us to be very cautious in clinical testing of anti-HIV drugs. A drug that is effective in the laboratory may be ineffective in patients and may produce dangerous side effects.

Zidovudine (formerly called azidothymidine or AZT) is the first drug against HIV that has showed clear benefits in slowing progression of disease. Recently approved for commercial release under the brand name Retrovir (Burroughs Wellcome), zidovudine is a modification of thymidine. It is thought to inhibit DNA synthesis and prevent replication of HIV. Zidovudine requires only 2.3 micromolar concentration to inhibit HIV reverse transcriptase compared with much higher concentrations required to inhibit cellular DNA polymerase.

In 1986, zidovudine was tested in 140 AIDS patients and 140 patients with symptomatic ARC in a multi-center, double-blind, placebo-controlled clinical trial (38). The first patients were enrolled February 18; by September 10, the Data Safety Monitoring Board decided that evidence of the drug's effectiveness was substantial enough to warrant stopping the trial at that time. Of 17 subjects who died during the trial, 16 were receiving placebo and one was receiving zidovudine. The difference between the two groups was highly significant (P=<.001). In addition, zidovudine seemed to decrease the frequency of complications of AIDS. After the first 6 weeks of the trial, the placebo and drug groups differed markedly in terms of frequency of serious events (opportunistic infections, Kaposi's sarcoma, lymphomas, death). Although some disease progression occurred in both groups, the placebo group progressed much more rapidly, with a higher rate of opportunistic infections and death.

The effects of zidovudine on the immune system are unclear. In patients with ARC who received the drug, T4 cells increased during 24 weeks of treatment compared with patients receiving placebo. In AIDS patients who received zidovudine, T4 cells increased early in the study, but by the end of the trial there were no significant differences between the drug group and the placebo group. HIV antigen levels were decreased in patients who received the drug compared to those who received placebo (39).

Zidovudine has considerable toxicity. Hemoglobin levels decreased dramatically in patients in the treatment group. Forty patients who received zidovudine required blood transfusions compared to 11 patients who received placebo. Twenty-two patients in the zidovudine group were transfused more than once, compared with only 3 in the placebo group. About 20-30% of patients with AIDS become transfusion dependent, requiring about one unit of red cells per week in order to continue taking zidovudine. If we consider the possibility that zidovudine might be taken by thousands of people who might then become transfusion dependent, the nation's blood supply could be adversely affected.

It is possible that hematologic toxicity from zidovudine is lower in less symptomatic people. Patients with ARC needed fewer blood transfusions during the clinical trial. This suggests that less risk and possibly greater benefit may be expected if the drug is used in infected people who have few or no symptoms of disease.

Other drugs still in clinical trials may prove useful for treatment of HIV. These include ribavirin and dideoxycitadine. Dideoxycitadine, a new drug now in Phase I testing at the National Institutes of Health, inhibits HIV in vitro at much lower micromolar concentration than zidovudine (.5 micromolar compared with 2.3 micromolar for zidovudine). However, it may not penetrate the central nervous system as well as zidovudine.

Some antiviral drugs may be more effective in combination. Zidovudine and acyclovir, now being tested in asymptomatic seropositive men at the University of California, San Francisco, may act at a similar site in the body and potentiate each other's effectiveness. In combination with probenicid, the half-life of zidovudine may be prolonged. Some drug combinations might enable us to inhibit the virus and facilitate immune recovery simultaneously in patients who have not yet advanced to AIDS.

Although it is unlikely that existing antiviral agents will reduce the magnitude of the AIDS epidemic within the next few years, there is reason for optimism. It is already possible to inhibit replication of HIV in the laboratory and to some degree in people with established infection. Of the three goals of antiviral therapy, we may be closest to achieving the most important, prevention of disease progression in people with established infection.

REFERENCES

1. Centers for Disease Control (1985). "The Case Definition of AIDS Used by the CDC for National Reporting." Document No. 0312S. Atlanta: Centers for Disease Control.
2. Barre-Sinoussi F, Chermann JC, Rey F, Nugeyre MT, Chamaret S, Gruest J, Daugier C, Axler-Blin C, Vezinet-Brun F, Rouzioux C, Rozenbaum W, Montagnier L (1983). Isolation of a T-lymphotropic retrovirus from a patient at risk for acquired immune deficiency syndrome (AIDS). Science 220:868-71.
3. Gallo RC, Salahuddin SZ, Popovic M, Shearer GM, Kaplan M, Haynes BF, Palker TJ, Redfield R, Oleske J, Safai B, White G, Foster P, Markham P(1984). Frequent detection and isolation of cytopathic retroviruses (HTLV-III) from patients with AIDS and at risk for AIDS. Science 224:500-3.
4. Levy JA, Hoffman AD, Kramer SM, Landis JA, Shimabukuro J, Oshiro LS (1984). Isolation of lymphocytopathic retroviruses from San Francisco patients with AIDS. Science 225:840-2.
5. Pinn-Wiggins VW (1985). Follow-up at 4 1/2 years on homosexual men with generalized lymphadenopathy. N Engl J Med 313:1542.
6. Sirianni MC, Rossi P, Scarpati B, Ragona G, Seminara R, Bonomo G, Aiuti F (1985). Immunological and virological investigation in patients with lymphadenopathy syndrome in a population at risk for acquired immunodeficiency syndrome (AIDS); with particular focus on the detection of antibodies to human T-lymphotropic retroviruses (HTLV-III). J Clin Immunol 5:261-8.
7. Abrams DI, Mess T, Volberding PA. Lymphadenopathy: Endpoint or prodrome? Update of a 36-month prospective study. Adv Exp Med Biol 187:73-84.
8. Morris L, Distenfeld A, Amorosi E, Karpatkin S. (1982). Autoimmune thrombocytopenic purpura in homosexual men. Ann Intern Med 96:714-7.
9. Abrams DI, Kiprov DD, Volberding PA (1985). Isolated thrombocytopenia in homosexual men - longitudinal follow-up. Adv Exp Med Biol 187:117-22.

10. Gottlieb GJ, Ragaz A, Vogel JV, Friedman-Kien A, Rywkin AM, Weiner EA, Ackerman AB (1981). A preliminary communication on extensively disseminated Kaposi's sarcoma in young homosexual men. Am J Dermatopathol 3:111-4.
11. Rivin BE, Monroe JM, Hubschman BP, Thomas PA (1984). AIDS outcome: A first follow-up. N Engl J Med 311:857.
12. Jaffe HW, Bregman DJ, Selik RM (1983). Acquired immunodeficiency syndrome in the United States: First 1,000 cases. J Infect Dis 148:339-45.
13. Abrams DI, Kiprov DD, Goedert JJ, Sarngadharan MG, Gallo RC, Volberding PA (1986). Antibodies to human T-lymphotropic virus type III and development of the acquired immunodeficiency syndrome in homosexual men presenting with immune thrombocytopenia. Ann Intern Med 104:47-50.
14. Centers for Disease Control (1987). AIDS Weekly Surveillance Report - United States. May 11.
15. National Academy of Sciences, Institute of Medicine (1986). "Confronting AIDS." Washington D.C.: National Academy Press, p 8.
16. Moss AR, McCallum G, Volberding PA, Bacchetti P, Dritz S. (1984). Mortality associated with mode of presentation in the acquired immune deficiency syndrome. JNCI 73:1281-4.
17. Hardy A, Rauch K, Echenberg DF, Morgan WM, Curran JW (1986). The economic impact of the first 10,000 cases of AIDS in the United States. JAMA 225:209-11.
18. Kizer KW, Rodreguez J, McHolland GF, Weller W (1986). "A Qualitative Analysis of AIDS in California." Sacramento: Department of Health Services.
19. Scitovsky AA, Rice DP, Showstack J, Lee PR (1986). "Estimating the Direct and Indirect Economic Costs of the Acquired Immune Deficiency Syndrome, 1985, 1986, and 1990." Task order 282-85-0061. Atlanta: Centers for Disease Control.
20. Volberding PA (1985). The clinical spectrum of the acquired immunodeficiency syndrome: Implications for comprehensive patient care. Ann Intern Med 103:729-33.
21. Scitovsky AA, Cline M, Lee PR. (1986). Medical care costs of patients with AIDS in San Francisco. JAMA 256:3103-6.
22. Wofsy C. (1987). Human immunodeficiency virus infection in women. JAMA 257:2074-5.
23. McCray E (1986). Occupational risk of the acquired immunodeficiency syndrome among health care workers. N Engl J Med 314:1127-32.

24. Moss A, Osmond D, Bacchetti P, Gerberding J, Sande M, Volberding P, Levy JA, Carlson J, Casavant C, Conant M (1986). Risk of seroconversion for the acquired immune deficiency syndrome (AIDS) in San Francisco health workers. J Occup Med 28:821-4.
25. Henderson DK, Saah AJ, Zak BJ, Kaslow RA, Lane HC, Folks T, Blackwelder WC, Schmitt J, LeCamera DJ, Masur HH, Fauci AS (1986). Risk of nosocomial infection with human T-cell lymphotropic virus type III/lymphadenopathy-associated virus in a large cohort of intensively exposed health care workers. Ann Intern Med 104:644-7.
26. Friedland GH, Saltzman BR, Rogers MF, Kahl PA, Lesser ML, Mayers MM, Klein RS (1986). Lack of transmission of HTLV-III/LAV infection to household contacts of patients with AIDS or AIDS-related complex with oral candidiasis. N Engl J Med 314:344-49.
27. Mann JM, Quinn TC, Francis H, Nzilambi N, Bosenge N, Bila K, McCormick JB, Ruti K, Asila PK, Curran JW (1986). Prevalence of HTLV-III/LAV in household contacts of patients with confirmed AIDS and controls in Kinshasa, Zaire. JAMA 256:721-24.
28. Fischl MA, Dickinson GM, Scott GB, Klimas N, Fletcher MA, Parks W (1987). Evaluation of heterosexual partners, children, and household contacts of adults with AIDS. JAMA 257:640-4.
29. Gabuzda DH, Ho DD, de la Monte SM, Hirsch MS, Rota TR, Sobel RA (1986). Immunohistochemical identification of HTLV-III antigen in brains of patients with AIDS. Ann Neurol 20:289-95.
30. Melbye M (1986). The natural history of human T lymphotropic virus III infection: The cause of AIDS. Br Med J 292:5-12.
31. Cooper DA, Gold J, Mclean P, Donovan B, Finlayson R, Barnes TG, Michelmore HM, Brooke P, Penny R (1985). Acute AIDS retroviral seroconversion. Lancet 1:537-40.
32. Groopman JE, Gottlieb MS, Goodman J, Mitsuya RT, Conant MA, Prince H, Fahey JL, Derezin M, Weinstein W, Casavant C, Rothman J, Rudnick SA, Volberding PA (1984). Recombinant alpha 2 interferon therapy of Kaposi's sarcoma associated with acquired immunodeficiency syndrome. Ann Intern Med 100:671-6.

33. Broder S, Yarchoan R, Collins JM, Lance HC, Markham PP, Klecker RW, Redfield RR, Mitsuya H, Hoth DF, Gellman E, Groopman JE, Resnick L, Gallo RC, Myers CE, Fauci AS (1985). Effects of suramin on HTLV-III/LAV infection presenting Kaposi's sarcoma or AIDS-related complex: clinical pharmacology and suppression of virus in vivo. Lancet 2:627-30.

34. Levine AM, Gill PS, Cohen J, Hawkins JG, Formenti SC, Aguilar S, Meyer PR, Krailo M, Parker J, Rasheed S (1985). Suramin antiviral therapy in the acquired immunodeficiency syndrome. Clinical, immunologic, and virologic results. Ann Intern Med 105:32-7.

35. Rouvroy D, Bogaerts J, Habyarimana JB, Nzaramba O, Van de Perre P (1985). Short-term results with suramin for AIDS-related conditions. Lancet 1:878-9.

36. Stein CA, Saville W, Yarchoan R, Broder S, Gellman EP (1986). Suramin and function of the adrenal cortex. Ann Intern Med 104: 286-7.

37. Kaplan LD, Wolfe PR, Volberding PA, Feorino P, Levy JA, Abrams DI, Kiprov D, Wong R, Kaufman L, Gottlieb MS (1987). Lack of response to suramin in patients with AIDS and AIDS-related complex. Amer J Med 82:615-19.

38. Fischl MA, Richmond DD, Grieco MH, Gottlieb MS, Volberding PA, Laskin OL, Leedom JM, Groopman JE, Mildvan D, Schooley RT, Jackson GG, Durack DT, King D, The AZT Collaborative Working Group (1987, in press). The efficacy of 3'-azido-3'-deoxythymidine (azidothymidine) in the treatment of patients with AIDS and AIDS-related complex: A double-blind placebocontrol trial. N Engl J Med.

39. Chaisson RE, Allain J-P, Leuther M, Volberding PA (1986). Significant changes in HIV antigen level in the serum of patients treated with azidothymidine. N Engl J Med 315:1610-1.

Human Retroviruses, Cancer, and AIDS: Approaches to Prevention and Therapy, pages 393–406

TREATMENT OF HUMAN IMMUNODEFICIENCY VIRUS-ASSOCIATED NEUROLOGICAL DISEASE WITH 3'-AZIDO-2',3'-DIDEOXYTHYMIDINE

Robert Yarchoan, Rose V. Thomas, Margaret A. Fischl, Jordan Grafman, Alison Wichman, Marinos Dalakas, Freda K. Jacobsen, Nanette McAtee, Carlo Federico Perno, Bijan Safai, Raymond W. Klecker, Jerry M. Collins, Gary Berg, Arturo Brunetti, Peter J. Schmidt, Pim Brouwers, A. Robert Spitzer, Steven M. Larson, Charles E. Myers, and Samuel Broder

National Cancer Institute, Bethesda, MD; University of Miami, FL; National Institute of Neurological and Communicative Disorders and Stroke, Bethesda; Memorial Sloan-Kettering Cancer Center, New York, NY; National Institute of Mental Health, and Depertment of Nuclear Medicine, Clinical Center, National Institutes of Health, Bethesda.

ABSTRACT Human immunodeficiency virus (HIV) can infect cells in the nervous system, and neurological dysfunction is frequently noted in patients with HIV infection. We have administered 3'-azido-2',3'-dideoxythymidine (AZT), a potent _in vitro_ inhibitor of HIV replication, to 7 patients with HIV-associated neurological disorders: 4 with dementia, 2 with peripheral neuropathy, 1 with dementia and peripheral neuropathy, and 1 with a T10 paraplegia. Five of the 7 patients had a substantial improvement in their neurological symptoms over a 3 to 8 week period of time, while a sixth patient had minimal improvement. Clinical improvement was corroborated by improvement in neuropsychometric testing, nerve conduction studies, and in two patients, positron emission tomographic (PET) scans. In 3 of the patients, the improvement was transient, and 2 of them expired from pneumonia 6 to 8 months after the start of therapy. Three of the patients have had sustained improvement 4 to 18 months after the initiation of AZT. These results suggest that certain HIV-associated neurological abnormalities are at least partially reversible following the administration of antiretroviral chemotherapy.

INTRODUCTION

Patients with acquired immunodeficiency syndrome (AIDS) and related disorders can develop a variety of neurological disturbances including progressive dementia, peripheral neuropathy, and myelopathy. The central nervous system (CNS) is an important site of HIV replication (1-3), and this neurotropism is one of several features that link HIV to animal lentiviruses (1). Some patients with AIDS may develop neurological dysfunction as a result of secondary infections or neoplasms. However, much of the neurological dysfunction in patients with HIV infection is a direct consequence of the retroviral infection (1-3).

3'-azido-2',3'-thymidine (AZT) is a dideoxynucleoside analogue which has been found to be a potent inhibitor of HIV infection _in vitro_ (4). Phase I studies of AZT in patients with AIDS and related disorders demonstrated that concentrations which inhibited HIV _in vitro_ were attainable in patients and that the drug effectively crossed the blood brain barrier (5-7). In addition, these studies showed that some patients with HIV infection had evidence of immunologic and clinical improvement upon receiving AZT for a 6 week period of time. One of the patients on this Phase I study had improvement in peripheral neuropathy while receiving AZT (5). With this background, we administered AZT to 6 additional patients with HIV-associated neurological disease. Preliminary results obtained in 4 of these patients have been previously reported (7); the present manuscript represents an extension of that report.

PATIENTS AND METHODS

Seven patients with HIV-related neurological abnormalities were studied. Each patient was assessed clinically, immunologically, and neurologically as described below and gave informed consent. The patients then started receiving AZT. Subsequent evaluations were done periodically. The protocol for this study was approved by the institutional review board of the National Cancer Institute.

A battery of standard tests were utilized for the neuropsychological evaluation of the patients. These included the trailmaking and WAIS-R digit-symbol substitution tests as measures of attention; the Wechsler memory stories test and Kimura's recurring figures test as measures of memory; and the Purdue or grooved pegboard test as a measure of motor coordination (7). Nerve conduction tests were done with standard methods and with the limbs at a constant temperature.

Positron emission tomography (PET) was done with 2-[18]fluoro-2-deoxy-d-glucose (FDG) and a standardized protocol (7). Briefly, subjects were given an intravenous injection of 5 mCi FDG (1 mCi = 3.7×10^7 Bq), and arterial blood samples were taken from a radial artery catheter at timed intervals. After 45 min of radionuclide uptake, during which the patient rested on the scanner bed with both eyes covered, PET scans were obtained with the NIH 'Scanditronix PC-1024' scanner. The images were corrected for attenuation of emitted radiation with the ellipse border method.

RESULTS

During the first 3 to 8 weeks of therapy, each of the 4 patients with HIV-associated dementia had a substantial improvement in their neuropsychiatric function. Two of these patient have had a sustained improvement for 4 and 6 months respectively; the other two expired 6 and 8 months after the initiation of therapy after a 5 to 6 month period of sustained neuropsychiatric improvement. One patient with a T10 paraplegia failed to improve during a 3 week period during which he received AZT. Of the 3 patients with peripheral neuropathy (including one who also had dementia), two had substantial improvements for 6 and 18 months respectively, while the third had minimal improvement. These cases are detailed below.

Case 1.

A 32-year old designer developed numbness of his feet, impotence, and oral candidiasis and was found to have antibodies to HIV. Over the next several months, his symptoms worsened and he developed mild memory loss; 5 months after his initial presentation he developed *Pneumocystis carinii* pneumonia which responded to treatment. By 7 months after his initial presentation, he could only walk short distances and was unable to draw because of weakness, incoordination, and lack of concentration. Neurological examination showed upper and lower extremity weakness, a wide-based gait, and reduced pinprick sensation in the legs. Nerve conduction studies showed a decreased amplitude and nerve conduction velocity indicative of a mixed demyelinating and axonal pattern (Table 1).

TABLE 1
NERVE CONDUCTION STUDIES IN PATIENT 1

Nerve	Week 0	Week 8	Week 14
Left ulnar			
sensory			
Amplitude	6 microV	21 microV	17 microV
Velocity	33.4 m/sec	43.0 m/sec	40.0 m/sec
Right ulnar			
motor (proximal)			
Amplitude	2.5 mV	5.7 mV	6.6 mV
Velocity	44.5 m/sec	38.4 m/sec	39 m/sec

On psychometric assessment, he had decreased attention and coordination, and memory was less than expected for a person of his educational background (Figure 1). Analysis of his cerebrospinal fluid (CSF) showed 42 mg/dl protein, 46 mg/dl glucose, and 2 white blood cells/mm^3; no mycobacterial, fungal, or bacterial organisms grew in culture. He was profoundly immunosuppressed with 43 CD4+ cells/mm^3 (normal range 540-1170).

He was started on 250 mg of AZT every 4 hrs. As shown in Figure 2, the concentration of AZT in his CSF 4 hours after an oral dose was 0.47 microM. A PET scan shortly after starting on AZT showed a heterogeneous pattern with a relative decrease in glucose metabolism in the posterior temporal, posterior occipital, and thalamic regions as compared to the frontal region. Over the next 10 weeks, he had a striking improvement in his neurologic and immunologic function (Table 1, Figure 1). His memory improved, his muscle strength increased (dominant hand grip strength increased from 17 to 26 kg), his gait became less ataxic and he was able to walk unassisted, he resumed drawing, and he was able to sustain an erection for the first time in 8 months. On nerve conduction studies, he had an increase in three of four parameters studied (Table 1). His CD4+ cells increased to 228/mm^3 and <u>in vitro</u> proliferation and gamma interferon in response to PHA increased. His anemia

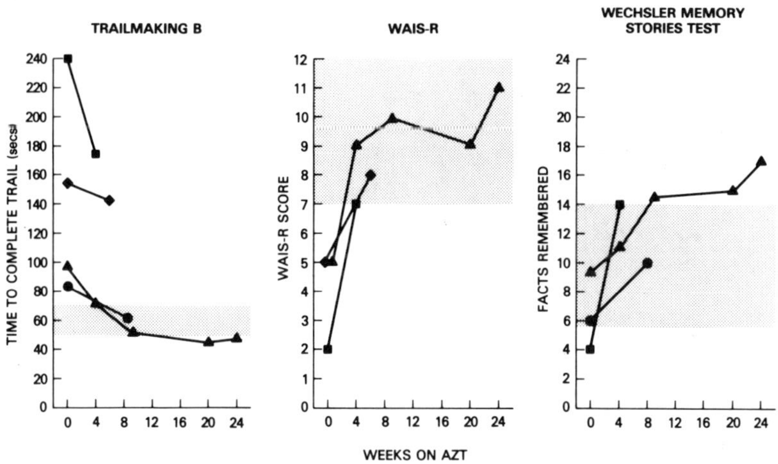

FIGURE 1. Results of psychometric testing in the 4 patients with HIV-induced dementia. Each symbol depicts the results obtained with one patient at the initiation of therapy and after various times on AZT: circles, pt. 1; squares, pt. 2; triangles, pt. 5; diamonds, pt. 6. The shaded areas show the normal range for each test. In the trailmaking test, decreased times to complete the test depict improvement. In the WAIS-R and Wechsler memory stories test, increased scores depict improvement.

worsened, however, and he required several blood transfusions. After 4 months, his helper $CD4^+$ cells decreased to $20/mm^3$ and he became thrombocytopenic; because of the latter, his dose of AZT was reduced to 250 mg every 8 hrs. He maintained his neurologic improvement on this reduced dose; however, 6 months after starting on therapy, he developed Pneumocystis carinii pneumonia and expired.

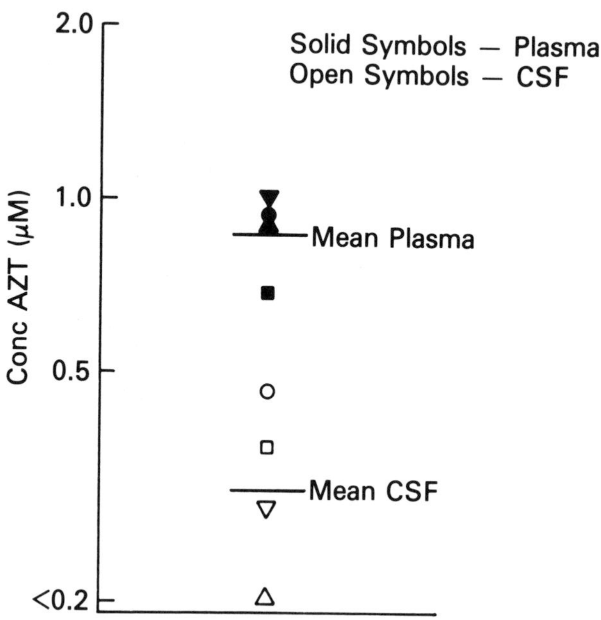

FIGURE 2. Plasma and CSF levels of AZT in 4 patients with HIV-associated dementia. Solid symbols depict plasma levels and open symbols depict simultaneously obtained CSF levels. The symbols are as follows: (●,O) pt. 1, 4 hrs after 250 mg AZT orally; (■,□), pt. 2, 4 hrs after 162 mg AZT given intravenously; (▼,▽), pt. 5, 4 hrs after 250 mg AZT given orally; (▲,△), pt. 6, 2 hrs after 250 mg AZT given orally.

Case 2.

A 58-year old male professional was diagnosed as having AIDS with Kaposi's sarcoma (KS) confined to the skin and was given recombinant interferon alpha over a 7 month period of time. Starting while he was receiving the interferon, he developed fatigue, memory loss, ataxia, and tremulousness; he had difficulty in walking unassisted. These symptoms did improve upon reducing the dose of interferon and subsequently stopping it. A computerized tomographic scan of the head showed moderate cerebral atrophy. Analysis of his CSF showed 79 mg/dl protein, 41 mg/dl glucose, and 4 white blood cells/mm^3; cultures for mycobacteria, fungi, and bacteria were negative. He had 90 CD4$^+$ cells/mm^3.

He was started on 162 mg of AZT intravenously every 4 hrs; 4 hrs after a dose of AZT, he had 0.36 microM AZT in his CSF. After 2 weeks he was switched to 324 mg and later 250 mg orally every 4 hrs. He had minimal change in his immunologic status. However, over a 4 to 6 week period of time, he had a substantial improvement in his mentation and improvement in his formal psychometric testing (Figure 2). He was able to resume some professional activities. He also had a complete resolution of his KS lesions.

While on the AZT he developed anemia with a hypocellular bone marrow and required periodic transfusions. Five months after being started on AZT, his dose was reduced to 250 mg every 8 hrs because of neutropenia, and 3 months later it had to be stopped. Over the next 4 weeks, his mentation progressively deteriorated to the point where his verbal output was confined to simple phrases, and he died from bacterial pneumonia.

Case 3

A 31 year old male developed oral candidiasis, fatigue, lymphadenopathy, and lower extremity numbness and tingling with difficulty ambulating and was found to have antibodies to HIV. He used a cane for support. A computerized tomographic scan of the head was normal. CSF contained 49 mg/dl protein, 61 mg/dl glucose, and 1 white blood cell/mm^3. Cultures of the CSF failed to grow mycobacteria, fungi, or bacteria. He had 365 CD4$^+$ cells/mm^3.

He was started on 156 mg AZT every 8 hrs intravenously for 2 weeks, followed by 312 mg AZT orally every 8 hrs;

after 16 weeks, this was changed to 250 mg every 8 hrs. Over the first 6 weeks of therapy, he had a resolution of his lower extremity numbness and difficulty ambulating; he no longer used a cane, his gait became normal, and he could climb stairs without difficulty. He remains on AZT 18 months after the initiation of therapy and maintains his clinical improvement.

Case 4

A 39-year old man with AIDS-associated KS had progressive T10 paraplegia and bladder and bowel dysfunction. Myelographs, magnetic resonance imaging, and computerized tomographic studies did not reveal evidence of a space-occupying lesion in the spinal cord or brain. Cultures of the CSF revealed HIV and cytomegalovirus. His paraplegia was attributed to HIV and/or cytomegalovirus infection. He was started on oral AZT, 250 mg every 4 hrs. On this regimen, he developed nausea and vomiting and was switched to intravenous AZT, 125 mg every 4 hrs. Over the next 3 weeks, his KS progressed but he had no significant change in his paraplegia. His AZT therapy was stopped after three weeks, and the patient expired approximately 4 months later.

Case 5

A 32-year old graduate student had an episode of pneumonia and was found to have antibodies to HIV. His pneumonia was presumed to be due to *Pneumocystis carinii* (although a bacteriologic diagnosis was not made) and he responded to trimethoprim-sulfamethoxazole. Six months later, he noticed the onset of progressive difficulty with memory, concentration, and handwriting; he was unable to read full magazine articles. He had 13 $CD4^+$ cells/mm^3. Psychometric tests showed impariment in attention, memory, and coordination (Figure 2, and below-normal performance on pegboard test). On magnetic resonance imaging of the head, there were bilateral periventricular white matter lesions that were not seen on a computerized tomographic scan. Positron emission tomography revealed heterogeneity of glucose metabolism in the parietal region. CSF contained 122 mg/dl protein, 39 mg/dl glucose, 8 white blood cells per mm^3. HIV was isolated from the CSF, but mycobacteria, fungi, and bacteria were not found.

He was given AZT orally, 250 mg every 4 hrs. There was excellent penetration of the drug into the CSF (Figure 1). For the first week on AZT, he had moderately severe headaches which subsequently resolved. Within 3 weeks, the patient appeared more alert and by 8 weeks, there was substantial improvement in his mental status; he reported that his memory was improved and that he could now read and comprehend novels. His performance on formal psychometric testing also improved (Figure 2; also his performance on the Purdue pegboard improved from 21 to 40 pegs in 120 secs, and his score on Kimura recurring figures increased from 13 to 44 [nl mean = 35]). His $CD4^+$ cells increased slightly to $40/mm^3$. A follow-up PET scan revealed improved glucose metabolism in the previously hypometabolic parietal cortex. After three months, he became anemic and neutropenic; his dose of AZT was reduced to 250 mg every 8 hrs. One month later, he developed *Pneumocystis carinii* pneumonia which responded to treatment with trimethoprim-sulfamethaxozale. He continued on AZT and maintained his improved cognitive functioning when last tested 5 1/2 months after starting on AZT (Figure 2).

Case 6

A 35-year old Spanish-speaking male developed fatigue and difficulty with his memory and was found to have antibodies to HIV. He found it difficult to drive because of difficulty in concentrating, and has increasing difficulty in speaking English (which was a second language for this patient). His CSF had 99 mg/dl protein and 40 mg/dl glucose; cultures of the CSF failed to grow mycobacteria, fungi, or bacteria. Psychometric tests (done with the assistance of a translator) revealed impaired performance on the Trailmaking and WAIS-R tests (Figure 2) and on the Purdue pegboard test (8 pegs in 30 seconds using the dominant hand; a normal person would be expected to place 15 pegs).

He was started on 250 mg every 4 hrs of AZT. CSF levels of AZT in this patient 2 hrs after an oral dose were less than 0.2 microM, compared to a plasma level of 0.95 microM (Figure 1). During his first 8 weeks on AZT, he became more alert and improved in his ability to speak English. Repeat psychometric testing showed improvement in his Trailmaking and WAIS-R tests (Figure 2) and he also improved in his performance on the Purdue pegboard test (13 pegs in 30 seconds). He continues on AZT as of this writing 4 months after the start of therapy and continues to maintain his neurological improvement.

Case 7

A 72 year old diabetic woman received several units of blood during an aortic valve operation; 3 years later, she became profoundly weak so that she was unable to sit unassisted and could not lift her legs off the bed. At this time, she was found to have antibodies to HIV and 330 $CD4^+$ cells/mm^3. Nerve conduction studies and an electromyelogram showed very low amplitude and no recruitment of muscle axon potentials in the lower extremities. After an extensive evaluation, no other etiology for her severe neuropathy could be found, and it was felt to be due to HIV infection with possible a contribution from her diabetes.

She was started on AZT 250 mg orally every 4 hrs. Over the first two months, she had a slight improvement in her strength and could lift her right leg unassisted. In addition, she was able to stand with assistance. A repeat electromyelogram and nerve conduction showed increased amplitude of the sensory neurons and detectable recruitment of muscle axon potentials in the lower extremities. She became anemic while on AZT and required several blood transfusions. In addition, she had a decrease in her $CD4^+$ cells to 180/mm^3. After three months, she developed localized herpes zooster. Her improvement continued for a total of five months. After this time, she developed nausea and stopped taking AZT; over the next two weeks, she became weaker and lost the improvements that she had made.

DISCUSSION

Since the observation that the brain is an important site of HIV replication (1), nervous system dysfunction in patients with HIV infection has increasingly been recognized as an important clinical problem (2,3,8,9). In the absence of treatment, this syndrome carries an extremely poor prognosis; in one recent study, the median survival after the diagnosis of HIV-associated dementia was 4.2 months (8). As we gain experience in the treatment of the opportunistic infections in patients with AIDS, it is likely that neurologic manifestations of the disease will become relatively more important. Because of this neurotropism of HIV, treatments that do not address the infection in the CNS will probably not in themselves be adequate since the brain is a target organ and because HIV in the CNS is likely to reinfect other sites continuously.

The pathogenesis of the disorder is at the time of this writing uncertain and indeed, there is some controversy as to which cells in the CNS are the main sites of HIV infection. Pathologic studies of patients with AIDS-related dementia have shown pallor and vacuolation of the white matter and microglial nodules (9). There is evidence at this time that some cells in the CNS may express CD4 or a similar antigen and could potentially be infected with HIV (10,11); the exact nature of these cells, however, is at present unclear. It has recently been shown that monocyte-derived cells can be infected with HIV and there is evidence that these cells may comprise at least one target population in the CNS (12,13,14).

From a therapeutic viewpoint, an important question is whether the neurologic dysfunction caused by HIV infection is reversible. Cerebral atrophy is found in some of these patients (8), and this suggests that once advanced, the disease may have some irreversible component. The results observed in the present study, however, suggest that this disease is at least in part reversible; 6 of 7 patients studied had at least some short term improvement in neurologic or neuropsychiatric function upon being administsred AZT, and in 5 of those patients, the improvement was substantial.

This reversibility with antiretroviral therapy must be addressed in considering possible pathogenic mechanisms for HIV-induced nervous system disease. As shown here, AZT crosses the blood-brain barrier and therefore can potentially protect cells in the CNS from <u>de novo</u> infection by HIV. The question remains, however, how reversibility of neurologic dysfunction (as opposed to stabilization of disease) would result within the 3 to 8 week period observed from such a protective effect. One possibility is that HIV or HIV-encoded proteins may cause an encephalitis, and that administration of AZT will reduce the viral load within the CNS. In this regard, a neuroactive protein called "neuroleukin" has recently been described which increases growth of certain neural cells and which has substantial sequence homology with HIV envelope glycoprotein (gp120) (15). It is possible that HIV gp120 produced within the CNS of infected persons competes with the neuroleukin binding site and starves cells for this factor; decreasing the load of HIV may reverse this effect.

It is also possible that some of the neurological symptoms may be caused by toxic lymphokines produced by infected cells (either within or outside the nervous system) and that AZT administration reduces such factors. It is important to stress that an anti-retroviral agent could work in the periphery and secondarily effect an improvement in central nervous function. Patients with AIDS have been found to have increased plasma levels of an unusual acid-labile alpha interferon (16). In collaboration with Dr. Olivia T. Preble, we have found that these levels are reduced substantially over a 6 week period of time after the patients start taking AZT (O. Preble, R. Yarchoan, and S. Broder, unpublished observation).

It should be noted that the results presented here only represent treatment of a small number of patients and in some cases, bone marrow toxicity necessitated discontinuing the drug, the patients did not respond, or the patients died of intercurrent opportunistic infections. In addition, it should be noted that all but two of the patients in this study had relatively early neurological disease, and the two patients with more advanced neurological syndromes responded minimally or not at all. Finally, it should be stressed that AZT may not influence secondary neurological disorders found in AIDS such as lymphoma, progressive multifocal leukoencephalopathy, or toxoplasmosis. With these caveats, however, the results suggest that AZT can induce improvements in patients with HIV-associated neurological disease, and they form the basis for a larger study in patients with this disorder.

As a final note, there is some evidence linking viruses other than HIV to certain neurological disorders; tropical spastic paraparesis and a similar myelopathy found in Japan have both been linked to HTLV-I infection (17,18), and it has been suggested that certain patients with multiple sclerosis may be infected with a retrovirus related both to HTLV-I and HIV (19). Dideoxy-pyrimidines such as AZT are effective inhibitors of HTLV-I replication (20), and if continued viral replication is implicated in the symptomatology of these disorders, then it is possible that AZT and related drugs may be worth exploring in these conditions.

ACKNOWLEDGEMENTS

The authors thank Dr. H. Mitsuya, Dr. A. Buchbinder, Dr. S. Tay, Dr. M. Lange, and the clinical staff of the National Cancer Institute for their help. In addition, they thank the Wellcome Research Laboratories for providing the AZT utilized in this study.

REFERENCES

1. Shaw GW, Harper ME, Hahn BH, et al. (1985). HTLV-III infection in brain of children and adults with AIDS encephalopathy. Science 227:177.
2. Resnick L, DiMarzo-Veronese F, Schupbach J, et al. (1985). Intra-blood brain synthesis of HTLV-III-specific IgG in patients with neurologic symptoms associated with AIDS or AIDS-related complex. New Engl. J. Med. 313:1498.
3. Ho DD, Rota TR, Schooley RT, et al. (1985) Isolation of HTLV-III from cerebrospinal fluid and neural tissues of patients with neurologic syndromes related to the acquired immunodeiciency syndrome. New Engl. J. Med. 313: 1493.
4. Mitsuya H, Weinhold KJ, Furman PA, et al. (1985) 3'-azido-3'-deoxythymidine (BW A509U): an anti-viral agent that inhibits the infectivity and cytopathic effect of human T-lymphotropic virus type III/ lymphadenopathy-associated virus in vitro. Proc. Natl. Acad. Sci. USA 82:7096.
5. Yarchoan R, Klecker RW, Weinhold KJ, et al. (1986) Administration of 3'-azido-3'-deoxythymidine, an inhibitor of HTLV-III/LAV replication, to patients with AIDS or AIDS-related complex. Lancet 1:575.
6. Klecker RW, Colline JM, Yarchoan R, et al. (1987). Plasma and cerebrospinal fluid pharmacokinetics of 3'-azido-3'deoxythymidine: a novel pyrimidine analog with potential application for the treatment of AIDS and related diseases. Clin. Pharm. Ther. In press.
7. Yarchoan R, Berg G, Brouwers P, et al. (1987). Response of human-immunodeficiency-virus-associated neurological disease to 3'-azido-3'-deoxythymidine. Lancet 1: 132.
8. Navia BA, Jordan BD, Price RW (1986). The AIDS dementia complex: I. Clinical features. Ann. Neurol. 19:517.

9. Navia BA, Cho E-S, Petito CK, Price RW (1986) The AIDS dementia complex: II. Neuropathology. Ann. Neurol. 19:525.
10. Maddon PJ, Dalgleish AG, McDougal JS, Clapham PR, Weiss RA, Axel R (1986) The T4 gene encodes the AIDS virus receptor and is expressed in the immune system and the brain. Cell 47:333.
11. Pert CB, Hill JM, Ruff MR, et al. (1986) Octapeptides deduced from the neuropeptide receptor-like pattern of antigen T4 in brain potently inhibit human immunodeficiency virus receptor binding and T-cell reactivity. Proc. Natl. Acad. Sci. USA 83:9254.
12. Gartner S, Markovits P, Markovitz DM, et al. (1986) The role of mononuclear phagocytes in HTLV-III/LAV infection. Science 233:215.
13. Ho DD, Rota TR, Hirsch MS (1986) Infection of monocyte/macrophages by human T lymphotropic virus type III. J. Clin. Invest. 77:1712.
14. Koenig S, Gendelman HE, Orenstein JM, et al. (1986) Detection of AIDS virus in macrophages in brain tissue from AIDS patients with encephalopathy. Science 233:1089.
15. Gurney ME, Heinrich SP, Lee MR, Yin H-S (1986) Molecular cloning and expression of neuroleukin, a neurotrophic factor for spinal and sensory neurons. Science 234:566.
16. Eyster ME, Goedert JJ, Poon M-C, Preble OT (1983) Acid-labile interferon. A possible preclinical marker for the acquired immunodeficiency syndrome in hemophelia. New Engl. J. Med. 309:583.
17. Gessain A, Barin F, Vernant JC, et al. (1985) Antibodies to human T-lymphotropic virus type-I in patients with tropical spastic paraparesis. Lancet 2:407.
18. Osame M, Usuku K, Izumo S, et al. (1986) HTLV-I associated myelopathy, a new clinical entity. Lancet 1:1031.
19. Koprowski H, DeFreitas EC, Harper ME, et al. (1985) Multiple sclerosis and human T-cell lymphotropic viruses. Nature 318:154.
20. Matsushita S, Mitsuya H, Reitz M, Broder S (1987) Pharmacological inhibition of *in vitro* infectivity of human T-lymphotropic virus type I (HTLV-I). J. Clin. Invest. In Press.

Human Retroviruses, Cancer, and AIDS: Approaches to Prevention and Therapy, pages 407–421

2',3'-DIDEOXYNUCLEOSIDES: BROAD SPECTRUM ANTIRETROVIRAL ACTIVITY AND MECHANISM OF ACTION

Hiroaki Mitsuya*, John E. Dahlberg†, Zachary Spigelman§, Shuzo Matsushita*, Ruth F. Jarrett¶, Makoto Matsukura*, Michael J. Currens*, Stuart A. Aaronson†, Marvin S. Reitz¶, Ronald S. McCaffrey§, and Samuel Broder*

*The Clinical Oncology Program, †Laboratory of Cellular and Molecular Biology, ¶ Laboratory of Tumor Cell Biology, National Cancer Institute, Bethesda, Maryland, 20892; §Section of Medical Oncology, Boston University Medical School, Massachusettes 02118.

ABSTRACT 2',3'-Dideoxynucleoside analogues can significantly inhibit the *in vitro* replication and/or cytopahtogenicity of a wide range of human and animal retroviruses following anabolic phosphorylation in target cells. We have learned that didexoynucleoside analogues including 3'-azido-2',3'-dideoxythymdiine (AZT) can block the infectivity of human immunodeficiency virus (HIV) and human T-lymhotropic virus type I (HTLV-I) against helper/inducer T-cells *in vitro*. These analogues also inhibit the infectivity of animal lentiviruses (caprine arthritis-encephalitis virus, CAEV; equine infectious anemia virus, EIAV) as well as C-type murine leukemia viruses. 2',3'-Dideoxynucleoside-5'-triphosphates more strongly inhibit HIV reverse transcriptase activity than mammalian DNA polymerase alpha. These results suggest that dideoxynucleoside analogues could be promising agents for further studies in the treatment of retrovirus-related disorders.

INTRODUCTION

In the relatively short time since the first clinical recognition of acquired immunodeficiency syndrome (AIDS), a great deal has been learned about the biochemistry and molecular biology of the causative retrovirus, human immuno deficiency virus (HIV)(1-4), as well as the treatment of the disease (5). When AIDS was found to represent a retroviral infection, there was a serious question as to whether an antiretroviral drug could even be shown to provide a practical benefit to patients. One agent which we have studied, the erythro version of 3'-azido-2',3'-dideoxythymidine (AZT)(6-8), has been shown to confer a significant survival advantage to patients with AIDS in a multi-center, randomized, double-blind, placebo-controlled trial and has recently been approved as a prescription drug. However, the chronic nature of infection and the propensity of the virus to infect the brain (9-11) has prompted a search for additional classes of drugs which have the potential for oral administration, penetrate the blood-brain barrier, and are less toxic. We have recently reported that essentially every purine and pyrimidine nucleoside with a 2',3'-dideoxy-ribose moiety blocks the infectivity of HIV *in vitro* (12). In this paper, we describe the capacity of 2',3'-dideoxynucleoside derivatives to inhibit the *in vitro* replication and/or cytopathogenicity of a wide range of human and animal retoviruses. We also describe the most likely mechanism of antiviral effect of 2',3'-dideoxynucleoside derivatives.

MATERIALS AND METHODS

HIV Cytopathic Effect Assay

HIV cytopathic effect inhibition assays were performed as described earlier (6, 12). $HTLV-III_B$ was obtained from the culture supernatant of $HTLV-III_B$-producing H9 cells (3). Briefly, $2x10^5$ ATH8 cells were exposed to $HTLV-III_B$ in the form of cell-free virions (2,000 virus particles per cell) and cultured in the presence and absence of 2',3'-dideoxynucleoside derivatives. At various time points, the total viable cells were counted.

HTLV-I Infectivity Inhibition

Clonal tetanus-toxoid-specific helper/inducer T-cells (TM11) were obtained from a volunteer and served as target T-cells as described elsewhere (14). Briefly, tetanus-toxoid-activated TM11 cells were cocultured with irradiated HTLV-I-producing cells and viable cells were counted at various time points. On day 19, high molecular DNA was extracted and tested for the level of HTLV-I proviral DNA.

Animal Lentivirus Infectivity Assays

For measurement of CAEV and EIAV infectivity, Himalayan tahr (goat) ovary and equine dermis cells, respectively, were exposed to serial 10-fold dilutions of the virus, and cultured for 2 weeks. The replication of CAEV and EIAV was monitored by determining the levels of purified gag protein (p28 and p15 respectively) present in clarified culture supernatants obtained from drug-treated and control cultures by using radioimmunoasaays as previously described (15).

Assay for HIV Reverse Transcriptase and DNA Polymerase alpha Activity

An M13 clone of Bam HI/Kpn I DNA fragment of a cloned HIV probe, HXB2, following annealing with an M13 universal primer, served as a template. Conditions used were described elsewhere. Purified HIV reverse transcriptase was kindly provided by Drs. Anthony Devico and M.G. Sarngadharan.

RESULTS AND DISCUSSION

Dideoxynucleoside Derivatives Inhibitors of Retroviral Infection.

We have previously shown that a broad family of 2',3'-dideoxynucleoside derivatives are potent inhibitors of infectivity and cytopathic effect of HIV. The structures of 2',3'-dideoxynucleoside derivatives discussed in this report are provided in Figure 1. *In vitro* these analogues can inhibit the replication of HIV and its capacity to destroy helper/inducer T-cell cultures at concentrations that are 10-20 fold lower than those that impair the proliferation, survival, and immune functions of target cells (12). It should be noted that 2',3'-dideoxynucleoside analogues under discussion are not new chemicals, and pioneering studies on these compounds were initiated in 1960's and 1970's, before human retroviruses

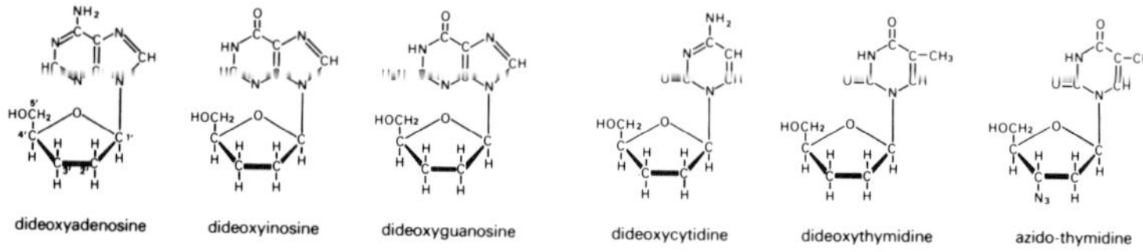

Figure 1. Structures of 2',3'-dideoxynucleoside derivatives discussed in this paper. The primed numbers for 2',3'-dideoxyadenosine (left end) refer to positions in the sugar moiety.

were proven to exist (16-19). These analogues have long been familar to molecular biologists as reagents for the Sanger DNA-sequencing procedure (20). However, application to human anti-retroviral therapy demands a new perspective. These dideoxynucleoside derivatives are of special interest because they prove that a simple chemical modification of the sugar moiety can predictably convert a normal substrate for nucleic acid synthesis into a compound with a potent capacity to inhibit the replication and cytopathic effect of HIV, at least *in vitro* (12).

Certain relationships between the structure and activity of adenosine analogues are explored in Figure 2. This figure summarizes the capacity of six congeners of adenosine to act as inhibitors of HIV. In these experiments, the adenine portion of the nucleoside analogue is kept constant whereas several simple changes in the sugar moiety are tested as variables. The reference agent is 2'-deoxyadenosine, a normal building block for DNA which, as expected, has no anti-retroviral activity in this system. But a simple reduction (removal of the oxygen) at the 3'-carbon of the sugar, creates a potent inhibitor of the retrovirus, 2',3'-dideoxyadenosine (Figure 2, top). A further reduction at the 5'-carbon, creating 2',3',5'-trideoxyadenosine (Figure 2, bottom) nullifies the anti--viral effect, and neither 3'-deoxyadenosine (cordycepin), an *arabinosyl* derivative (Ara-A), nor 2',3'-epoxyadenosine inhibits the virus. It is important to note that these experiments were performed under conditions of high estimated multiplicity of infection (6, 12, 13).

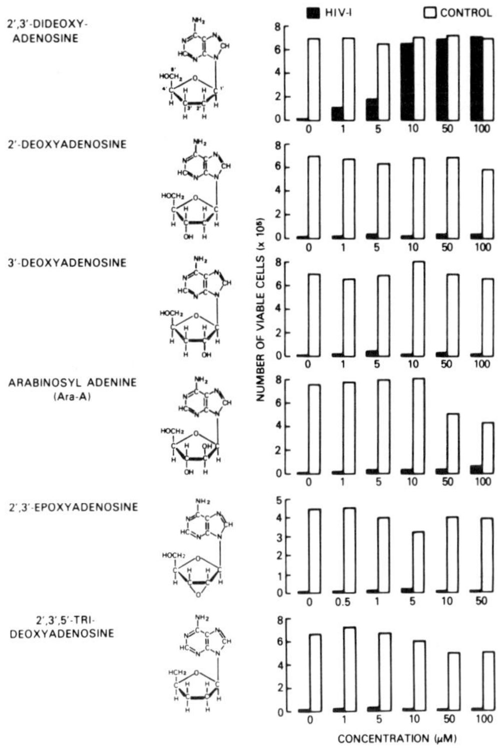

Figure 2. Activity of adenosine congeners against the cytopathic effect of HIV.

ATH8 cells ($2x10^5$) were preexposed to polybrene, exposed to HTLV-III_B (2,000 virus per cell), resuspended in cuture tubes (solid column) in the presence or absence of various amounts of adenosine congeners. 2',3'-Epoxyadenosine was kindly provided by Drs. Don Jerina and Nashaat Nashed. On day 5, the total viable cells were counted by dye expclusion method (12).

We are currently developing 2',3'-dideoxycytidine as a possible agent for treating patients infected with HIV. On a molar basis, dideoxycytidine is the most potent antiviral nucleoside that we have tested. We have found that concentrations of ≥ 0.5 μM 2',3'-dideoxycytidine completely protect target helper/inducer T-cells against HIV infection and enable them to survive and grow (12). Under conditions of low multiplicity of infection, concentrations ≥ 10 nanomolar 2',3'-dideoxycytidine can suppress the virus (Figure 3). This agent has been selected for clinical development because of its *in vitro* potency against HIV (12), relative resistance to cytidine deaminase (a major catabolic enzyme for cytidine analogues)(21), good oral bioavailability, straight-forward pharmacokinetic

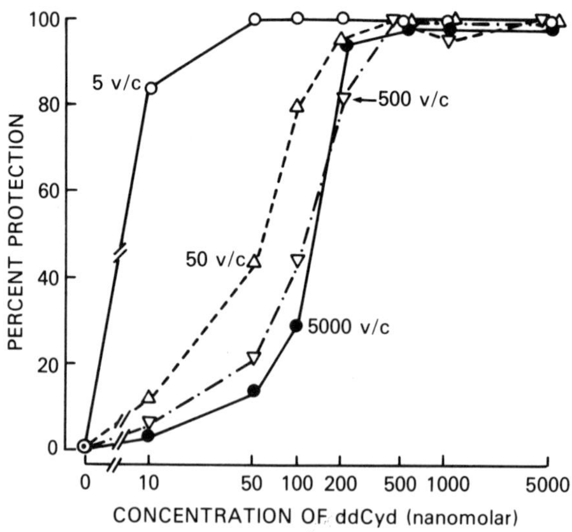

Figure 3. Anti-HIV activity of 2',3'-dideoxycytidine at various multiplicities of infection.

$2x10^5$ ATH8 cells were preexposed to polybrene, exposed to the indicated numbers of HTLV-III_B virus particles per cell, resuspended in culture tubes in the presence or absence of various amounts of 2',3'-dideoxycytidine. On day 6, viable cells were counted by a dye exclusion method.

clearance by the kidney, failure to reduce normal intracellular pyrimidine pools, and comparative lack of toxicity when administered to animals.

Several issues related to the anti-retroviral effects of 2',3'-dideoxynucleosides are as yet not resolved, but it seems that as they are successively phosphorylated in the cytoplasm of a target cell to yield 2',3'-dideoxynucleoside-5'-triphosphates, they become analogues of the 2'-deoxynucleoside-5'-triphosphates that are the natural substrates for cellular DNA polymerases and reverse transcriptase. Such analogues could compete with the binding of normal nucleotides to DNA polymerases, or could be incorporated into DNA and bring about DNA chain termination because normal 5'→3' phosphodiester linkages cannot be completed. In this context, the lack of activity against HIV that was observed using 2',3',5'-trideoxyadenosine (Figure 2, bottom) probably relates to the unavailability of the 5'-site to undergo initial phosphorylation. We have recently demonstrated that as expected, 2',3'-dideoxynucleoside-5'-triphosphates serve as substrates for HIV reverse transcriptase to elongate a DNA chain by one residue, after which the chain is terminated (22). Anabolic phosphorylation of 2',3'-dideoxynucleoside to the corresponding 5'-triphosphate products occurs in animal and human cells, and in the case of 2',3'-dideoxycytidine we know that the relative intracellular concentrations in cultured cells exceed those needed to bring about the DNA-chain termination (21, 22). It should be noted that the retrovirus does not provide its own enzymes for phosphorylation, and therefore, unlike *Herpes* viruses, cannot develop drug resistance via mutations of a kinase gene. Of course, mutations in the *pol* gene that alter binding to the relevant nucleotide could theoretically confer drug resistance to the virus.

Dideoxynucleoside Derivatives Suppress the In Vitro Replication of a Range of Human and Animal Retroviruses.

Now we believe that 2',3'-dideoxynucleosides could potentially have an effect against virtually any retroviruses if the target cells have appropriate kinases for anabolic phospharylation of the dideoxynucleosides. We have recently found that two dideoxynucleosides, 2',3'-dideoxycytidine and 3'-azido-2',3'-dideoxythymidine can block the infectivity of another human retrovirus, human T-lymphotropic virus type I (HTLV-I), against helper/inducer T-cells _in vitro_ (23). Both 2',3'-dideoxynucleoside analogues inhibited the over-growth of target T-cells which results from virally-mediated transformation when they were exposed to both HTLV-I and the compounds. Moreover, we observed that the amount of proviral DNA detected in high molecular DNA isolated from the target T-cells was substantially reduced when the cells were cultured with the compounds, and that at certain drug concentrations, the synthesis of viral DNA was completely suppressed (23).

2',3'-Dideoxynucleoside analogues can also inhibit the _in vitro_ replication and pathogenic effects of a range of animal retroviruses, even when the pathogenic effect being monitored (transformation) requires only a single round of replication (15). Figure 4 shows the properties of 2',3'-dideoxyadenosine, 2',3'-dideoxycytidine, and AZT to suppress the replication of two animal lentiviruses, CAEV, and EIAV (15). In these experiments, the drugs were added to endpoint titration assays and the presence or absence of replication in each well was determined by radioimmunoassay. It was noted that 2',3'-dideoxyadenosine and 2',3'-dideoxycytidine were very potent agents against CAEV when tahr ovary cells were used as target cells. CAEV _gag_ production in these assays was suppressed by these compounds by more than 5 orders of magnitude. In contrast, AZT was not effective at all in these cells. The most likely explanation for AZT failing to suppress the replication of CAEV in tahr cells is that an adequate level of AZT-5'-triphosphate was not formed in tahr cells. Indeed, in comparison to the human helper/inducer T-cells we have tested, tahr cells contain a very low level of 5'-triphosphate form of AZT (unpublished, J. Balzarini et al.). In contrast, when dideoxynucleosides were tested in EIAV-exposed equine dermis cells, all of these agents were potent in suppressing the replication of EIAV. Indeed, we have not as yet observed any type or strain of retrovirus that is resistant to

Figure 4. Activity of 2',3'-dideoxyadenosine and 2',3'-dideoxycytidine against the replication of animal lentiviruses *in vitro*.

Himalayan tahr ovary cells and equine dermis cells grown in 24 wells microtiter plates were pretreated with 2',3'-dideoxynucleosides, exposed to serial dilutions of caprine arthritis-encephalitis virus (CAEV) and equine infectious anemia virus (EIAV) respectively, and cultured in the presence of the indicated dideoxynucleosides. On day 14, the culture supernatants were tested for *gag* protein, indicating virus replication, by radioimmunoassay (15).

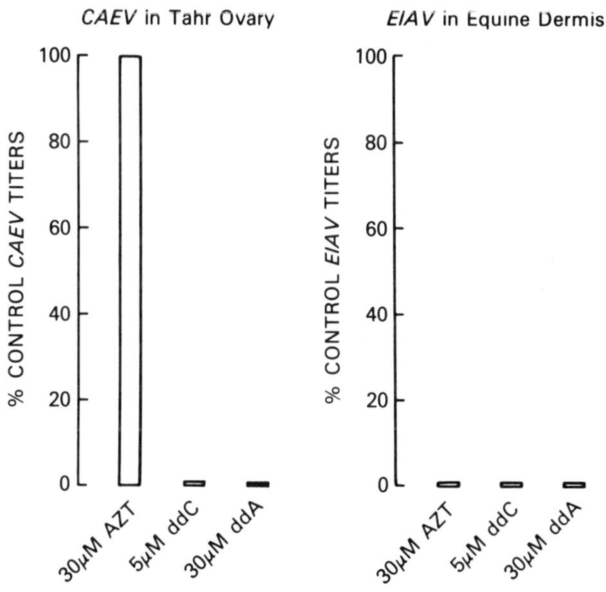

2',3'-dideoxynucleosides in appropriate target cells; however, the emergence of drug-resistant mutants must always be considered possible.

HIV Reverse Transcriptase is Susceptible to 2',3'-Dideoxynucleoside-5'-triphosphate.

We then tested if 2',3'-dideoxycytidine-5'-triphosphate could inhibit HIV DNA synthesis which was mediated by purified HIV reverse transcriptase. In this experiment, we used an M13-clone of HIV 3'-*orf* DNA fragment as a template. Figure 5 shows that the HIV reverse transcriptase is much more susceptible to the inhibitory ef-

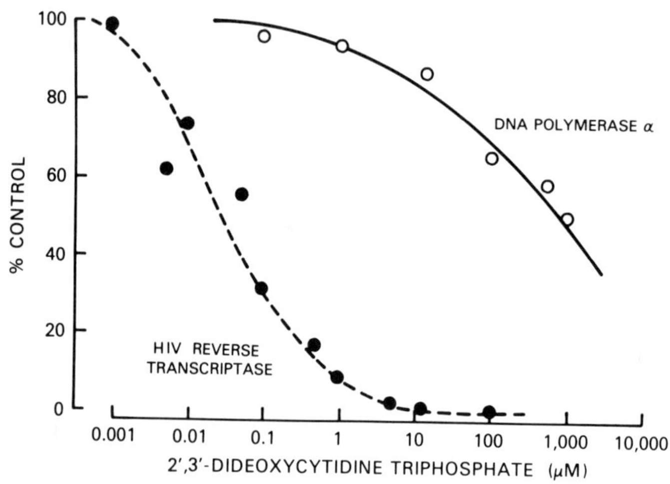

Figure 5. Inhibitory effect of 2',3'-dideoxycytidine-5'-triphosphate on the activity of HIV reverse transcriptase and mammalian DNA polymerase alpha. An M13 clone of a Bam HI/Kpn I DNA fragment of cloned HIV probe, HXB2, following annealing with an M13 universal primer, served as a template (22). Conditions used were described elsewhere (29). Purified HIV reverse transcriptase was kindly provided by Drs. Anthony Devico and M.G. Sarngadharan. Note HIV reverse transcriptase activity was profoundly inhibited by 2',3'-dideoxycytidine-5'-triphosphate, while DNA plymerase alpha activity was over 1000-fold less sensitive.

fects of 2',3'-dideoxycytidine as a 5'-triphosphate than is mammalian DNA polymerase alpha, an enzyme which has key DNA synthetic and repair functions in the life of a cell. Our finding and others (24, 25) that the reverse transcriptase has a higher affinity for dideoxynucleotides than normal substrates parallel what had been learned in animal retroviral systems (26-29). Although 2',3'-dideoxynucleoside-5'-triphosphates can inhibit mammalian DNA polymerase beta (a repair enzyme), and DNA polymerase gamma (a mitochondrial enzyme)(26), we have observed that dideoxynucleosides can suppress HIV replication and protect sensitive helper/inducer T cell target cells _in vitro_ for long periods without interfering with the function and survival of target T cells (22). As discussed above, our working explanation for the activity of these drugs against pathogenic retroviruses is that following anabolism to nucleoside-5'-triphosphates, they terminate DNA synthesis during reverse transcription. Since RNase H will digest any RNA present in the RNA-DNA hybrid, the virus dos not have a second chance. Thus, one explanation for the selective anti-retroviral activity of these compounds is that the viral DNA polymerase more readily accepts the dideoxynucleotide than the corresponding cell enzyme. Alternatively (or additionally) the viral DNA may have less likelihood of being repaired following the incorporation of the false nucleotide. In some cases, however, such drugs may perturb normal nucleoside metabolism or exert other effects that result in drug-related toxicity (5, 7).

These properties of 2',3'-dideoxynucleosides, taken together, suggest that at least several 2',3'-dideoxynucleosides are attractive candidates for further development for treatment of human retrovirus-related diseases and may also have an important role in veterinary medicine. At this point, the question is no longer whether drugs that inhibit retroviruses can confer a clinical benefit in certain diseases; the question now is how many such drugs will be found and what is the best way to select candidate drugs for clinical trials.

ACKNOWLDGEMENT

The authors thank Drs. Anthony Devico and Sarngadharan for providing purified HIV reverse transcriptase and Drs. Mikulus Popovic and Robert C. Gallo for providing the $HTLV\text{-}III_B$ virus.

REFERENCES

1. Gottlieb, M.S., Schroff, R., Schanker, H.M., Weisman, J.D., Fan, P.T., Wolf, R.A., & Saxon, A. (1981) Pneumocystis carinii pneumonia and mucosal candidiasis in previously healthy homosexual men. Evidence of a new acquired cellular immunodeficiency. New Engl. J. Med. 305, 1425-1431.
2. Barré-Sinoussi, F., Chermann, J.C., Rey, F., Nugeyre, M.T., Chamaret, S., Gruest, J., Dauguet, C., Axler-Blin, C., Vézinet-Brun, F., Rouxioux, C., Rozenbaum, W., & Montagnier, L. (1983) Isolation of a T cell lymphotropic virus from a patient at risk for acquired immunodeficiency syndrome (AIDS) Science, 220, 868-871.
3. Popovic, M., Sarngadharan, M.G., Read, E., & Gallo, R. C. (1984) Detection, isolation, and continuous production of cytopathic retrovirus (HTLV-III) from patients with AIDS and pre-AIDS. Science, 224, 497-500.
4. Wong-Staal, F. & Gallo,R.C. (1985) Human T-lymphotropic retroviruses. Nature, 317, 395-403.
5. Mitsuya, H. & Broder, S. (1987) Strategies of antiviral therapy in AIDS. Nature, 325, 773-778.
6. Mitsuya, H., Weinhold, K.J., Furman, P.A., St. Clair, M.H., Lehrman, S.N., Gallo, R.C., Bolognesi, D., Barry, D.W., & Broder, S. (1985) 3'-Azido-3'-deoxythymidine (BW A509U): An antiviral agent that inhibits the infectivity and cytopathic effect of human T-lymphotropic virus type III/lymphadenopathy-associated virus in vitro. Proc. Natl. Acad. Sci. USA. 82, 7096-7100.
7. Yarchoan, R., Klecker, R.W., Weinhold, K.J., Markham, P.D., Lyerly, H.K., Durack, D.T., Gelmann, E., Lehrman, S.N., Blum, R.M., Baryy, D.W., Shearer, G.M., Fischl, M.A., Mitsuya, H., Gallo, R.C., Collins, J.M., Bolognesi, D.P., Myers, C.E., and Broder, S. (1986) Administration of 3'-azido-3'-deoxythymidine, An inhibitor of HTLV-III/LAV replication, to patients with AIDS

or AIDS-related complex. Lancet, i, 575-580.
8. Yarchoan, R. and Broder, S. (1987) Development of anti-retroviral therapy for the acquired immunodeficiency syndrome and related disorders. New Engl. J. Med. 316, 557-564.
9. Shaw, G.M., Harper, M.E., Hahn, B.H., Epstein, L.G., Gajdusek, D.C., Price, R.W., Navia, B.A., Petito, C.K., O'Hara, C.J., Groopman, J.E., Cho, E.-S., Oleske, J.M., Wong-Staal, F., & Gallo, R.C. (1985) HTLV-III infection in brains of children and adults with AIDS encephalopathy. Science, 227, 177-182.
10. Ho, D.D., Rota, T.R., Schooley, R.T., Kaplan, J.C., Allan, J.D., Grropman, J.E., Resnick, L., Felsenstein, D., Andrews, C.A., & Hirsch, M.S. (1985) Isolation of HTLV-III from cerebrospinal fluid and neural tissue of patients with neurologic syndromes related to the acquired immunodeficiency syndrome. New. Engl. J. Med. 313, 1493-1497.
11. Koenig, S., Gendelman, H.E., Orenstein, J.M., Dal Canto, M.C., Pezeshkpour, G.H., Yungbluth, M., Janotta, F., Aksamit, A., Martin, M.A., & Fauci, A.S. Science, 233, 1089-1093.
12. Mitsuya, H. & Broder, S. (1986) Inhibition of the *in vitro* infectivity and cytopathic effect of human T-T-lymphotropic virus type III/lymphadenopathy-associated virus (HTLV-III/LAV) by 2',3'-dideoxynucleosides. Proc. Natl. Acad. Sci. U.S.A. 83, 1911-1915.
13. Mitsuya, H., Matsukura, M. and Broder, S. (1987) Rapid in vitro systems for assessing activity of agents against HTLV-III/LAV. In AIDS: modern concepts and therapeutic challenges" (ed. Broder, S.) p.303-333, Marcel Dekker, Inc., New York.
14. Mitsuya, H., Guo, H.-G., Cossman, J., Megson, M., Reitz, M.S. Jr., and Broder, S. (1984) Functional properties of antigen-specific T cells infected by human T-cell luekemia-lymphoma virus (HTLV-I). Science, 225, 2484-2486.
15. Dahlberg, J.E., Mitsuya, H., Blam, S.B., Broder, and Aaronson, S.A. (1987) Broad spectrum antiretroviral activity of 2',3'-dideoxynucleosides. Proc. Natl. Acad. Sci. USA. 84, 2469-2473.
16. Robins, M.J. & Robins, R.K. (1964) The synthesis of 2',3'-dideoxyadenosine from 2'-deoxyadenosine. J. Am. Chem. Soc. 86, 3585-3586.

17. Horwitz, J.P., Chua, J. & Noel, M. (1964) Nucleosides. V. The monomesylates of 1-(2'-deoxy-β-D-lyxofuranosyl) thymine. J. Org. Chem. 29, 2076-2078.
18. Horwitz, J.P., Chua, J., Noel, M., & Donatti, J.T. (1967) Nucleosides. XI. 2',3'-dideoxycytidine. J. Org. Chem. 32, 817-818.
19. Toji, L. and Cohen, S.S. (1970) Termination of deoxyribonucleic acid in Escherichia coli by 2',3'-dideoxyadenosine. J. Bacteriol. 103, 323-328.
20. Sanger, F., Nicklen, S., and Coulson, A.R. (1977) DNA sequencing with chain-terminators. Proc. Natl. Acad. Sci. USA. 74, 5463-5467.
21. Cooney, D.A., Dalal, M., Mitsuya, H., McMahon, J.B., Nadkarni, M., Balzarini, J., Broder, S., and Johns, D.G. (1986) Initial studies on the cellular pharmacology of 2',3'-dideoxycytidine, an inhibitor of HTLV-III infectivity. Biochem. Pharmacol. 35, 2065-2068.
22. Mitsuya, H., Jarrett, R.F., Matsukura, M., Di Marzo Veronese, F., DeVico, A.L., Sarngadharan, M.G., Johns, D.G., Reitz, M.S., and Broder, S. (1987) Long-term inhibition of human T-lymphoctropic virus type III/ lymphadenopathy-associated virus (human immunodeficiency virus) DNA synthesis and RNA expression in T cells protected by 2',3'-dideoxynucleosides in vitro. Proc. Natl. Acad. Sci. USA. 84, 2033-2037.
23. Matsushita, S., Mitsuya, H., Reitz, M.S., & Broder, S. (1987) Pharmacological inhibition of human T-lymphotropic virus type 1 (HTLV-I). J. Clin. Invest. (in press).
24. Furman, P.A., Fyfe, J.A., St.Clair, M.H., Weinhold, K., Rideout, J.L., Freeman, G.A., Lehrman, S.N., Bolognesi, D.P., Broder, S., Mitsuya, H., and Barry, D.W. (1986) Phosphorylation of 3'-azido-3'-deoxythymidine and selective interaction of the 5'-triphosphate with human immunodeficiency virus reverse transcriptase. Proc. Natl. Acad. Sci. USA. 83, 8333-8337.
25. Starnes, M.C. and Cheng, Y.-C. (1987) Cellular metabolism of 2',3'-dideoxycytidine, a compound active against human immunodeficiency virus in vitro. J. Biol. Chem. 226, 988-991.
26. Waqar, A., Evans, M.J., Manly, K.F., Hughs, R.G., and Huberman, J.A. (1985) Effects of 2',3'-dideoxynucleo-

sides on mammalian cells and viruses. J. Cell. Physiol. 121, 402-408.

27. Atkinson, M.R., Deutscher, M.P., Kornberg, A., Russel, A.F., and Moffat, J.G. (1969) Enzymatic synthesis of deoxyribonucleic acid. XXXIV. Termination of chain growth by a 2',3'-dideoxyribonucleotide. Biochemistry, 8, 4897-4904.

28. Smoler, D., Molineux, I., and Baltimore, D. (1971) Direction of polymerization by the avian myeloblastosis virus deoxyribonucleic acid polymerase. J. Biol. Chem. 246, 7697-7700.

29. Di Marzo Veronese, F., Copeland, T.D., Devico, A.L., Rahman, R., Oroszlan, S., Gallo, R.C., and Sarngadharan, M.G. (1986) Characterization of highly immunogenic p66/p51 as the reverse transcriptase of HTLV-III/LAV. Science, 231, 1289-1291.

Human Retroviruses, Cancer, and AIDS:
Approaches to Prevention and Therapy, pages 423–438

INHIBITION OF REPLICATION AND EXPRESSION OF HIV-I TISSUE CULTURE BY OLIGODEOXYNUCLEOTIDE HYBRIDIZATION COMPETITION[1]

J. Goodchild, R.L. Letsinger[2], P.S. Sarin[3]
M. Zamecnik, and P.C. Zamecnik,

Worcester Foundation for Experimental Biology
Shrewsbury, MA 01545

ABSTRACT Oligodeoxynucleotides (12-26mers) complementary to critical conserved regions of the primary structure of HTLV III/LAV (HIV-I) were synthesized and tested for capacity to inhibit replication and expression of this virus in tissue cultures of H9 cells. Inhibition of viral replication, as measured by reverse transcriptase, and of P17 and P24 protein expression was found. Degree of inhibition was related to choice of hybridization site, with splice donor, acceptor, and primer binding regions being most effective. Unmodified oligodeoxynucleotides appeared to enter cells, and uptake was linear with time up to ten minutes at 37°, with 10^{-6} molar external concentration being taken up to approximately a 5 percent level internally ($\sim 5 \times 10^{-8}$ molar). Uptake was inhibited by 5×10^{-4}M dinitrophenol, indicating an endergonic transport process. Modification of a 12mer oligomer by addition of two internucleotide trichloromethyldimethylethyl phosphotriester groups resulted in enhancement of survival of the oligomer extracellularly and intracellularly in a tissue culture system.

1 This work was supported by a grant from the Mathers Foundation (to PCZ), a Cooperative Grant from the NIH (to PCZ and R.L.), and Contract FOD-0756-01 from the Frederick Cancer Research Facility (to PCZ).

2 Northwestern University, Evanston, IL 60201
3 National Cancer Institute, Bethesda, MD 20892

INTRODUCTION

Early Work on Rous Sarcoma Virus.

Some years ago it became clear that elucidation of the genetic code of a pathogenic virus might provide clues to its control. The Rous sarcoma virus (RSV) was the first animal retrovirus to become available in sufficient quantity to make sequencing of its primary structure feasible. It was first determined that the 3' end of the virus ended in an A residue, then that the 3' end was in fact a poly A tail (1), with the first residue internal thereto a C. With this information, an oligo dT with a 3' terminal C was synthesized and used as a primer for synthesis of a cDNA transcript of the 3' end of the RSV genome. By means of wandering spot analysis, the first 21 residues internal to the poly A tail were specified (2). At this time (1976), Walter Gilbert showed us the new unpublished sequencing technique of Maxam and Gilbert. To our astonishment, we found that this powerful new method had in a few months, unbeknown to us, elucidated the sequence of 101 residues (3) at the 5' end of the same retrovirus (RSV) which our laboratory had been sequencing at the 3' end for at least two years. Equally surprising was the finding that 21 residues at the 5' end, and just internal to the poly A tail at the 3' end, were identical and in the same polarity. Thus, since the replication process began near the 5' end of the virus with a tRNA as a primer, and was followed by destruction by ribonuclease H of the viral RNA just copied, a single-stranded DNA complement of the 3' end of the virus became available for base pairing hybridization, with this event resulting in a circular intermediate. DNA copying of the viral RNA could then continue from the 3' end of the virus. The above data provided an explanation for the circular proviral intermediate which had been observed by electron microscopy in retroviral replication, and was the first evidence for the existence of long terminal repeat areas at the 5'- and 3'-ends of retroviruses.

It occurred to us that a synthetic piece of DNA identical to the reiterated terminal sequences might interfere with the circularization step, and thus bring viral replication to a halt. We had a 13-mer oligomer synthesized, and tested this possibility in a tissue culture system consisting of chick embryo fibroblast (CEF) cells, RSV, and oligomer. Replication of the virus was inhibited, as measured by reverse transcriptase assay of virus secreted into the culture medium (4). <u>Focus formation in the tissue culture cells was also inhibited, a finding which encouraged us to consider that the 13-mer oligodeoxynucleotide was traversing the CEF external membrane and entering the cytosol of the infected cell</u> (4). In a cell-free protein synthesizing system, employing the RSV RNA as mRNA, addition of this 13-mer to the system resulted in inhibition of translation (5). Oligomers of other sequences did not produce translation inhibition, attesting to the specificity of the translation inhibition. Blockade of the 3'- and 5' termini of the 13-mer as the isourea derivatives enhanced the inhibition of viral replication ten fold, at 10^{-5}M concentration, in comparison with the natural, unblocked oligomer (4). This we regarded as probably due to inhibition of exonuclease activities.

Thus, the stage was set to test the possibility, termed the "hybridon" approach (4), that a human oncogenic retrovirus, if such were to be found (and we thought the possibility likely (6)), might be similarly inhibited. A hybridon was defined as a synthetic oligomer which hybridized with a complementary sequence of a viral or cell genome, producing a metabolic effect. It was also considered at that time that activity of a human gene might be inhibited by hybridization competition, with possible inhibition, for example, of the gene(s) responsible for overproduction of erythrocytes in polycythemia vera. This was a new concept, not received with enthusiasm at the time, since it was widely held that oligonucleotides did not enter cells due to their negative charge.

Studies on HIV-I.

<u>Background</u>. When the primary nucleotide sequence of HTLV-I became known (7), Dr. Gallo's laboratories and ours planned a collaboration to test the possibility of inhibiting replication of this virus by the hybridon approach. At this same time, the primary structure of HTLV-III (HIV-I) was also being determined, and was soon completely elucidated (8-11). The latter virus seemed to be a more promising and urgent target than HTLV-I. There was considerable variability in the primary structure of clones from HIV-I, but certain areas among the primary sequences of HTLV-I to HTLV-IV (HIV-IV) had invariant

sequences or only single base variations. One such region was the initiation site of DNA synthesis, at which a sequence of 14 nucleotides at the 3'-end of $tRNA^{Lys}_3$ hybridized with the viral RNA and served as a primer for the nascent DNA chain. The reason for the choice of tRNAs as primers is certainly an intriguing mystery. Later studies indicated splice donor and acceptor sites for the tat III gene to be highly conserved regions of the viral genome and promising targets, in view of the great stimulation of viral synthesis induced by the tat gene translation product (12,13).

RESULTS

Inhibition of HIV-I Replication and Expression in Tissue Culture.

Experimental details of the tissue culture studies have been published (14), and the results are shown in Table I, taken from this publication. Three independent measures of viral inhibition were used: 1) assay of reverse transcriptase as an indication of whole virus secretion into the tissue culture medium, 2) P15 (or more accurately P17) and 3) P24 immunofluorescent antibody assays of the presence of these viral proteins in the H9 cells used in the tissue culture assay system. There was inhibition of production of all three viral proteins in the presence of specific hybridons. A control sequence consisting of the same nucleotides as in an inhibitory sequence, but in random order, had no inhibitory effect. Detailed studies on cell toxicity were not carried out, but there was no loss of cells in hybridon treated H9 cells. Some years previously we had injected ten one-day old chicks with 0.4 mg of a tridecamer deoxynucleotide every day for five days, and had not observed any toxic effects (15). A limitation in the present studies was the shortage of supplies of oligonucleotides, synthesized by solid state machine methods (Biosearch, Sam II). While it would have been desirable to renew the oligomer (at 10^{-5}M concentration) daily until the 96 hour assay due to continual nuclease degradation of oligomer, the quantity of oligomer available was insufficient in most instances to do so. Thus our current goal is to synthesize and purify oligomers (12-20 mers) in the multimilligram range for more detailed dose-response and toxicity studies. Results to date strongly suggest that end blocking and greater length (20 mers vs. 12 mers) of oligomers enhance their inhibitory effect. Since there is one chance in four of having a particular nucleotide at a single position in a random oligomer, in a 16 mer there are 4^{16} chances of a given sequence occurring at random, or one chance in 4×10^9. The latter approximates the number of base pairs in the human genome. A specific oligomer over 16 residues in length is therefore seldom likely to occur at random in the human genome. This situation gives rise to the hope that a possible hybridon therapy will involve a high order of specificity as well as a low level of toxicity.

Apparent Cellular Uptake of Labeled Oligomers.

The inhibitory effects of hybridons on RSV and HIV-I replication are most readily explained by uptake of these oligomers into the cytosol of the cell. Early studies on uptake of oligonucleotide homopolymers into cells (16,17) left open the possibilities that the oligomers entered the cells, alternatively were bound to the cell membranes, or that both situations were occurring. An unequivocal answer however rests with the results of electron microscopy of ^{3}H-labeled oligomers, as described later in this text. Our current studies strongly suggest that cell membrane penetration does occur. Persuasive results come from electroporation. In these studies we have labeled 20-mer oligodeoxynucleotides internally with ^{32}P (14), and incubated HeLa cells in suspension in 10^{-6}-10^{-7}M labeled oligomers in Dulbecco's medium for 15' at 37°. Then we have washed the labeled incubation medium away by repeated centrifugations, with addition of fresh unlabeled medium at each centrifugation step, the process being carried out at 0-2° as rapidly as possible. The washed cells in unlabeled medium were then subjected to electroporation, centrifuged, and radioactivity determined in the external medium, into which cell leakage had occurred. The results showed radioactivity in the incubation medium, which came apparently from the interior of cells as a result of holes produced in the external cell membrane by the electroporation process. These results were very similar to other experiments in which cell membrane leakage was induced by hypotonicity or by addition of formic acid to either cell suspension or cell monolayer media. The radioactivity released thereby was subjected to polyacrylamide gel electrophoresis, and the internally labeled ^{32}P oligomers were found by radioautography to be 94-97 percent intact after the 15' incubation.

We have also carried out time course studies on CEF and HeLa cells in monolayers, with internally labeled ^{32}P-20 mers in the incubation medium. The apparent internal concentration of labeled oligomer rises as a straight line from time zero to 10 minutes at 37°, gradually reaching a plateau within a few hours, and in CEF cells declines to approximately ten percent of its maximal value, after overnight incubation. In HeLa cells, the rate of degradation is more rapid, both internally and in the serum-free incubation medium. 5'-end labeled oligomer radioactivity declines much more rapidly than does internally labeled oligomer, due to phosphomonoesterase activity secreted extracellularly into the incubation medium (Dulbecco's medium without serum), and also due to intracellular phosphomonoesterases.

A comparison was carried out on the apparent cellular uptake and survival of an internally labeled 20-mer deoxynucleotide, and the same molar concentration of internally labeled 20 mer of the same sequence, but with lipophilic groups on the internucleoside phosphates as phosphotriesters. At the present time it can only be stated that the presence of lipophilic groups modifies the behavior of the oligomers, and that more work must be done to reach firm conclusions.

Electron Microscope Studies.

These studies were designed to provide a more definitive answer to the question of whether an external unmodified deoxynucleotide oligomer actually enters the cytosol of a living cell. We therefore added to the 3' end of a 10-mer oligodeoxynucleotide ^{3}H-labeled thymidine monophosphate, using ^{3}H TTP (20 Ci/m mol). Approximately ten TMP residues were added using deoxynucleotidyl terminal transferase. The labeled oligomer was purified and shown to travel on PAGE as a family of closely related bands. This gave a specific activity of 209 Ci/m mol.

To each of two nearly confluent monolayer cultures of HeLa cells, grown under sterile conditions in Nunc 4-welled dishes, containing approximately 200,000 cells per well, 50 μl of Dulbecco's medium were added, containing 1 x 10^7 dpm of radioactivity at 5 x 10^{-7}M concentration of oligomer. One well was used as a zero time control, then the medium was immediately removed, and the well washed ten times with ice cold Dulbecco's medium, all within 30 seconds. After exposure to silver emulsion for a week, the electron micrograph sections showed, in the zero time control, silver grains in the microvilli of the external membranes of the cell. In the HeLa cell monolayer which was incubated 15' at 37°, and then washed as above, most of the silver grains were located just inside the nuclear membrane. There were also occasional silver grains in the cytosol, and some embedded in the microvilli of the external membranes. Thus the externally added, labeled oligomer appeared to have entered the HeLa cells (18). One reservation to this interpretation remains. During the 15' incubation 3-6 percent of the oligomer was determined to be degraded, presumably to the monomer or deoxynucleoside level. We have yet to run controls on this point.

Target Sites in HIV-I.

Optimal containment of the AIDS virus may require agents that protect uninfected as well as infected cells. In uninfected cells, for example, it may be best to inhibit synthesis of DNA in incoming virus to prevent integration into the host genome. In cells already infected, it would be desirable to prevent synthesis of viral proteins, for example, in order to prevent spread of the virus.

The hybridon approach blocks the functions of single-stranded nucleic acid, and in the case of HIV, these include DNA synthesis, RNA processing, protein synthesis and RNA packaging. We have concentrated on the first three; as yet, there is scant information on the mechanism of packaging of the virus.

In model studies using β-globin mRNA, the capped 5'-end and the initiator AUG codon were found to be the most susceptible sites for inhibition of translation by complementary oligonucleotides (19). Oligomers binding to other regions of the translated or 5'-untranslated regions of the messenger were more easily displaced during translation and gave less inhibition. In choosing targets, therefore, we have concentrated on binding or recognition sites on the viral RNA.

DNA synthesis by reverse transcriptase is initiated at the $tRNA^{Lys}_{3}$ primer bound near the 5' end. This might be disrupted in two ways. Firstly, an oligonucleotide could be used that competed with the tRNA for the binding site on the viral RNA. It is not known what effect replacing the tRNA with an oligodeoxynucleotide might have. If the oligomer itself could serve as a primer, then it might be necessary to block the 3'-end.

Secondly, an oligomer could be used that bound immediately upstream of the tRNA to block physically initiation by the polymerase. Again, it may prove necessary to block the 3'-end of such an oligonucleotide, as we have done in one of the compounds in Table I.

TABLE 1
INHIBITION OF HIV-I REPLICATION AND PROTEIN EXPRESSION BY COMPLEMENTARY OLIGODEOXYNUCLEOTIDES[a]

Sequence	Conc. g/ml	HIV binding Site *	Cells	HIV	% Inhibition RT	p17	p24
None	--	--	H9	--	0	0	0
None	--	--	H9	+	0	0	0
CCCCAACTGTGTACT	5	--	H9	+	0	0	0
	10	--	H9	+	0	0	0
CTGCTAGAGATddt	5	5' to primer	PB	+	20	0	17
	10	5' to primer	PB	+	36	0	50
	20	5' to primer	PB	+	40	35	36
	5	5' to primer	H9	+	10	15	35
	10	5' to primer	H9	+	17	15	30
	10	5' to primer	H9	+	0	10	12
	29	5' to primer	H9	+	0	28	38
CTGCTAGAGATTTTCCACAC	50	5' to primer	PB	+	50	50	50
	10 (x3)	5' to primer	H9	+	50	75	75
	50	5' to primer	H9	+	23	27	30
TTCAAGTCCCTGTTC-GGGCGCCAAAA	50	At primer §	H9	+	80	4	8
GCGTACTCACCAGTCGCCGC	50	Splice donor site	H9	+	85	40	60
CTGCTAGAGATTAA	50	5' to primer ¶	H9		75	8	11
ACACCCAATTCTGAAAATGG	50	Splice acceptor site ∏	H9	+	67	95	88

RT, reverse transcriptase activity; p17, viral 17 protein; p24, viral p24 protein; H9, transformed immortalized human T-cell line; PB, peripheral human blood cells.

*, "5' to primer", indicates 5'-vicinal to primer binding site for $tRNA^{Lys}_{3}$; "At primer" indicates directly competing at primer binding site.

HIV, protein expression was measured by an immunofluorescence technique using monoclonal antibodies to HTLV-III p17 and p24. Percent inhibition is based on comparison to control values obtained for cells incubated without oligodeoxynucleotide. No deoxynucleotide cytotoxicity for cells was observed in any of the experiments as monitored by phase-contrast microscopy and cell counts. Oligodeoxynucleotides were added at time zero, at the same time as virus, unless otherwise indicated. Assays of inhibition were carried out at 96 hr.

+, Addition of 10μg/ml on days 1,2, and 3 from time of virus infection.

§, Has three noncomplementary bases at 3' end.

¶, Has two noncomplementary bases at 3' end.

∏, Computer search of all known sequences did not reveal any similar 20-nucleotide sequence with fewer than seven mismatches. This is the splice acceptor site for the _tat_-III gene.

a, data from (14), reproduced courtesy of PNAS.

HIV-I is particularly rich in splice sites. There are five acceptor and four donor sites, most of them clustered in the middle of the RNA around _sor_. Current views on the mechanism of splicing suggest that these are recognized by snRNP's or other splicing factors and so are targets for the hybridon approach, as might also be the polyadenylation signal. We have tested oligomers complementary to two of the splice acceptor and one of the donor sites. All three were active in our viral inhibition screen and one of them, that complementary to the first acceptor site for the _tat_ mRNA, was particularly so (14). The group of Miller and Ts'o have found splice sites in herpes simplex virus to be targets for their modified oligonucleotides (20).

Although a family of mRNA's is produced using the multiple splice sites, all of them use the same cap site from the 5'-end of the parent RNA. From our findings with β-globin (19), this is a potential target site as are the six AUG initiator codons for _gag_, _sor_, _tat_, _art_, _env_ and 3'-_orf_. The _pol_ mRNA does not have an initiator codon. It is contiguous with _env_ mRNA but uses a different reading frame and so requires a frameshift signal for initiation. This signal too might be a target.

We have synthesized oligonucleotides complementary to all the above target sites and these are currently being evaluated (Table II). Of those for which we have

TABLE 2

Binding Site	Sequence
Cap	5' CTG CTC TAA CCA GAG AGA CC
Next to PBS	5' CTG CTA GAG ATT TTC CAC AC
PBS	5' AAG TCC CTG TTC GGG CGC CA
Splice Donor 300	5' GCG TAC TCA CCA GTC GCC GC
gag initiator AUG	5' CTC GCA CCC ATC TCT CTC CT
pol frame shift site	5' TCT TCC CTA AAA AAT TAG CC
Splice Acceptor 4493	5' TCT GCT GTC CCT GTA ATA AA
Splice Donor 4543	5' GCC CCT TCA CCT TTC CAG AG
sor initiator AUG	5' CTC TTT TCC ATA ATC CCT AA
Splice Acceptor 4970	5' ATA GCA GAG TCT GAA AAA CA
Splice Donor 5045	5' GAG ATC CTA CCT TGT TAT GT
Splice Acceptor 5359	5' ACA CCC AAT TCT GAA AAT GG
tat initiator AUG	5' ACT GGC TCC ATT TCT TGC TC
Splice Donor 5626	5' TAC TAC TTA CTG CTT TGA TA
env initiator AUG	5' TTC ACT CTC ATT GCC ACT GT

Binding site numbers refer to location in sequence, as described in (11).
PBS = prime binding site.

results, all compounds complementary to viral RNA were active to some degree, whereas two non-complementary controls tested at the same concentration were inactive. At present, we are testing mainly 20-mers. After identifying the most promising target sites, we plan to optimize chain length. Currently, we are synthesizing larger quantities of our most active compound to establish dose response curves.

Chemically Modified Oligonucleotides.

It is generally considered that highly charged species do not readily cross lipophilic cell membranes (21, and references therein). We have presented evidence that cellular uptake of unmodified oligonucleotides occurs, and may be an energy requiring process. Furthermore, we have shown that undegraded 20-mer can be recovered from cells after overnight incubation. However, it may well be possible to enhance antiviral activity by chemical modifications. In this, we have been joined by Dr. R. L. Letsinger who made the triester derivative discussed later.

In order to promote uptake and survival Miller and Ts'o pioneered the approach of blocking the negative charges on the internucleoside phosphates using first phosphotriesters and later phosphonates (for reviews see 23 and 24). In cell-free translation of globin mRNA, they found similar inhibition by complementary oligonucleotides or their methylphosphonate analogues (25 and 26). They have reported inhibition of replication of both vesicular stomatitis virus (26) and herpes simplex virus type 1 (20) by complementary oligonucleoside methyphosphonates.

We have tested a derivative of our most active compound in which several of the internucleoside phosphates were blocked as triesters of (1,1)-dimethyl-(2,2,2)-trichloroethyl alcohol 1 (22). The effect of the modification in HeLa cells was to alter both the rate of uptake and of survival of the oligomer. These effects vary with the number and chain position of the substituents, and more data are necessary before a firm evaluation of the effects can be made.

Dr. S. Agrawal, in our group, has synthesized various oligomers containing mixed phosphate and methylphosphonate internucleoside linkages 2. In degradation studies with snake venom phosphodiesterase, he finds that the enzyme can jump over one phosphonate linkage to release a

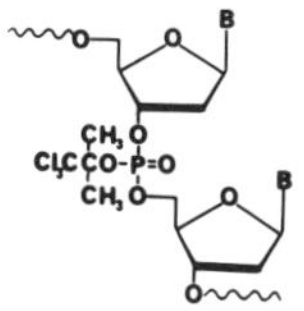

1

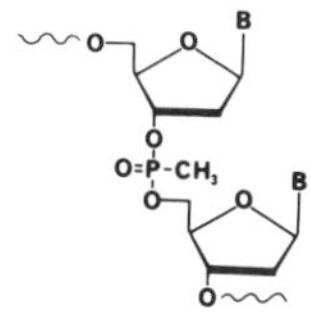

2

dinucleoside methylphosphonate but that two consecutive phosphonate linkages constitute a severe barrier to the enzyme. Thus, it may be possible to protect oligomers from degradation using just two modified linkages at each end of the molecule (27).

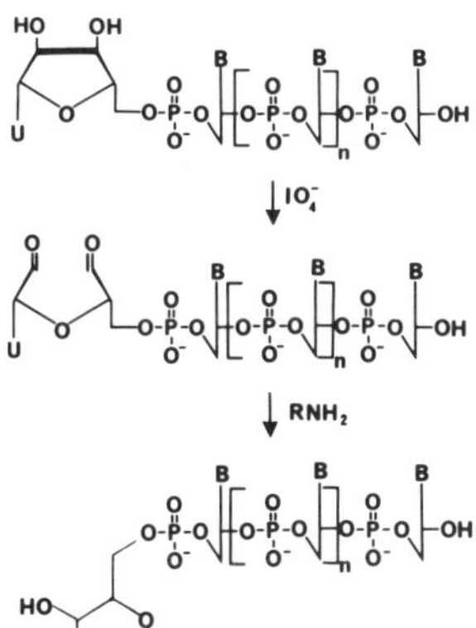

FIGURE 1. Coupling of polylysine to an oligonucleotide. RNH_2 = Polylysine

Another approach to increasing cellular uptake is to attach oligolysine or polylysine covalently to the 5' (Fig. 1) (28) or 3' end of an oligonucleotide (29). The latter resulted in inhibition of vesicular stomatitis virus using very low concentrations of compound (29). In our own laboratory, Dr. Agrawal has attached long chain alcohols to the 5' end of oligomers, in an effort to promote uptake and possibly inhibit degradation by 5' exonucleases (Fig. 2). We plan to augment this with substi-

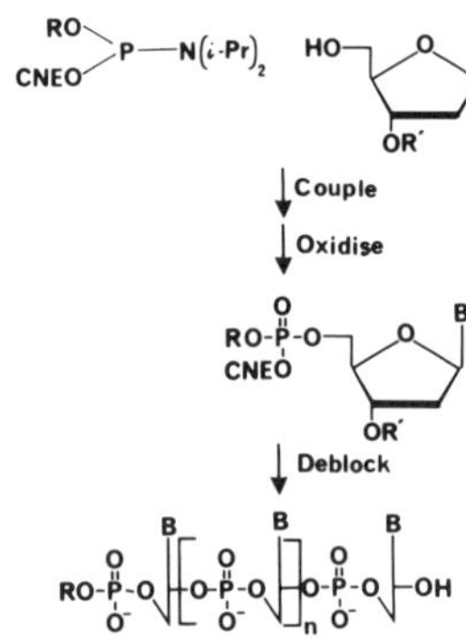

FIGURE 2. Coupling of lipophilic groups to 5'-end of an oligonucleotide on a solid support.
Pr - Propyl; CNE = Cyanoethyl

tution of the natural linkage by two consecutive internucleoside phosphonate groups at the 3' end to protect against 3' exonucleases. Another phosphate modification we are building into our compounds is thiophosphate 3. This is also known to confer stability against nuclease degradation (30) but does not alter the charge on the molecule.

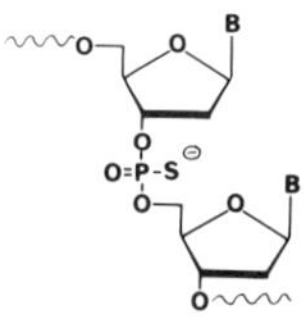

3

A different effort to improve the hybridon approach is to join intercalating agents covalently to the oligomers to stabilize interaction with the target RNA. This has been shown to improve inhibition of mRNA translation *in vitro* (31). Alternatively, groups may be incorporated that cause chain breakage or alkylation in the target site (32-36) or confer covalent linkage with the target. A novel approach we are considering may be termed "missplicing". It has been shown that an alternative splice acceptor site may be substituted for a natural acceptor site (37,38). Thus, if a "sense" oligomer identical to an HIV acceptor site were to compete with the natural acceptor site, an abortive splice might result, with foreshortening of the viral genome and loss of the viral phenotype specified thereby.

The hybridon approach has been shown to work against several viruses in tissue culture. It has not been tried in whole animals, and considerable progress in the scale-up of oligonucleotide synthesis must first be achieved. It is also unclear as to the optimal form the oligomer should take - the length, lipophilicity, charge density and so forth that are required for uptake, stability and hybridization that will determine the overall biological activity. It may be that combinations of different internucleoside linkages and terminal adducts may prove beneficial. There is also a possibility of enhanced inhibitions by simultaneous employment of more than one hybridon, each positioned at a different target site.

It is encouraging that at this symposium, two reports from other laboratories (39,40) provide independent evidence that the use of oligonucleotides of defined sequence or their modifications inhibit the replication of HIV-I in tissue culture systems.

ACKNOWLEDGMENTS

We would like to thank Drs. G. Witman and J. Aghajanian for electron microscopy studies and Sandra Johnson for expert work on the manuscript.

REFERENCES

1. Stephenson ML, Scott JF, Zamecnik PC (1973). Evidence that the polyadenylic acid segment of "35" RNA of avian myeloblastosis virus is located at the 3'-OH terminus. Biochem Biophys Res Commun 55:8.
2. Schwartz DE, Zamecnik PC, Weith HL (1977). The Rous sarcoma virus genome is terminally redundant: the 3' sequence. Proc Natl Acad Sci USA 74:994.
3. Haseltine WA, Maxam A, Gilbert W (1977). Rous sarcoma virus genome is terminally redundant: The 5' sequence. Proc Natl Acad Sci USA 74:989.

4. Zamecnik PC, Stephenson ML (1978). Inhibition of Rous sarcoma virus replication and transformation by a specific oligoneoxynucleotide. Proc Natl Acad Sci USA 75:280.
5. Stephenson ML, Zamecnik PC (1978). Inhibition of Rous sarcoma viral RNA translation by a specific oligodeoxyribonucleotide. Proc Natl Acad Sci USA 75:285.
6. Zamecnik PC (1966). The mechanism of protein synthesis and its possible alteration in the presence of oncogenic RNA viruses. Cancer Res 26:1.
7. Seiki M, Hattori S, Hirayama Y, Yoshida M (1983). Human T-cell leukemia virus: Complete nucleotide sequence of the provirus genome integrated in leukemia cell DNA. Proc Natl Acad Sci USA 80:3618.
8. Ratner L, Haseltine W, Patarca R, Livak KJ, Starcich B, Josephs SF, Doran ER, Rafalski JA, Whitehorn EA, Baumeister K, Ivanoff L, Petteway Jr SR, Pearson ML, Lautenberger JA, Papas TS, Ghrayeb J, Chang NT, Gallo RC, Wong-Staal F (1985). Complete nucleotide sequence of the AIDS virus, HTLV-III. Nature 313:277.
9. Wain-Hobson S, Sonigo P, Danos O, Cole S, Alizon M (1985). Nucleotide sequence of the AIDS virus, LAV. Cell 40:9.
10. Sanchez-Pescador R, Power MD, Barr PJ, Steimer KS, Stempien MM, Brown-Shimer SL, Gee WW, Renard A, Randolph A, Levy JA, Dina D, Luciw PA (1985). Nucleotide sequence and expression of an AIDS-associated retrovirus (ARV-2). Science 227:484.
11. Muesing MA, Smith DH, Cabradilla CD, Benton CV, Lasky LA, Capon DJ (1985) Nucleic acid structure and expression of the human AIDS/lymphadenopathy retrovirus. Nature 313:450.
12. Sodroski J, Rosen C, Goh WC, Haseltine WA (1985). A transcriptional activator protein encoded by the X-lor region of the human T-cell leukemia virus. Science 228:1430.
13. Arya SK, Guo C, Josephs SF, Wong-Staal F (1985). Trans-activator gene of human T-lymphotropic virus type III (HTLV-III). Science 229:69.
14. Zamecnik PC, Goodchild J, Taguchi Y, Sarin PS (1986). Inhibition of replication and expression of human T-cell lymphotropic virus type III in cultured cells by exogenous synthetic oligonucleotides complimentary to viral RNA. Proc Natl Acad Sci USA 83:4143.

15. Zamecnik PC, Zamecnik M, Beard D, Beard J (1978) Unpublished experiments.
16. Schell PL (1971) Uptake of polynucleotides by intact mammalian cells VIII. Synthetic homoribopolynucleotides. Biochim Biophys Acta 240:472.
17. Schell PL (1974). Uptake of polynucleotides by mammalian cells XIV. Stimulation of the uptake of polynucleotides by poly (l-lysine). Biochim Biophys Acta 340:323.
18. Unpublished data from this laboratory.
19. Goodchild J, Carroll E, Greenberg J. Inhibition of Rabbit -Globin Synthesis by Complementary Oligonucleotides: Identification of mRNA Sites Sensitive to Inhibition. In preparation.
20. Smith CC, Aurelian L, Reddy MP, Miller PS, Ts'o POP (1986). Antiviral effect of an oligo(nucleoside methylphosphonate) complementary to the splice junction of herpes simplex virus type 1 immediate early pre-mRNAs 4 and 5. Proc Natl Acad Sci USA 83:2787.
21. Westheimer FH, (1987). Why nature chose phosphates. Science 235:1173.
22. Letsinger RL, Groody EP, Tanaka T (1982). Use of trichlorodimethylethyl as a protecting group and tributylphosphine as a deprotecting agent in oligonucleotide synthesis. J Am Chem Soc 104:6805.
23. Miller PS, Agris CH, Blake KR, Murakauri A, Spitz SA, Reddy MP, Ts'o POP (1983). Nonionic oligonucleotide analogs as new tools for studies on the structure and function of nucleic acids inside living cells. In Pullman B, Jortner J, (eds): "Nucleic Acids: The Vectors of Life," D. Reidel Publishing Co.
24. Miller PS, Agris CH, Aurelian L, Blake KR, Murakami A, Reddy MP, Spitz SA, Ts'o POP (1985). Control of ribonucleic acid function by oligonucleoside methylphosphonates. Biochimie 67:769.
25. Blake IR, Murakami A, Miller PS (1985) Inhibition of rabbit globin mRNA translation by sequence-specific oligodeoxyribonucleotides. Biochem 24:6132.
26. Blake KR, Murakami A, Spitz SA, Glave SA, Reddy MP, Ts'o POP, Miller PS (1985) Hybridization arrest of globin synthesis in rabbit reticulocyte lysates and cells by oligodeoxyribonucleoside methylphosphonates. Biochem 24:6139.
27. Agrawal S. <u>et al</u>. Unpublished data.

28. Agrawal S, Christodoulou C, Gait MJ (1986) Efficient methods for attaching non-radioactive labels to the 5' ends of synthetic oligodeoxyribonucleotides. Nucleic Acids Res 14:6227.
29. Lemaitre M, Bayard B, Lebleu B (1987) Specific antiviral activity of a poly(L-lysine)-conjugated oligodeoxyribonucleotide sequence complementary to vesicular stomatitis virus N protein mRNA initiation site. Proc Natl Acad Sci USA 84:648.
30. Eckstein F (1985). Nucleoside phosphorothioates. Ann Rev Biochem 54:367.
31. Toulme JJ, Krisch HM, Loreau N, Thuong NT, Helene C (1986). Specific inhibition of mRNA translation by complementary oligonucleotides covalently linked to intercalating agents. Proc Natl Acad Sci USA 83:1227.
32. Knorre DG, Vlassov VV (1985). Complementary-addressed (sequence-specific) modification of nucleic acids. Prog Nucl Acid Res Mol Biol 32:291.
33. Chu BCF, Orgel LE (1985). Nonenzymatic sequence-specific cleavage of single-stranded DNA. Proc Natl Acad Sci USA 82:963.
34. Dreyer GB, Dervan PB (1985). Sequence-specific cleavage of single-stranded DNA: Oligodeoxynucleotide-EDTA-Fe(II). Proc Natl Acad Sci USA 82:968.
35. Doan TL, Perronault L, Helene C, Chassignol M, Thuong NT (1986). Targeted cleavage of polynucleotides by complementary oligonucleotides covalently linked to iron-porphyrins. Biochem 25:6736.
36. Webb TR, Matteucci MD (1986). Hybridization triggered cross-linking of deoxyoligonucleotides. Nucl Acid Res 14:7661.
37. Solnick D (1985). Trans splicing of mRNA precursors. Cell 42:157.
38. Konarska MM, Padgett RA, Sharp PA (1985). Trans splicing of mRNA precursors _in vitro_. Cell 42:165.
39. Zaia JA, Cantin E, Rossi JJ, Spallone PA, Murakawa G, Erijta R, Kaplan B, Wallace RB (1987) Inhibition of hujan immunodeficiency virus (HIV) using an oligonucleoside mehtylphosphonate. J Cell Biochem, Supp 11D, Abstract p 72.
40. Matsukura M, Shinozuka K, Zon G, Mitsuya H, Cohen JS, Border S (1987). Phosphorothioate analogs of oligodeoxynucleotides: Novel inhibitors of replication and cytoplthic effects of HTLV-III/LAV (Immunodeficiency virus). J Cell Biochem, Supp 11D, Abstract p 67.

Human Retroviruses, Cancer, and AIDS: Approaches to Prevention and Therapy, pages 439–445

A FUSION ASSAY FOR THE DETECTION OF HIV INFECTED CELLS

George N. Pavlakis, Barbara K. Felber and Connie M. Wright

NCI-Frederick Cancer Research Facility
BRI-Basic Research Program
P.O. Box B
Frederick, Maryland 21701

Human immunodeficiency virus (HIV) encodes two activators of viral gene expression, the transactivator or tat and the art or trs protein (1-9). The transactivator is an essential viral protein that increases the steady-state level of viral mRNA. One of the methods we, and others, have used to study the function of tat was the generation of hybrid genes containing HIV sequences. The LTR promoter and parts of the transcribed R region were ligated to the chloramphenicol acetyl transferase (CAT) or other indicator genes and the effect of tat was conveniently monitored at the protein level by CAT enzyme assays and other methods. In human cells the amount of protein produced by the HIV LTR-CAT constructs is greatly increased in the presence of tat (500- to 1000-fold activation). In Figure 1 we compare the expression of three different viral LTRs ligated to the CAT gene in human cells (HeLa) and in mouse 3T3 cells in the presence or in the absence of their homologous viral transactivators. In both cell types the activation of HTLV-I and HTLV-II promoters by their homologous transcriptional activators was similar. On the contrary, HIV activation by tat is prominent in human cells (~ 500-fold activation) but not in mouse cells (~ 5- to 10-fold activation). Upon stable integration of the HIV LTR in human or mouse cells, the extent of transactivation remains the same (4, unpublished results).

We took advantage of the great activation of the LTR promoter by tat in human cells to develop a fusion assay for the detection of tat. Since tat is an essential viral pro-

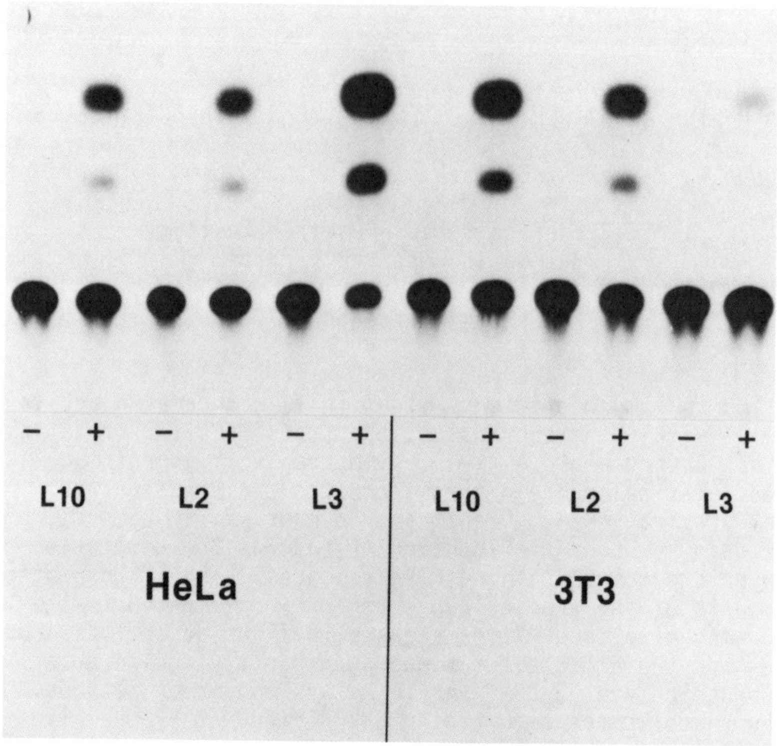

Figure 1. Activation of different LTR-CAT constructs in HeLa and NIH/3T3 cells. LTR-CAT plasmids containing the LTR of HTLV-I (L10), HTLV-II (L2) or HIV (L3) were transfected into HeLa or NIH/3T3 cells either alone (-) or with (+) the homologous transactivator-producing plasmid pMAXneo, pMAX2neo or pMX3Nneo, respectively. Two days later, the cells were harvested and assayed for CAT. In both cell types, the activation of HTLV-I or HTLV-II LTR is similar. On the contrary, HIV LTR transactivation is prominent only in human cells.

tein expressed early after infection, virus-infected cells can also be detected by this assay. An outline of the assay is shown in Figure 2. HL3T1 cells contain integrated LTR-CAT sequences and were selected as the indicator cells on the basis of their great inducibility in the presence of tat protein (4). Cells containing tat protein were fused to the HL3T1 cells by polyethylene glycol (PEG). We used this assay for the detection of tat in several different cells: B2MX3 is a mouse cell line that produces high levels of tat (4). These cells were plated together with HL3T1 cells, and the next day the cells (which should be close to confluency) were fused by PEG (50% w/v in serum-free RPMI medium) for 3 min. Another cell line, ψAM-GVL3CAT, that contains integrated copies of LTR-CAT was also used in fusion experiments with B2MX3 cells. The result of these experiments are shown in Table 1 and suggest that the activation phenotype of human cells is dominant in mouse-human heterocaryons.

To verify that this assay can be used for the detection of HIV-infected cells, we fused line HL3T1 in suspension to different numbers of human lymphoid cells infected by HIV ($H9/HIV_{IIIB}$). HL3T1 cells were mixed with the infected cells, washed, resuspended in the PEG solution (50% w/v PEG in RPM1 medium) for 3 min, centrifuged for 3 min at 1200 rpm, washed and grown for 2 days in RPM1 + 10% FCS. After two days in culture, the activation of HIV LTR was measured by CAT assays (Figure 3). The quantitation of these assays demonstrate that the activation of CAT enzyme is dependent on the number of HIV-infected cells. In the present form, this assay can detect approximately 300 cells infected by the AIDS virus in a population of 10^6 cells.

The stable indicator cell line HL3T1 was also examined for activation by other viruses such as Herpes simplex virus-1 (HSV-1), HTLV-I, HTLV-II and equine infectious anemia virus (EIAV) in transfection, fusion or infection experiments as detailed in Table 2. In agreement with other investigators (10,11), it was found that HSV-I can activate the expression of CAT after infection of HL3T1 cells but this activation was one order of magnitude lower than the one caused by HIV tat (Figure 4). Several lines of evidence suggest that the HSV-1 activates the LTR via a different mechanism (unpublished results). Although the activation

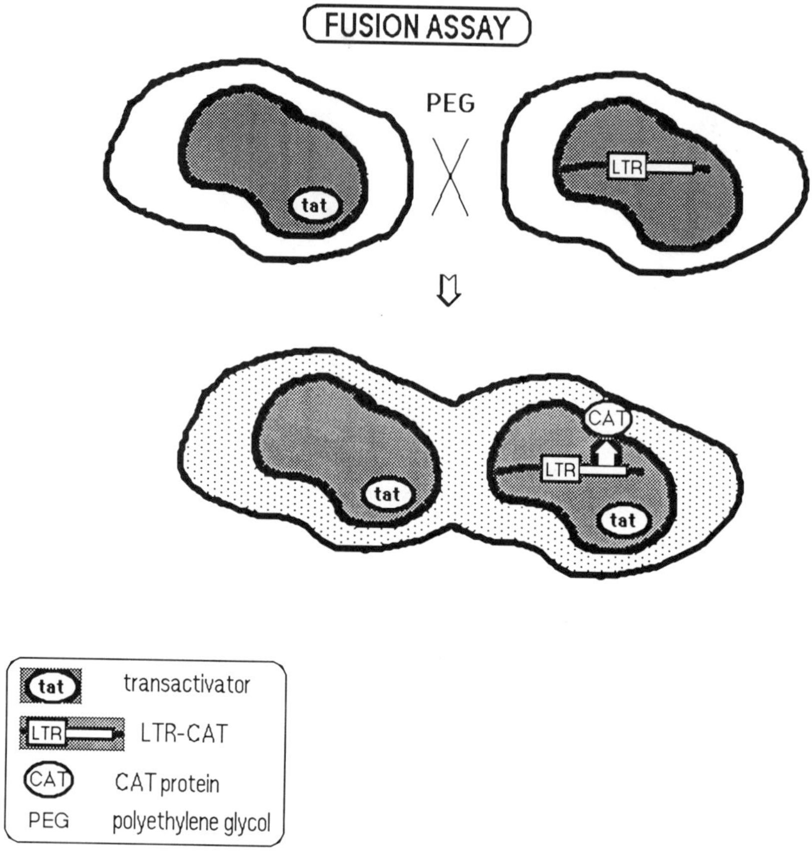

Figure 2. Schematic representation of the fusion assay.

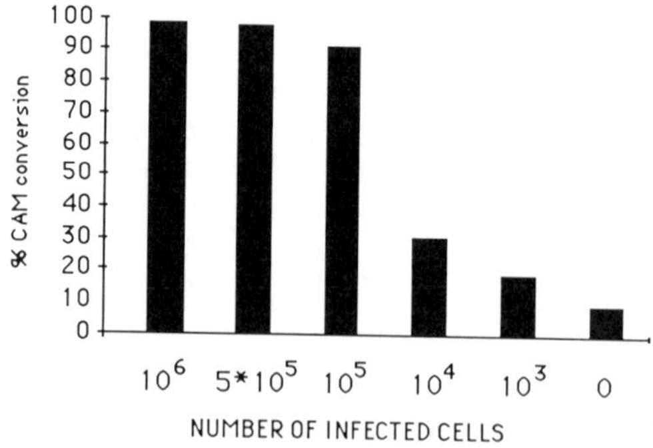

Figure 3. Quantitation of CAT assays after fusion of HL3T1 to different numbers of HIV-infected cells ($H9/HIV_{IIIB}$).

Table 1

Activation of LTR-CAT by fusion.

HIV LTR-CAT indicator cell line	*tat* producer cell line	Activation
HL3T1	B2MX3	> 500 X
"	$H9/HIV_{IIIB}$	> 500 X
"	HeLa/MX3Bneo	> 500 X
ψ_{AM}GVL3CAT	B2MX3	10 X

Cells containing integrated LTR-CAT copies (left column) were fused to cells expressing HIV *tat* protein (middle column) and the CAT enzyme was quantitated after two days.

Table 2

Activation of HL3T1 cells by other viruses

Virus	Method	Activation
HTLV-I	- transfection of transcriptional activator DNA	-
	- fusion to HTLV-I-infected cells (HUT102, MT2)	-
HTLV-II	- transfection of transcriptional activator DNA	-
EIAV	- fusion to EIAV-infected cells (CF2, EFK)	-
HSV-1	- infection	+
HIV	- transfection	+++
	- fusion to $H9/HIV_{IIIB}$ or H9/HIV RF	+++

HL3T1 cells were either transfected with DNA, fused to virus-infected cells or infected with the indicated virus.

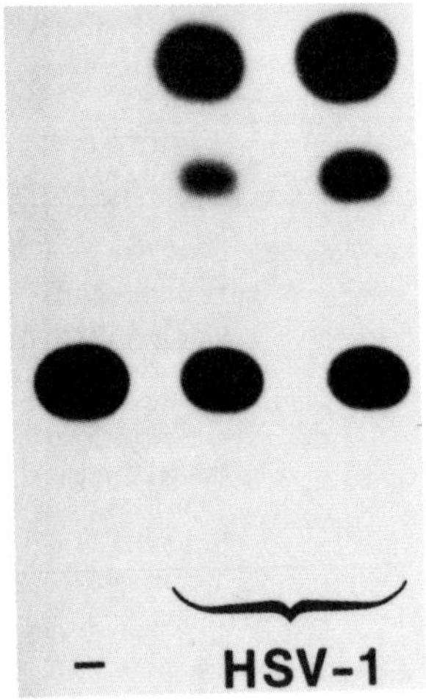

Figure 4. Infection of HL3T1 cells by Herpes virus (HSV-1). Cells were infected with 2 x 10^6 pfu (middle lane) or with 2 x 10^7 pfu of HSV-1. Uninfected cells are shown in the left lane. The cells were assayed for CAT enzyme two days post-infection.

by HSV-1 is low, the presence of HSV-1 may confuse the interpretation of this fusion assay when applied to the detection of HIV infected cells. To overcome this limitation, we assayed several other human indicator cell lines for activation in the presence of HIV. We have now identified cell lines which are very specific for the HIV transactivator and are not activated by HSV-1.

More recently, we have constructed cell lines containing the LTR-CAT indicator gene that express the T4 cell surface receptor, which is required for viral infection (12,13). These cell lines can be infected by HIV and, therefore, greatly simplify the detection and quantitation of both cell-free virus and virally infected cells. A fusion assay may still be very helpful for the detection of latent HIV that exists in a non-permissive cellular environment.

Acknowledgements

We thank Tony Tse for expert technical assistance and Hilda Marusiodis for expert editorial assistance. Barbara K. Felber was supported by a senior fellowship from the Swiss National Science Foundation. Research sponsored by the National Cancer Institute, DHHS, under contract No. NO1-CO-23909 with Bionetics Research, Inc.

REFERENCES

1. S.K. Arya, C. Guo, S.F. Josephs, F. Wong-Staal. Science 229:69, 1985.

2. L.J. Siegel, L. Ratner, S.F. Josephs, D. Derse, M.B. Feinberg, G.R. Reyes, S.J. O'Brien, F. Wong-Staal. Virology 148:226, 1986.

3. J. Sodroski, R. Patarca, C. Rosen, F. Wong-Staal, W. Haseltine. Science 229:74, 1985.

4. C.M. Wright, B.K. Felber, H. Paskalis, G.N. Pavlakis. Science 234:988, 1986.

5. B. Cullen, Cell 46:973, 1986.

6. C.A. Rosen, J.G. Sodroski, W. Chun Goh, A.I. Dayton, J. Lippke, W.A. Haseltine. Nature (London) 319:555, 1986.

7. M.B. Feinberg, R.F. Jarrett, A. Aldovini, R.C. Gallo, F. Wong-Staal. Cell 46:807, 1986.

8. M.A. Muesing, D.H. Smith, D.J. Capon. Cell 48:691, 1987.

9. B.M. Peterlin, P.A. Luciw, P.J. Barr, M.D. Walker. Proc. Natl. Acad. Sci. USA 83:9734, 1986.

10. J.D. Mosca, D.P. Bednarik, N.B.K. Raj, C.A. Rosen, J.G. Sodroski, W.A. Haseltine, P.M. Pitha. Nature 325:67, 1987.

11. H.E. Gendelman, W. Phelps, L. Feigenbaum, J.M. Ostrove, A. Adachi, P.M. Howley, G. Khoury, H.S. Ginsberg, M.A. Martin. Proc. Natl. Acad. Sci. USA 83:9759, 1986.

12. A.G. Dalgleish, P.C.L. Beverley, P.R. Clapham, D.H. Crawford, M.F. Greaves, R.A. Weiss. Nature 312:763, 1984.

13. D. Klatzmann, E. Champaign, S. Chamaret, J. Gruest, D. Guetard, T. Hercend, J.-C. Gluckman, L. Montagnier. Nature 312:767, 1984.

Human Retroviruses, Cancer, and AIDS:
Approaches to Prevention and Therapy, pages 447–461

THERAPY AGAINST NEUROTROPIC RETROVIRUSES: A RAPID MURINE MODEL INVOLVING TRANSPLACENTAL OR NEONATAL INFECTION[1]

Ruth M. Ruprecht,[2] Arlene H. Sharpe[3], Janet Andersen[2] and Rudolf Jaenisch[3]

[2]Dana-Farber Cancer Institute, Boston MA 02115 and
[3]Whitehead Institute, Cambridge MA 02142

ABSTRACT The severe neurologic deficits caused by HTLV-III/LAV/HIV call for prompt study of retroviral neurovirulence and treatment strategies. The increasing frequency of perinatal infections necessitates specific examination of therapy during gestation and in the perinatal period. To address these important issues, we have developed murine models involving infection of SWR/J mice either as midgestation embryos or on postnatal day 1 with the neurotropic retrovirus Cas-Br-E that causes hind limb paralysis. *In utero* infection dramatically shortened the time to full paralysis as compared to neonatal infection (20 vs 112 days; $p<0.0001$). Treatment with 3'-azido-3'-deoxythymidine (AZT) significantly delayed development of neurologic disease and led to marked gains in survival in a dose-dependent fashion. AZT was given orally to pregnant and/or lactating females to treat infected embryos or pups. We conclude: 1) AZT is active in the CNS sanctuary and significantly ameliorates retroviral neurologic disease; 2) AZT is effective across the placental barrier; 3) AZT is secreted into milk; 4) our murine models are well-suited to study pathogenesis and therapy of neurotropic retroviral infections; and 5) perinatal infection and therapy can be evaluated readily. In summary, our model systems are well suited for *in vivo* analysis

[1]Supported by a contract from the Massachusetts Department of Public Health (RMR), a Lucille P. Markey Charitable Trust Scholarship (AHS), and NIH grants HD19015 and CA38497 (RJ).

of questions relevant to human neurovirulent retroviruses.

INTRODUCTION

Infection with HTLV-III/LAV/HIV (1-3), the causative agent of the acquired immune deficiency syndrome (AIDS), is spreading. In addition to severe depletion of T-helper cells resulting in loss of immune functions, HIV can attack the central nervous system (CNS) and induce neurological deficits ranging from mild personality changes to dementia and paralysis (4-7). The number of pediatric AIDS patients is rising due to perinatal infection of infants born to HIV-antibody positive mothers (8-13). No practical animal model systems exist to study retroviral neuro-virulence, transplacental and perinatal infection, as well as treatment strategies aimed at these clinical problems.

The murine retrovirus Cas-Br-E, isolated from a wild mouse population at Lake Casitas, California, induces a progressive lower motor neuron disease (14-16). As in some HIV-induced CNS syndromes, no inflammatory reaction is noted in the CNS of Cas-Br-E infected mice. These mice develop hind limb paralysis associated with spongiform changes in the anterior horns of the spinal cord, dentate nucleus of the cerebellum, and brain stem (17-21). Experimental infection of susceptible strains of mice, such as SWR/J, during the first few days of life induces hind limb paralysis in all infected mice with a latency period of 3 to 5 months. Here we show that infection during gestation markedly shortens the incubation time and hastens progression of disease from mild tremor to complete hind limb paralysis without changing the clinical presentation.

The neurotropic murine retrovirus model described appears ideally suited to test antiretroviral effects of candidate anti-AIDS drugs targeted at the CNS sanctuary. At the same time, therapeutic approaches for transplacental and neonatal infection can be studied.

To test the feasibility of this approach, we used SWR/J mice infected with the neurotropic Cas-Br-E virus as midgestation embryos or neonates to analyze the effects of therapy with 3'-azido-3'-deoxythymidine (AZT) (22-26), a thymidine analogue used for treating patients with AIDS (25-28). AZT acts as a reverse transcriptase inhibitor following intracellular conversion to AZT triphosphate, and is able to cross the blood-brain barrier (28).

Administration of AZT to AIDS patients with HIV-induced neurological deficits has led to clinical improvement (28). In addition, oral AZT therapy has been highly effective in suppressing viremia and prolonging life of BALB/c mice infected with the Rauscher MuLV complex (29). Here we show that AZT therapy markedly retarded progression of CNS disease in mice with Cas-Br-E viremia, resulting in highly significant gains in survival. This was true whether AZT was given to pregnant dams to treat embryos infected during midgestation, or to lactating females to treat postnatally infected pups.

MATERIALS AND METHODS

NIH 3T3 cells producing molecularly cloned Cas-Br-E (clone NE-8) were kindly provided by Dr. P. Jolicoeur (Montreal). SWR/J mice, initially obtained from Jackson Laboratories (Bar Harbor, ME), were bred in our facilities. AZT was a gift of Dr. S. Nusinoff-Lehrman, Burroughs Wellcome Co. (Research Triangle Park, NC).

XC plaque assays and plaque reduction assays were carried out as described (30). Cas-Br-E virus stocks were prepared by passing tissue culture supernatant obtained from virus-producing NIH 3T3 cells through a 0.22 μm Nalgene filter and quick-freezing and storing it in liquid nitrogen.

Neonatal SWR/J mice were infected during the first two days of life by injection of $2x10^4$ plaque-forming units (pfu) of Cas-Br-E virus in 0.1 ml. AZT therapy was started 4 hr post-inoculation by administering the drug in drinking water to lactating females at 0.1 mg/ml. Based on average fluid intake, weight and litter size of about 6 pups, this dose corresponds to approximately 50 mg/kg/day per female during the first week post-partum. This dose was well tolerated throughout the lactating period by both mothers and pups. After weaning, AZT was continued at 0.1 mg/ml in drinking water, unless stated otherwise.

Cas-Br-E was microinjected into midgestation embryos as described previously (31). Pregnant mice were anesthetized on embryonic day (E) 8.75 and 9.0 and laparotomy was performed by a long ventral incision. The uterus was held with sharp forceps and NIH 3T3 cells producing Cas-Br-E were microinjected into individual embryos by introducing the micropipet into the ventral third of the decidual swelling. Approximately 0.1 to 0.5 μl ($3x10^6$ cells/ml) was injected per embryo. AZT was started 12 hr postoperatively by giving the drug in drinking water at 0.1 mg/ml or 0.2 mg/ml to pregnant females. Approximate doses based on weight and fluid intake ranged from 32 to 63 mg/kg/day for mice receiving 0.2 mg/ml of AZT. At these doses no maternal morbidity or mortality was observed. Unless indicated otherwise, AZT treatment was continued throughout the life of the infected animals by first giving the drug at the same concentration to the lactating mothers after birth, followed by direct oral treatment of the infected offspring after weaning.

For *in vivo* testing of AZT, all experimental mice were examined regularly and were scored as fully paralyzed when no motion was observed in the hind limbs or when mice with known neurologic dysfunction of the hind limbs were found dead. Moribund or fully paralyzed mice were sacrificed for humane reasons. For statistical analysis, mice lost in the neonatal period due to maternal cannibalism were excluded. For experimental animal cohorts undergoing microinjection as midgestation embryos, only animals scoring positive for viremia as measured by radioimmunoassay (RIA) at age 2 to 3 weeks were entered into statistical analysis because of a success rate of 66% for microinjection. This procedure could represent a bias against the therapeutic benefits of AZT since animals that were successfully protected from infection because of AZT therapy, and consequently score RIA negative, were excluded.

Viremia was assessed by RIA using radioiodinated Moloney murine leukemia virus (MoMuLV) p30 (p30 was obtained from NCI) and rabbit anti-MoMuLV p30 serum as published (32). The p30 antigen is shared by numerous murine retroviruses including Cas-Br-E and MoMuLV.

AZT levels in tissues were analyzed by high performance liquid chromatography (Ruprecht and Trites, unpublished results).

RESULTS

AZT inhibits Cas-Br-E propagation *in vitro*.

First, the susceptibility of Cas-Br-E to AZT was analyzed *in vitro* in the XC plaque reduction assay. AZT was highly effective as shown by an inhibitory concentration$_{50}$ (IC_{50}) of 3 nM. No significant cytotoxicity was noted at AZT concentrations increased by several logs (Figure 1).

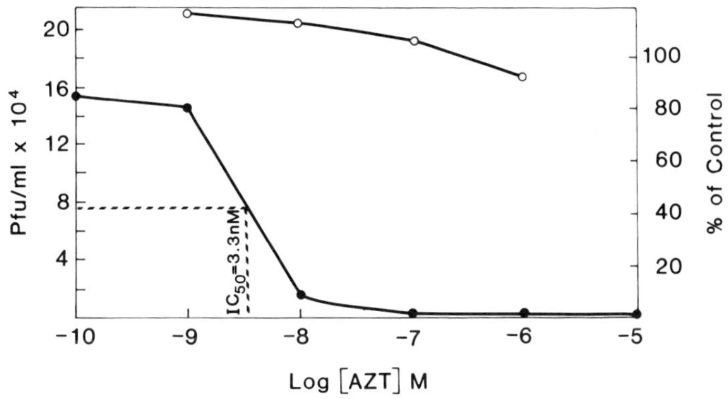

FIGURE 1. AZT inhibition of XC plaque formation by Cas-Br-E virus. The number of pfu/ml are shown (•). Parallel cultures were analyzed for cytotoxicity to AZT; the percentage of surviving cells compared to untreated controls is shown (o).

Infection of SWR/J Midgestation Embryos with Neurotropic Cas-Br-E.

Cas-Br-E virus was introduced into post-implantation SWR/J mouse embryos between embryonic day (E) 8.75 and 9.0 of gestation by microinjection of virus-producing cells into individual embryos with a micropipette (31). This is the time period during development in which complex patterns of cell migration and organogenesis occur. Specifically, neural tube closure begins on E 8 and is complete by E 9.5, and simultaneously, spinal cord development begins. Cell division is extremely rapid during midgestation, with cell number increasing from 800 on E7 to 15,000 over the next 24 hr period.

Approximately 63% of microinjected embryos survived to birth (Table 1) and were born without obvious signs of disease or developmental anomaly. Animals were bled at 2 to 3 weeks of age and serum was assayed for viremia by radioimmunoassay (RIA) for the group-specific antigen p30. Viremia was used to assess the success of the microinjection technique because it is a highly sensitive indicator of viral infection and replication (32). The RIA results indicate that 59% to 66% of microinjected embryos surviving after birth were successfully infected. This success rate as well as the percentage of microinjected embryos surviving to birth (44% to 74%) are similar to previous studies with MoMuLV (31). The numbers of animals surviving to birth and developing viremia may be underestimated because of cannibalism of neonates by SWR/J mothers. The Fv-1 N restriction for Cas-Br-E is maintained during infection at midgestation; no animals derived from BALB/c or C57BL/6J embryos (Fv-1 B) infected with Cas-Br-E became viremic (Table 1).

TABLE 1
MICROINJECTION OF MOUSE EMBRYOS IN UTERO

Strain	Injected with	# born/# injected		# viremic/# alive at 2 wk	
		- AZT	+ AZT	- AZT	+ AZT
SWR/J	Cas-Br-E[a]	46/73 (63%)	89/120 (74%)	21/32 (66%)	32/54 (59%)
SWR/J	Mock[b]	8/15 (53%)	40/63 (63%)	0/8 (0%)	0/40 (0%)
BALB/c	Cas-Br-E[a]	13/22 (59%)	---	0/11 (0%)	---
C57BL	Cas-Br-E[a]	12/27 (44%)	---	0/10 (0%)	---

[a]Cas-Br-E virus-producing NIH 3T3 cells were injected.
[b]Uninfected NIH 3T3 cells were injected.

Viremic SWR/J mice derived from embryos infected at midgestation began to show mild tremor between 8 to 14 days of age. These animals often were smaller and weighed less than uninfected age-matched controls. Neurologic disease progressed over the course of 1 to 2 weeks to complete hind limb paralysis associated with prominent tremor. Infected animals also exhibited atrophy of hind limb musculature, ruffled hair, and bladder incontinence. Disease never involved the upper limbs. Animals died between postnatal day 19 and 25.

Histopathologic analysis of infected animals revealed spongiform changes in the CNS similar in location to the disease produced in animals infected postnatally (Sharpe and Jaenisch, unpublished observations). Thus, infection of SWR/J mice as midgestation embryos results in neurologic disease clinically and histopathologically similar to disease occurring in mice infected after birth. The course of disease, however, is telescoped in time. Whereas animals infected postnatally develop tremor at about 3 months of age followed by paralysis and death by 6 months, mice derived from infected midgestation embryos develop tremor and paralysis by 2 weeks of age and die of neurologic disease at $3\frac{1}{2}$ to 4 weeks (Figure 2; $p<0.0001$ by log rank).

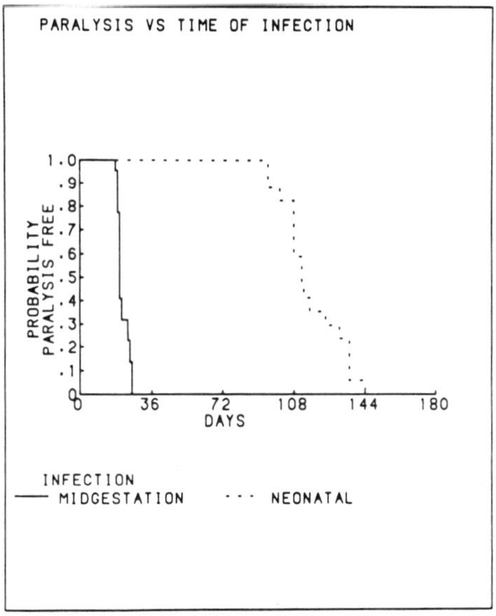

FIGURE 2. Development of full hind limb paralysis as a function of age of infection. SWR/J mice were infected either as midgestation embryos (—, 22 mice) or during the first two days after birth (- - -, 17 mice) as described in METHODS. The probability of remaining free of complete hind limb paralysis is shown in a Kaplan-Meier plot. The median time to full hind limb paralysis was 20 days for midgestation infection and 112 days for neonatal infection ($p<0.0001$ by log rank).

AZT Therapy of Mice Infected as Midgestation Embryos with Cas-Br-E.

The rapid development of neurologic disease in mice infected as midgestation embryos prompted the examination of this mode of infection for use in the study of biological efficacy of candidate antiviral agents targeted against neurovirulent retroviruses. AZT was chosen for initial studies because it is known to penetrate the blood-brain barrier, leading to CNS levels reaching 50% of serum levels (28).

AZT therapy dramatically altered the onset and progression of neurologic disease in SWR/J mice infected as post-implantation embryos between E 8.75 and 9.0. AZT therapy was begun within several hours after viral inoculation and was continued throughout the life of infected mice. Initially, AZT was administered to the infected embryos via pregnant females which received the drug dissolved in drinking water at 0.1 mg/ml or at 0.2 mg/ml. At the latter concentration, the AZT level in embryonic tissues at E 12, as determined by high performance liquid chromatography, was 0.23 μg/g, indicating effective penetration of the placental barrier (Ruprecht and Trites, unpublished observation). AZT did not affect embryo survival to birth ($p >> 0.05$ by Fisher Exact Test for all comparisons) (Table 1), and no gross malformations were seen in AZT-treated offspring. Postnatally, AZT therapy was continued via lactating females followed by direct oral treatment of infected animals after weaning.

In viremic mice infected at midgestation, the onset of hind limb tremor was delayed from a median of 14 days in untreated viremic control animals to a median of 27 days in animals given 0.1 mg/ml of AZT ($p=0.01$ by log rank) and a median of 50 days in mice given 0.2 mg/ml of AZT ($p<0.0001$ by log rank) (Figure 3A). To analyze dose effect, the AZT doses were ranked in increasing order (control=1, 0.1 mg/ml=2, 0.2 mg/ml=3), and dose rank was entered into a Cox regression program as covariate. Dose rank was highly associated with time to tremor ($p=0.00008$) and with survival ($p<0.00001$).

Most AZT-treated mice progressed from mild to more pronounced tremor over several months. Only at 6 months after birth have some of the AZT-treated mice begun to develop hind limb paralysis. Median survival has not yet been reached for AZT-treated mice and is longer than 5 months, in sharp contrast to a median survival of only 20 days for viremic untreated controls (Figure 3B). Mock infected control animals treated with AZT or receiving no treatment remained clinically well.

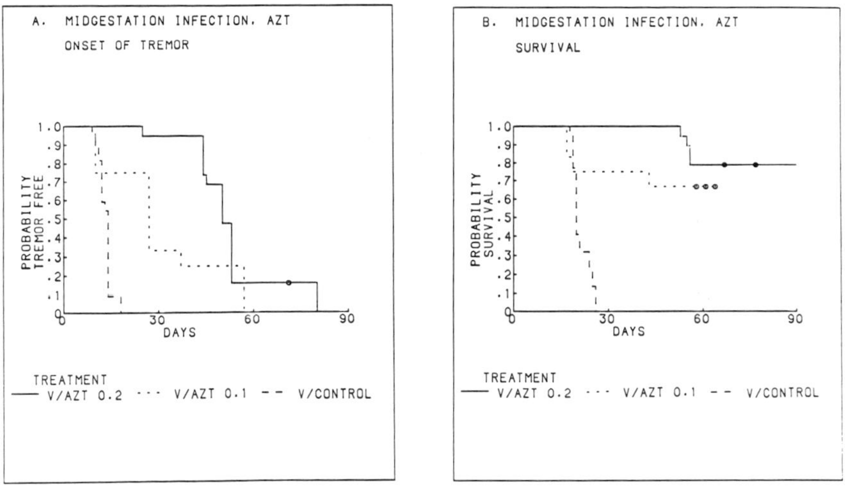

FIGURE 3. Effect of AZT on onset of tremor and survival of mice infected as midgestation embryos, as shown by Kaplan-Meier analysis. 3A: The probability to remain tremor-free is shown for SWR/J mice infected _in utero_. (— — —, 22 mice): untreated animals; (•••••, 12 mice): animals on 0.1 mg/ml AZT; and (——— , 19 mice): animals on 0.2 mg/ml AZT. AZT was given orally as described in METHODS. One RIA positive mouse on 0.2 mg/ml AZT was symptom free on day 71 (-•-). 3B: Same as 3A, but showing the probability of survival. Animals alive at the time of analysis are shown by (-•-) (15 mice on 0.2 mg/ml; 8 mice on 0.1 mg/ml).

When animals infected _in utero_ received AZT from their mothers transplacentally only until birth, onset and progression of disease was significantly delayed. In contrast to infected untreated mice that had a median time to tremor of 14 days, these mice began to develop tremor on postnatal day 32 with a median of day 38 (p=0.01 by log rank) (Figure 4A), and survived until postnatal day 99 to

127. Untreated mice had a median survival of only 21 days (p=0.005 by log rank) (Figure 4B). This clearly shows that transplacental treatment with AZT resulted in improved clinical outcome for offspring infected at midgestation. Because of small numbers of experimental animals, the effects of continuous AZT treatment as compared to transplacental treatment alone yielded no significant differences.

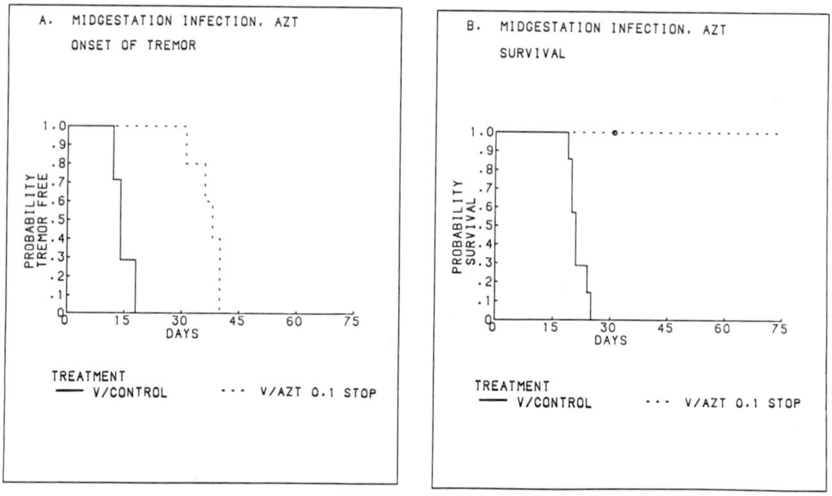

FIGURE 4. Effect of AZT given only prior to birth, on onset of tremor and survival of mice infected at midgestation with Cas-Br-E. 4A: Probability to remain tremor-free is shown by Kaplan-Meier plot (——, 7 mice): infected, untreated animals; (- - -, 5 mice): infected animals undergoing only prenatal AZT treatment. The pregnant female received 0.1 mg/ml AZT in drinking water. 4B: Same as 4A, but showing the probability of survival. —⊖— : One mouse censored on day 32 due to accidental death.

AZT Therapy of Mice Infected as Neonates with Cas-Br-E.

Mice inoculated with virus postnatally also showed a remarkable alteration in disease course when given AZT via the milk of lactating females receiving 0.1 mg/ml AZT, followed by 0.1 mg/ml in drinking water after weaning. These mice developed complete hind limb paralysis with a median onset of 181 days in contrast to viremic, untreated controls that developed paralysis at a median of 112 days ($p<0.0001$ by log rank) (Figure 5). When AZT treatment was stopped at weaning, infected mice still had a delayed onset of hind limb paralysis as compared to infected controls (median, 148 days versus 112 days, $p=0.04$ by log rank). However, continuous AZT therapy led to significantly longer paralysis-free survival ($p=0.003$ by log rank). There was no difference in the time to development of full paralysis by sex nor any influence of sex on AZT therapy.

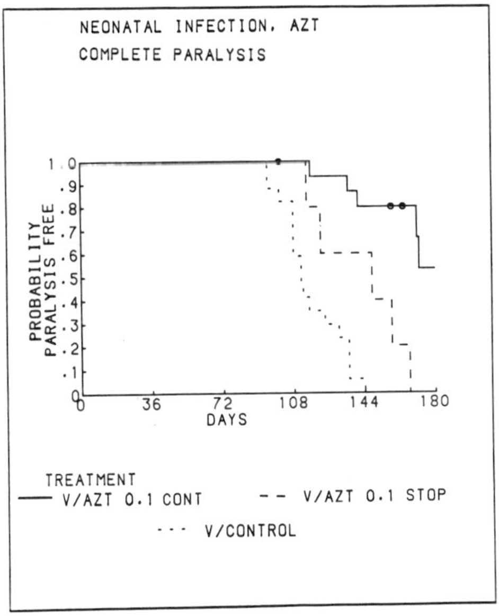

FIGURE 5. Probability to remain free of complete paralysis versus time is shown for SWR/J mice infected as neonates during the first two days of life. (-----, 17 mice): untreated animals; (—— , 16 mice): animals on 0.1 mg/ml AZT continuously as described in METHODS; (— — —, 5 mice): animals on 0.1 mg/ml AZT until weaning only. (-⊕-): 1 animal censored at 108 days due to accidental death, 8 animals without complete paralysis at time of analysis.

DISCUSSION

Using *in utero* infection of midgestation mouse embryos, we have developed a rapid model that permits analysis of retroviral neurovirulence and the development of therapeutic approaches to CNS disease. By one month after birth, the effects of a candidate antiviral agent on CNS disease and survival can be evaluated. Non-effective agents can be quickly eliminated and promising ones studied in more detail. Prodrugs (i.e. drugs depending on *in vivo* conversion to the active form) aimed at the CNS sanctuary can be screened in a relatively short time.

We have shown that AZT dramatically alters the onset and progression of retrovirus-induced neurologic disease. AZT effectively crosses the placental barrier and ameliorates the disease in offspring infected *in utero* when treatment is given during gestation to the pregnant female. Similarly, AZT therapy led to significant clinical benefits for animals infected during the neonatal period.

The therapeutic effects of AZT on retrovirus-induced neurologic disease were highly dose-dependent. Thus, the murine neurotropic disease model described permits quantitative assessment of treatment strategies for therapy of neurologic manifestations of human retrovirus infections rapidly and cost effectively. Because AZT alters the onset and course of disease due to transplacental and perinatal retrovirus infection, we can also evaluate the efficacy of treatment during gestation and in the perinatal period, an important issue considering the increasing prevalence of pediatric AIDS (8-13).

ACKNOWLEDGEMENTS

We thank Dr. P. Jolicoeur for Cas-Br-E producing cells, Dr. S. Nusinoff-Lehrman (Burroughs Wellcome Co.) for AZT, L.G. O'Brien, P. Chassler, R. Curry and D. Grottkopp for excellent technical assistance, and K. Elliott for preparation of this manuscript. RMR is the recipient of a Faculty Development Award from the Pharmaceutical Manufacturers Asociation Foundation, and AHS is a Lucille P. Markey Scholar.

REFERENCES

1. Popovic M, Sarngadharan MG, Read E, Gallo RC (1984). Detection, isolation and continuous production of cytopathic retroviruses (HTLV-III) from patients with AIDS and pre-AIDS. Science 224:497.
2. Barré-Sinoussi F, Chermann JC, Rey F, Nugeyre MT, Chamaret S, Gruest J, Dauguet C, Axler-Blin C, Vezinet-Brun F, Rouzioux C, Rozenbaum W, Montagnier L (1983). Isolation of a T-lymphotropic retrovirus from a patient at risk for Acquired Immune Deficiency Syndrome (AIDS). Science 220:868.
3. Coffin J, Haase A, Levy JA, Montagnier L, Oroszlan S, Teich N, Temin H, Toyoshima K, Varmus H, Vogt P, Weiss R (1986). Human immunodeficiency viruses. Science 232:697.
4. Shaw GM, Harper ME, Hahn BH, Epstein LG, Gajdusek DC, Price RW, Navia BA, Petito CK, O'Hara CJ, Groopman JE, Cho E-S, Oleske JM, Wong-Staal F, Gallo RC (1985). HTLV-III infection in brains of children and adults with AIDS encephalopathy. Science 227:177.
5. Ho DD, Rota TR, Schooley RT, Kaplan JC, Allan JD, Groopman JE, Resnick L, Felsenstein D, Andrews CA, Hirsch MS (1985). Isolation of HTLV-III from cerebrospinal fluid and neural tissues of patients with neurologic syndromes related to the aquired immunodeficiency syndrome. N Engl J Med 313:1493.
6. Navia BA, Jordan BD, Price RW (1986). The AIDS dementia complex: I. Clinical features. Ann Neurol 19:517.
7. Navia BA, Cho E-S, Petito CK, Price RW (1986). The AIDS dementia complex: II. Neuropathology. Ann Neurol 19:525.
8. Cowan MJ, Hellman D, Chudwin D, Wara DW, Chang RS, Ammann AJ (1984). Maternal transmission of acquired immune deficiency syndrome. Pediatrics 73:382.
9. Lapointe N, Michaud J, Pekovic D, Chausseau JP, Dupuy J-M (1985). Transplacental transmission of HTLV-III virus. N Engl J Med 312:1325.
10. Jovaisas E, Koch MA, Schäfer A, Stauber M, Löwenthal D (1985). LAV/HTLV-III in a 20-week fetus. Lancet 2:1129.
11. Ziegler JB, Cooper DA, Johnson RO, Gold J (1985). Postnatal transmission of AIDS-associated retrovirus from mother to infant. Lancet 1:896.
12. Scott GB, Fischl MA, Klimas N, Fletcher MA, Dickinson

GM, Levine RS, Parks WP (1985). Mothers of infants with the acquired immunodeficinecy syndrome. JAMA 253:363.
13. Pahwa S, Kaplan M, Fikrig S, Pahwa R, Sarngadharan MG, Popovic M, Gallo RC (1986). Spectrum of human T-cell lymphotropic virus type III infection in children. JAMA 255:2299.
14. Gardner MB, Henderson BE, Officer JG, Rongey RW, Parker JC, Oliver C, Estes JD, Huebner RJ (1973). A spontaneous lower motor neuron disease apparently caused by indigenous type-C RNA tumor virus in wild mice. J Natl Cancer Inst 51:1243.
15. Gardner MB (1978). Type C viruses of wild mice: characterization and natural history of amphotropic, ecotropic and xenotropic MuLV. Curr Top Microbiol Immunol 79:215.
16. Gardner MB (1985). Retroviral spongiform polioencephalomyelopathy. Rev Infect Dis 7:99.
17. Petito CK, Navia BA, Cho E-S, Jordan BD, George DC, Price RW (1985). Vacuolar myelopathy pathologically resembling subacute combined degeneration in patients with acquired immunodeficiency syndrome (AIDS). N Engl J Med 312:874.
18. Swarz JR, Brooks BR, Johnson RT (1980). Spongiform polioencephalomyelopathy caused by a murine retrovirus. II. Ultrastructural localization of virus replication and spongiform changes in the central nervous system. Neuropath Appl Neurobiol 7:365.
19. Brooks BR, Swarz JR, Johnson RT (1980). Spongiform polioencephalomyelopathy caused by a murine retrovirus. II. Pathogenesis of infection in newborn mice. Lab Invest 43:480.
20. Oldstone MBA, Jensen F, Dixon FJ, Lampert PW (1980). Pathogenesis of slow disease of the central nervous system associated with wild mouse virus. Virology 107:180.
21. Oldstone MBA, Lampert PW, Lee S, Dixon FJ (1977). Pathogenesis of the slow disease of the central nervous system associated with WM 1504 E virus. I. Relationship of strain susceptibility and replication to disease. Am J Pathol 88:193.
22. Horwitz JP, Chua J, Noel M (1964). Nucleosides. V. The monomesylates of 1-(2'-deoxy-β-D-lyxofuranosyl) thymine. J Org Chem 29:2076.
23. Mitsuya H, Weinhold KJ, Furman PA, St. Clair MH, Nusinoff-Lehrman S, Gallo RC, Bolognesi D, Barry DW,

Broder S (1985). 3'-Azido-3'-deoxythymidine (BW A509U): an antiviral agent that inhibits the infectivity and cytopathic effect of human T-lymphotropic virus type III/lymphadenopathy-associated virus in vitro. Proc Natl Acad Sci USA 82:7096.

24. Mitsuya H, Broder S (1987). Strategies for antiviral therapy in AIDS. Nature 325:773.
25. Yarchoan R, Broder S (1987). Development of anti-retroviral therapy for the acquired immunodeficiency syndrome and related disorders. N Engl J Med 316:557.
26. Furman PA, Fyfe JS, St. Clair MH, Weinhold K, Rideout JL, Freeman GA, Nusinoff-Lehrman S, Bolognesi DP, Broder S, Mitsuya H, Barry DW (1986). Phosphorylation of 3'-azido-3'-deoxythymidine and selective interaction of the 5'-triphosphate with human immunodeficiency virus reverse transcriptase. Proc Natl Acad Sci USA 83:8333.
27. Yarchoan R, Klecker RW, Weinhold KJ, Markham PD, Lyerly HK, Durack DT, Gelmann E, Nusinoff-Lehrman S, Blum RM, Barry DW, Shearer GM, Fischl MA, Mitsuya H, Gallo RC, Collins JM, Bolognesi DP, Myers CE, Broder S (1986). Administration of 3'-azido-3'-deoxythymidine, an inhibitor of HTLV-III/LAV replication, to patients with AIDS or AIDS-related complex. Lancet 1:575.
28. Yarchoan R, Berg G, Brouwers P, Fischl MA, Spitzer AR, Wichman A, Grafman J, Thomas RV, Safai B, Brunetti A, Perno CF, Schmidt PJ, Larson SM, Myers CE, Broder S (1987). Response of human immunodeficiency virus-associated neurological disease to 3'-azido-3'-deoxythymidine. Lancet 1:132.
29. Ruprecht RM, O'Brien LG, Rossoni LD, Nusinoff-Lehrman S (1986). Suppression of mouse viremia and retroviral disease by 3'-azido-3'-deoxythymidine. Nature 323:467.
30. Ruprecht RM, Rossoni LD, Haseltine WA, Broder S (1985). Suppression of retroviral propagation and disease by suramin in murine systems. Proc Natl Acad Sci USA 82:7733.
31. Jaenisch R (1980). Retroviruses and embryogenesis: microinjection of Moloney murine leukemia virus into midgestation embryos. Cell 19:181.
32. Nobis P, Jaenisch R (1980). Passive immunotherapy prevents expression of endogenous Moloney virus and amplification of proviral DNA in BALB/c mice. Proc Natl Acad Sci USA 77:3677.

Human Retroviruses, Cancer, and AIDS:
Approaches to Prevention and Therapy, pages 463–474

ANTIRETROVIRAL THERAPY OF HIV INFECTION

Michael S. Gottlieb, M.D.

The human retroviruses are now known to be important pathogens. Human immunodeficiency virus (HIV-1) is etiologic for the acquired immune deficiency syndrome (AIDS) and its associated conditions. HIV-2 is etiologic for severe immune deficiency in certain areas of West Africa. The need for developing effective antiretroviral therapy is urgent given that (a) millions are already infected with these agents, (b) the attack rate for AIDS is high in HIV infected populations, and (c) the disease has a high mortality rate. Significant progress in understanding the pathogenesis of HIV infection has opened doors to developing strategies for antiviral therapy. This review summarizes the state of the art as well as newly emerging rationales and approaches.

The Problem

HIV-1 infects thymus-derived (T) lymphocytes and blood monocytes via the specific binding of its envelope glycoprotein (gp 120) to CD-4 molecules on the cell surface [1,2]. Subsequent fusion of cell membranes with formation of syncitia and multinucleated giant cells occurs, a process which appears to be central to the induction of T cell injury. [3] This mechanism is supported by observations that some HTLV-III mutants fail to induce cytopathic effects in cultures of susceptible target cells [4]. T cell injury also appears to be related in some way to the rate of HIV replication, a process accelerated by transactivation [5].

Hybridization studies reveal a low frequency of infected cells *in vivo* [6]. This would on the surface appear encouraging, however any optimism must be tempered by recent information on non-cytopathic infection of blood monocytes which are long-lived and migrate widely [7]. Thus, chronic infection of monocytes establishes this cell type as a reservoir of the infection and vector for transmission to additional CD-4 T cells, as well as to additional target organs most notably the brain [8]. Current evidence implicates monocytes which have migrated to brain as the major site of productive viral infection in the nervous system. Addressing central nervous system HIV infection is an important priority in devising therapy. Treatment of CNS infection is complicated by the requirement for drugs to cross the blood brain barrier, and the probability that some proposed antiviral agents will prove to have neurotoxic properties.

A high attack rate for AIDS among HIV infected populations has been demonstrated in prospective and retrospective studies [9,10]. Progression to AIDS has been associated with a number of markers including absolute CD-4 cell number, persistence of plasma p24 antigen, and loss of serum antibody to p24. Thus it appears that among those infected immunity to HIV is rare. The current model of the pathogenesis of AIDS is that in most infected individuals ongoing HIV replication leads to progressive CD-4 lymphopenia which ultimately predisposes to opportunistic infections and/or malignancy. A major goal is to develop effective agents with high therapeutic ratios, suitable for use by patients in the early stages of HIV infection. The desirable characteristics of anti-HIV drugs are listed in Table I.

Table 1

Some Desirable Characteristics of Anti-HIV Agents
Penetrate lymphocytes and monocytes
Metabolized to active moieties by cellular enzymes (for dideoxynucleosides)
Cross the blood brain barrier
Non-toxic to host cells
Complete inhibition of viral replication
Elimination of virus shedding in genital secretions
Address the issue of integrated provirus
Inexpensive
Easily administered
Safe over long periods of administration

The definition of endpoints for therapeutic efficacy of antiviral agents in HIV infection requires careful consideration. Endpoints which are relatively "hard" for assessment of efficacy include prolongation of survival after diagnosis of AIDS, improved quality of life, decrease in the frequency and/or severity of infectious complications, and improved CNS function. Alteration in the attack rate of CDC-defined AIDS or the AIDS-related complex is a major objective of clinical trials in asymptomatic HIV carriers. At the present time the most central laboratory endpoints in clinical trials are effects on agents on alsolute CD-4 cell number, plasma antigenemia, and detection of HIV antigens or virus in lymphocytes by cocultivation.

Antiviral Approaches

Review of the biology of HIV reveals potential sites for attack with antiviral agents (Table 2). The virus first binds to CD-4 or a closely linked molecule via its envelope glycoprotein. After entering the cell it is uncoated and genomic RNA is transcribed into DNA by the reverse transcriptase enzyme. The DNA is circularized and integrated into host cell chromosomes as provirus. During active replication proviral DNA is transcribed to viral RNA which is processed before binding to ribosomes to initiate translation and synthesis of viral proteins in the rough endoplasmic reticulum. Subsequent processing includes cleavage to smaller forms and glycosylation. At the plasma membrane complete particles of protein and genomic RNA are assembled and released by budding through the membrane. HIV has at least eight genes including tatIII and art which code for transactivating factors which regulate viral gene expression. These regulatory factors represent potential targets for antiviral chemotherpy [11].

Table 2

Sites of action of potential HIV antivirals

REPLICATION STEP	AGENT
Binding to the target cell	anti-CD-4 antibody
Entry and uncoating	(hypothetical)
Reverse transcription	3'azido, 3'deoxythymidine (zidovudine, AZT)
	2',3'dideoxycytidine
	phosphonoformate
	HPA-23 suramin
Integration of DNA into host genome	agents which affect integrase (hypothetical)

(continued)

Transcription	(hypothetical)
Translation	ribavirin
	agents which affect tat-III, or art-trs
	"antisense" constructs
Component assembly and release	(hypothetical)
Viral budding	interferons

The findings that the nucleoside analog 3'-azido-3'-deoxythymidine (AZT, zidovudine) was a potent inhibitor of HIV *in vitro* [12,13] and of murine retroviruses *in vivo* prompted accelerated clinical trials of this agent. Cellular kinases phosphorylate azidothymidine to mono and triphosphate forms. The incorporation into DNA of the triphosphate by the reverse transcriptase leads to termination of chain elongation. This occurs because its 3' substitution prevents further 5' to 3' phosphodiester linkages. There is evidence that the reverse transcriptase is more susceptible to the inhibitory effects of phosphorylated nucleosides than the mammalian polymerase alpha. In phase I studies the drug was well absorbed by the oral route with plasma concentrations attained which inhibit HIV replication *in vitro.* Passage across the blood brain barrier was documented [14].

In a placebo controlled trial in patients with AIDS or advanced AIDS related complex zidovudine prolonged survival, improved neurological deficits, and reduced plasma HIV antigenemia [15,16]. The major adverse effects were on hematopoiesis, notably anemia and leukopenia. In March, 1987, zidovudine was approved by the Food and Drug

Administration for symptomatic HIV infected individuals (AIDS and ARC) with a proven episode of Pneumocytsis pneumonia or with fewer than 200 CD-4 cells per cubic millimeter.

Additional dideoxynucleoside analogs inhibit HIV replication in vitro. These include 2'3'-dideoxyadenosine [17], 3'azido-2'3'-dideoxy- 5-ethyluridine, 3'-azido-2'3'-dideoxyguanosine, 2'3'-dideoxythymidine, 2'3'-dideoxythymidinene, and 2'3'didexycytidinene [18,19]. Broder has emphasized the importance of testing multiple cell lines in screening for antiviral activity. The absence in a individual cell line of kinases required for phosphorylation of a specific nucleoside analog to its active form might lead to the erroneous conclusion of drug resistance [17].

Of the nucleoside analogs screened to date, the pyrimidine analog 2',3' dideoxycytidine (ddC) is the most potent on a molar basis [20]. Complete in vitro inhibition is seen at 0.5 micromolar. ddC is relatively resistant to cytidine deaminase which degrades cytidine analogs. Studies suggest that ddC triphosphate acts by inhibiting DNA chain elongation in a manner analogous to AZT. The effects can be reversed by deoxycytidine presumably by competition for deoxycytidine kinase [21]. ddC is currently in phase I trials assessing toxicity and pharmacokinetic properties.

Studies in progress of the the HIV reverse transcriptase could lead to the rational development of additional inhibitors. In preliminary studies using site-directed mutagenesis and a cell free assay system Larder and colleagues identified regions which are critical to enzyme function [22]. The methods of xray diffraction or computer generated modelling of proteins could be applied to the design of inhibitors of reverse transcriptase, or tat-III. In addition studies on structural (integrase, protease) and regulatory proteins (tat-III, trs) produced in large scale could lead to the development of specific inhibitors.

Yet another approach to therapy has been the synthesis of antisense oligonucleotides which are complementary to regions of HIV RNA or messenger RNA [23]. These could possibly block the expression of viral proteins through a "hybridization arrest" of messenger RNA or by inhibiting the binding of a regulatory protein (e.g. tat-III). Phosphorothioates [24] and methylphosphonates [25] of oligonucleotides have been shown to enhance their _in vitro_ activity.

One novel approach is to introduce "suicide inhibitors" into cells consisting of the gene for diptheria toxin A-chain linked to the viral long terminal repeat sequence (LTR) [26]. This scheme is based on the assumption that transactivation systems in HIV infected cells would act on the LTR and induce synthesis of the toxin leading to death of these specific infected cells. The prospects for utility of these approaches _in vivo_ remain doubtful.

Interferons appear to act late in the viral replication cycle at the stages of translation, assembly and budding. Beta and gamma as well as alpha interferon have been demonstrated to have _in vitro_ activity [27-29].

Ultimately the use of combinations of antiretroviral agents acting at multiple sites in the process of viral replication may prove feasible. This additive approach might facilitate the use of lower doses of compounds which might otherwise have toxicity at the doses required for use as single agents. In addition a multiagent approach could minimize the emergence of drug resistance among HIV isolates.

In summary, the discovery of HIV as the etiologic agent of AIDS has accelerated the identification and development of antiviral agents. Azidothymidine (AZT, zidovudine) is the first agent found to be clinically useful in the management anti-HIV infection. Within 3 years of the discovery of HIV a clinically useful drug was identified and approved. The impact of this development cannot be minimized. Recent progress in understanding the biology of HIV has greatly improved the prospects for developing even more effective antiviral regimens.

REFERENCES

1. Dalgleish AG, Beverley PCL, Clapham PR, Crawford DH, Greaves MF, Weiss RA. 1984. The CD-4 (T4) antigen is an essential component antigen of the receptor for the AIDS retrovirus. Nature 312:763-767.

2. Klatzmann D, Champagne E, Chamaret S, Gruest J, Guetard D, Hercend T, Gluckman JC, Montagnier L. 1984. T-lymphocyte T4 molecule behaves as the receptor for human retrovirus LAV. Nature 312:767-768.

3. Sodroski J, Goh WC, Rosen C, Campbell K, Haseltine WA. Role of the HTLV-III/LAV envelope in syncytium formation and cytopathicity. Nature 1986; 322:470-4.

4. Fisher AG, Ratner L, Mitsuya H, Marselle LM, Harper ME, Broder S, Gallo RC, Wong Staal F. 1986b. Infectious mutants of HTLV-III with changes in the 3' region and markedly reduced cytopathic effects. Science 233:655-659.

5. Fisher AG, Feinberg MB, Josephs SF, et al. The trans-activator gene of HTLV-III is essential for virus replication. Nature 1986; 320:367-71.

6. Harper ME, Marselle LM, Gallo RC, Wong-Staal F. Detection of lymphocytes expressing

HTLV-III in lymph nodes and peripheral blood from infected individuals by in site hybridization, Proc. Nat. Acad. Sci. PNAS 1986 83:772-776.

7. Ho DD, Rota TR, Hirsch MS, Infection of monocyte/macrophages by human T-lymphotropic virus type III J. Clin Invest. 1986. 77: 1712-1715.

8. Ho DD, Rota TR, Schooley RT, Kaplan JC, Allan JD, Groopman JE, Resnick L, Felsenstein D, Andrews CA, Hirsch MS. 1985. Isolation of HTLV-III from cerebro-spinal fluid and neural tissues of patients with neurologic syndromes related to the acquired immunodeficiency syndrome. N. Engl. J. Med. 313: 1493-1497.

9. Polk BF, Fox R, Brookmeyer R, Kanchanaraksa S, Kaslow R, Visscher B, Rinaldo C, Phair J. Predictors of the acquired immunodeficiency syndrome developing in a cohort of seropositive homosexual men. N Engl J Med 1987; 316:61-6.

10. Detels R, Fahey J, Sever J, Madden DL, Schwartz K, Dudley JP, English PA, Powers H, Clark VA, Gottlieb MS. Predictors of Clinical AIDS in Young Homosexual Men in a High Risk Area International Journal of Epidemiology. 16:271-276, 1987.

11. Hirsch MS, Kaplan J. Treatment of human immunodeficiency virus infections. Antimicrob. Agents. Chemother 1987; 31:839-43.

12. Mitsuya H, Broder S. 1986. Inhibition of the _in vitro_ infectivity and cytopathic effect of human T-lymphotropic virus type III/lymphadenopathy-associated virus (HTLV-III/LAV) by 2'3'-dideoxynucleosides. Proc. Natl. Acad. Sci. USA 83:1911-1915.

13. Mitsuya H, Weinhold KJ, Furman PA, St. Clair MH, Lehrman S, Gallo RC, Bolognesi D, Barry DW, Broder S. 1985. 3'Azido-3'deoxythymidine (BWA509U); an antiviral agent that inhibits the infectivity and cytopathic effect of human T-lymphotropic virus type III/lymphadenopathy-associated virus in vitro. Proc. Natl. Acad. Sci. USA 82:7096-7100.

14. Yarchoan R, Klecker RW, Weinhold KJ, Markham PD, etal. Administration of 3'azido-3'deoxythymidine, an inhibitor of HTLV-III replication, to patients with AIDS or AIDS related complex. Lancet I:575-580.

15. Fischl, MA, Richman DD, Grieco MH, Gottlieb MS, Volberding TA, Laskin OL, Leedom JM, Groopman JE, Mildvan D, Schooley RT, Jackson GA, Durack DT, King D, and the AZT Collaborative Group. The effect of Azidothymidine in the treatment of patients with AIDS and the AIDS-related complex: a double-blind placebo controlled trial. N Engl J. Med 1987; 317:185-191.

16. Fischl MA, Richman DD, Grieco MH, Gottlieb MS, Volberding TA, Laskin OL, Leedom JM, Groopman JE, Mildvan D, Hirsch M, Jackson GG, Durack DT, Nusinoff-Lehrman S. The toxicity of azidothymidine in the treatment of patients with AIDS and the AIDS-related complex: a double blind placebo controlled trial. N Engl J. Med 1987; 317:192-197.

17. Yarchoan R, Broder S. Development of Antiretroviral therapy for the acquired immunodeficiency syndrome and related disorders: a progress report. N Engl J Med 1987; 316:557-64.

18. Hartman H, Hunsmann G, Eckstein F. Letter. Lancet i:40-41, 1987.

19. Schinazi CK, Chu CK, Feorino P, Sommados JP. Program Abstract: 26th Interscience Conference Antimicrors. agents. cheomother. Abstract No. 1092. 1986.

20. Balzarini J, Mitsuya H, De Clercq E, Cooney DA, Kong CJ, Dalal M, Johns DG, Broder S. 1987. Potent and selective anti-HTLV-III/LAV activity of 2'3'-dideoxycytidinene, the 2'3'-unsaturated derivative of 2'3'-dideoxycytidine. Biochem. Biophys. Res. Commun. 140:735-742.

21. Cooney DA, Dalal M, Mitsuya H, McMahon JB, Nadkarni M, Balzarni J, Broder S, Johns DG. 1986. Initial studies on the cellular pharmacology of 2'3'-dideoxycytidine, an inhibitor of HTLV-III infectivity. Biochem. Pharmacol. 35:2065-2068.

22. Larder BA, Purifoy DJM, Powell, KJ, Darby G. Indentification of functional regions in the HIV reverse transcriptase by site-directed mutagenesis. J Celluar Biochem 11D, 1987 Abstracts; pg 72.

23. Zamecnik PC, Goodchild J, Taguchi Y, Sarin PS. 1986. Inhibition of replication and expression of human T-cell lymphotropic virus type III in cultured cells by exogenous synthetic oligonucleotides complimentary to viral RNA. Proc. Natl. Acad. Sci. USA 83:4143-4146.

24. Zaia J, Cantin E, Rossi JJ, Spallone PA, Murakawa G, Erijta R, Kaplan B, Wallace RB. Inhibition of Human immunodeficiency virus

(HIV) using an oligonucloside methylphosphonate. J Cell Biochem 11D, 1987 Abstracts; p72.

25. Matsukura M, Shinozuko K, Zon G, Mitsuya H, Cohen J, Broder S. Phosphorothioate analogs of oligodeoxynucleotides: novel inhibitors of replication and cytopathic effects of HTLV-II/LAV (Human Innunodeficiency virus). J Celluar Biochem 11D, 1987 Abstracts; pg67

26. Maxwell IH, Glode LM, Maxwell F, HTLV-regulated expression of a transfected diphtheria toxin gene. J Celluar Biochem 11D, 1987 Abstracts; pg67

27. Ho DD, Hartshorn KL, Rota TR, Andrews CA, Kaplan JC, Schooley RT, Hirsch MS. 1985. Recombinant human interferon alpha A suppresses HTLV-III replication in vitro. Lancet i:602-604.

28. Nakashima H, Toshida T, Harada S, Yamamoto N. 1986. Recombinant human interferon gamma suppresses HTLV-III replication in vitro. Int. J. Cancer. 38:433-436

29. Yamamoto JK, Barre-Sinoussi F, Bolton V, Pederson NC, Gardner MB. 1986. Human alpha- and beta-interferon but not gamma suppress the in vitro replication of LAV, HTLV-III, and ARV-2. J. Interferon Res. 6:143-152.

VIII. CLOSING REMARKS

**Human Retroviruses, Cancer, and AIDS:
Approaches to Prevention and Therapy, pages 477–489**

HIV 1987

David Baltimore

Whitehead Institute for Biomedical Research
Nine Cambridge Center
Cambridge, MA 02142

In which the author provides an idiosyncratic view of what took place in Keystone, Colorado when a group of experts convened to consider the present state of knowledge about the causation of AIDS.

Living through an AIDS meeting is inevitably a disturbing experience. The problem is so pressing that the usual scientific detachment is hard to maintain. The possible rewards from success are great enough to distort human relations among the participants. The eye of the press is always evident, reminding us that the whole world is watching (and praying for surcease). But no matter what the need, science takes its measured pace.

Not being a long-standing member of the AIDS research community, I look at the problem as a virologist and, sometimes, an immunologist. What follows are semi-random thoughts on selected aspects of the meeting. Because I am unsure of some facts, probably unaware of many subtleties and somewhat mixed up about who did what, I have left out reference to individual achievements. In that way the reader can decide for him or herself which comments seem relevant and which are off-the-wall without my giving the pretense of providing a scholarly opinion.

How many viruses?

The last few years has seen an explosion of knowledge about the various viruses isolated from AIDS patients. Striking differences in nucleotide sequence have been found leading to the view that HIV is a particularly mutable virus and that vaccine production may be difficult because of the variability. To provide some perspective, perhaps we should return to an earlier era when nucleotide sequence was not so easy to obtain and the definitions of virus types were done by serology. A serological definition is, of course, what we want because we are interested in knowing whether different isolates are immunologically cross-protective. The available data using human sera show that even though the neutralizing titers are low, the sera are generally cross-reactive. Even the serum from a chimpanzee is cross-reactive. Thus, by this definition, the enormous nucleotide sequence diversity of the virus may be a red herring. HIV1, at least, may be a single serotype. If it isn't, it is very important to get clear data on the question. The LAV2 isolate seems appropriately named HIV2 because it is probably a second serological type.

This perspective comes from looking at natural sera. Looking at serological reactions to purified viral glycoproteins, however, gives a very different perspective. These sera are highly type-specific with individual isolates showing very little cross-reaction. It may be that natural sera reflect infection by multiple serotypes. But, more likely, the difference comes from the different presentation of antigen in the form of virus as opposed to glycoprotein or polypeptide subunits. Viruses are the best natural immunogens about which we know and protein subunits have never been nearly as effective. Why subunits should give a highly type-specific reaction is not clear, but a good hypothesis is that the difference lies in the structure of the antigenic unit presented to the immune system.

Even if there is only one serotype of HIV1, there is yet no evidence that a vaccine against infection by HIV1 is going to be easy to produce. At the moment the obvious is being tried: subunit vaccines, either natural or synthetic. The preliminary data is not exciting and suggests that more imaginative approaches may be necessary. One approach that shows some signs of value is to induce the formation of antibodies that interfere with the interaction of the viral glycoprotein and the CD4 receptor molecule. Such antibodies could be against the CD4 molecule itself and apparently can be induced as anti-idiotypic antibodies.

Genetic interactions and the origin of HIV

No matter how many serotypes there actually are, there is no question that HIV is a highly variable virus. One clue to an origin for some of that variability comes from the observation, quite preliminary, that LAV2 may be a bit like a cross between HIV1 and SIV. Whether this is true or not, it raises the possibility that recombination may play a significant role in variability.

In his opening remarks, Howard Temin suggested that HIV probably arose from a non-human primate source in the recent past. While this position has a lot to recommend it, I still believe that we should consider the possibility that the virus has been within some human population for many years. The suggestion that a serum from 1959 had anti-HIV1 antibodies already takes us back well before the first reports of AIDS. Because infectious disease is a consequence of the interaction of the properties of an infectious agent with the social structure of communities, it seems likely that changes in social mores are what have made the virus so prevalent not changes in the infectious agent. We know that the 1970's brought to the homosexual and IV drug abuser populations major changes in terms of the number of interactions with other people where either semen or blood was transferred. It is not so obvious what happened in Africa, but a significant increase in prostitution seems a reasonable hypothesis. Even if the virus did arise *de novo* by modification of a primate virus, it was probably the fertile social structure that allowed the virus to take hold. Had the social structure altered many years before, the virus might well have appeared then. No matter where the virus came from, it is eerie that it waited until after the discovery of the reverse transcriptase to make its appearance. This remarkable apparent coincidence leads one to wonder whether the same sources of freedom that allow for unconventional thought also allow for unconventional behavior.

Another aspect of viral variation is the variants that can be isolated from a single individual. Apparently isolates from different portions of the body can have specific tropisms even though the viruses are obviously close relatives. If significant viral variation occurs over the course of a single person's infection, then we must consider whether the virus' ability to infect multiple cell types -- cells in the brain, macrophages, endothelial cells, T lymphocytes, B lymphocytes and other suggestions -- may not come about because the virus is able to mutate its regulatory sequences to allow for infection of different cell types. Given the long latent period of the infection, it is not unreasonable that the virus could take on multiple forms in its life cycle in one person much as happens with malaria and other parasites.

Natural history of HIV

We still have much to learn about the natural history of the virus. We know that it is spread by three routes: sexual contact, parenteral inoculation and perinatal transmission. In no case, however, do we know how much is transmitted by cells, how much by free virus and what cell is the initially infected cell in the recipient. Figure 1 provides a framework for thinking about the various steps that follow the initiation of infection. The first landmark after a person is initially infected is seroconversion, which occurs weeks later and implies that the synthesis of a sufficient antigenic load to stimulate the immune system requires a remarkably long time. Seroconversion presumably is accompanied by T-cell responses and strong CTL responses have been described. In fact, the only known deficit in the immune response is that the neutralizing antibody titers are low; otherwise the immune response might be quite conventional.

```
                                Infection (t=0)

                              ⎧ Seroconversion (weeks)
                              ⎪
Multiple immune               ⎪ Preliminary Phase (years)
responses                     ⎨
(neutralizing Ab Low)         ⎪    - Slow deterioration
                              ⎪      of immune function
                              ⎩    - Low virus load
                 ⎧                 - Lymphadenopathy
                 ⎪                  (oligoclonal expansion?)
                 ⎪  I
                 ⎪  N         ⎧ Accelerating Phase
                 ⎪  F         ⎪
Brain            ⎨  E         ⎪      - Increased virus load
Disease          ⎪  C         ⎪      - Massive loss of CD4's
                 ⎪  T         ⎨      - Majority of immune
                 ⎪  I         ⎪        function lost
                 ⎪  O         ⎪
                 ⎪  N         ⎩ Death
                 ⎩  S
```

FIGURE 1. The time-line of AIDS infections

Following seroconversion there is a period of years that we might call the Preliminary Phase of the infection cycle. During these years there is a slow deterioration of immune function, there is a relatively low virus load as indicated by the difficulty of isolating the virus and there is the development of lymphadenopathy. There have been recent suggestions that lymphadenopathy may be an oligoclonal expansion suggesting that it is more akin to a neoplastic than to an immune response. Following the relatively stable preliminary phase of the disease, at a period some five years or so later, there begins the Accelerating Phase of the disease. Around this time begin the infections that have been the hallmark of AIDS, there is an increased virus load, there is a massive loss of CD4 lymphocytes, there is finally a major deterioration in immune function. Even during the earlier phase there are the beginnings of brain disease and there may be the development of Kaposi's sarcoma. The various symptoms finally lead to a irremedial condition that becomes the cause of death.

This course of disease is very unusual. Most virus infections involve an initial acute phase, followed perhaps by a chronic virus-infected state, but not one that involves continued deterioration. Most RNA virus infections are completely cured by the immune response, most DNA virus infections lead to a chronic carrier state. There are occasional exacerbations in other viral infections, but only hepatitis virus causes progressive deterioration in a significant fraction of infected individuals. The uniqueness of HIV is that it virtually always wins the battle. As the data from the military show, it appears that progressive deterioration in an HIV infection is a consistent finding.

One hypothesis that might explain the course of the infection is that there is a continuing fight between the immune system and the virus. Initially the immune system holds the virus in check, but because the virus can insinuate itself into the nucleus as a provirus, the immune system cannot eradicate the infection and over years the infection slowly spreads widely enough to overwhelm the immune system. A different hypothesis, suggested above, is that the virus mutates and recombines continually so that the course of the infectious process is actually an evolutionary change in virus structure. This may require years, but ultimately leads to a sufficiently wide spread of the virus so that it takes over and kills the host. One problem with this notion is that as the virus spreads it should become more virulent and when it infects another individual the course of the infection should be much more rapid. Perhaps, however, this is not an appropriate analysis because as the virus mutates within an individual to adapt its growth to a wider range of cells it may become less effective in passing to another individual so that what really passes the infection is virus that has not significantly mutated.

Latency and Activation

The concept of latency is a crucial one in thinking about the biology of HIV. By latency we mean the ability of the virus to maintain itself in cells in a quiescent form over long periods of time. It is believed that there is a latent state, although it is unclear whether this involves the slow replication of the virus -- effectively a chronic infection -- or a true silent latency. The concept of viral latency raises the question of how the virus gets into cells in the first place. If it is like most other retroviruses, then it must need a growing cell to initially infect, the need for cell growth being apparently a necessity for DNA synthesis to provide sites for viral integration. HIV might not need to integrate, but other retroviruses certainly do and evidence presented at this meeting suggests that deletion of the integration machinery of the virus prevents infection.

Circulating T lymphocytes and macrophages are not dividing cells. To initiate an infection, the virus may, in fact, have to go to a lymph node where antigenically driven T lymphocytes are dividing. Other infections may provide the impetus for this division or HIV might itself. From what we know of HIV infections, they should be lytic in growing T cells, but perhaps a T cell that quickly returns to quiescence might be able to integrate a provirus, but not express the genetic potential of the provirus. If such a cell does not transcribe the provirus at all, then a true latent state will exist; if transcription is low, then perhaps a chronic state will ensue. For the virus-infected cell now to begin active virus synthesis, reactivation of the T cell must be necessary and that may require that the T cell return to the lymph node and encounter the same antigen that initially stimulated its growth. If this antigen is HIV itself, then this infection becomes a paradigm of the antigenic receptor driving proliferation under viral stimulation, as long championed by Dr. Irving Weissman, but the outcome here is cell death and not cancer.

A central question about the natural history of the virus is what role is played by the thymus. Studies of thymic function during HIV infection are desparately needed to understand this important potential aspect of the life cycle.

In the last year, my own laboratory has had occasion to study the interaction of antigenic stimulation with virus replication. These data, which were recently published (Nabel and Baltimore, Nature 326:711-713, 1987), show that a specific transcription factor is induced in T lymphocytes by mitogenic stimulation. This factor binds to a site in the HIV LTR involved in enhancement of transcription efficiency from the HIV promoter. We initially identified this factor as one stimulated in maturing B lymphocytes and involved in the regulation of kappa light chain immunoglobulin transcription. One important lesson from this work is that studies of parallel systems can often illuminate HIV function and that the study of AIDS will progress most rapidly if investigators from a wide range of backgrounds become aware of the problems posed by HIV.

The activation of HIV is not simply a matter of increased transcription under the influence of this cellular factor. The virus has designed itself for rapid, massive response to activation using internal regulation systems. In this way, HIV and related lentiviruses differ strikingly from other retroviruses. It is perhaps significant that the lentiviruses pass only by horizontal transmission from one infected individual to another and are not passed by genetic vertical transmission as is found with the classical retroviruses. The viral factors involved in amplification of viral mRNA are variously called *tat*, *art*, *trs*, x, etc. It remains debatable whether these factors affect transcription rate, processing of transcripts, stability of transcripts or translational rate. Presumably different factors act differently and the whole subject requires more intense investigation before a clear model will emerge. It is particularly striking that the 3'-*orf*, when deleted, upregulates viral gene expression. This shows that the virus has a calculated strategy of both inhibition and activation of transcription, presumably explaining the ability of the virus to be either latent or actively growing.

A major question about viral natural history is how a virus actually kills T lymphocytes. A simple answer is that the virus may subvert cellular metabolism so completely that the cell cannot maintain itself. This is not true of most other retroviruses, but they do not contain the genes for autoactivation. Most workers are not satisfied that this is the appropriate explanation and other suggestions have been made involving the interaction between the envelope and CD4. Another possibility is that the virus-infected cells release a toxic influence.

Therapy and Prevention

Turning from natural history and biology to therapy and prevention, we turn from one form of ignorance to another. Nothing said at this meeting suggests that either vaccines or totally effective drugs are going to be possible to produce. Only an optimism bred from the historic successes of biomedical research leads us to believe that these very important goals will be reached. Starting to think first about vaccines, it was striking that the whole range of immune reactions can be found in HIV-infected people. The major defect in the ordinary immune response appears to be the low neutralizing titers and no form of synthetic antigen has yet shown evidence of solving that problem. Rumors indicate that chimpanzees do not produce an effective immune response to either subunits or polypeptides representing the sequence of the envelope protein. The more we learn about the natural history of the virus, the clearer it becomes that designing a vaccine will be difficult. Such a vaccine must not only block the ordinary virus-to-cell transmission, but must also probably block cell-to-cell transmission. Furthermore, it is likely that a vaccine must block the initial infection of a person implying that IgA may play an important role where sexual transfer is involved. To protect against both parenteral and sexual transmission, both IgG and IgA responses will be needed.

The major advances at the meeting relevant to vaccines are the tentative identification of CD4 binding sites and the demonstration that the peptides covering this region can induce some level of neutralizing antibody. Although this antibody is highly type-specific, it indicates one possible route to a vaccine.

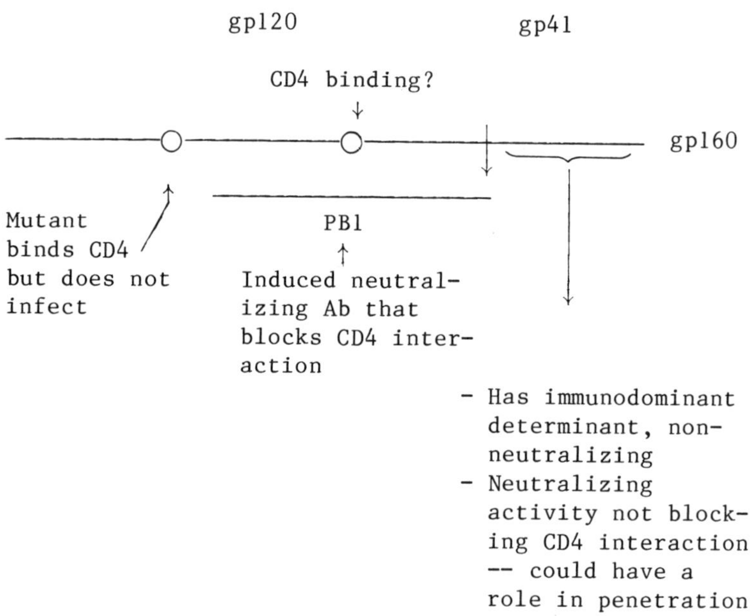

FIGURE 2. The organization of the HIV1 glycoprotein

The organization of the gp160 envelope precursor is becoming more evident (see Fig. 2). The gp120 portion has a segment in its C-terminal half that appears to be involved in CD4 binding. The peptide called PB1 that covers this region is one that will induce neutralizing antibody, antibody that will block the interaction between gp120 and CD4. At least one mutant outside of this region can block infection, but is not involved in the CD4 interaction. The gp41 component of the glycoprotein precursor has a very strongly immunodominant determinant which is non-neutralizing. There is neutralizing activity induced by the gp41, which does not involve blockade of CD4 interaction and could involve inhibition of the penetration reaction because the structure of gp41 suggests that it may have regions involved in viral penetration.

Turning from vaccines to drugs, the striking fact was that AZT is looking better, particularly during the earlier stages of HIV infection. There is significant hope that dideoxycytidine will be even better than AZT because of lower toxicity and it was surprising that more data on this potential new drug was not available. It is clear that if reverse transcriptase inhibitors will work, then they are going to be perfected in the next few years. The significant bone marrow toxicity of AZT, however, suggests that nucleic acid analogs may have only a limited effectiveness and that other types of drugs will have to be produced. At the moment there is no other part of the viral life cycle that offers a clear target, although the viral protease is one enzyme whose biochemistry is well enough understood that it may be an early candidate. Until we learn more about the function of the transactivating proteins, we will not be in a position to know how to block their function, although that remains a tantalizing hope.

Concluding Comments

I should like to conclude this personal summary by stepping back and making some general observations:

The first is that it is extremely impressive how much research is being done on HIV and how rapidly HIV has used up the base of existing virology. HIV research is now driving virology rather than living off the past. HIV research is equal to or better than research on other viruses in many areas including studies of virus-receptor interaction, regulation of gene expression, viral structure, reverse transcription and protease action. HIV virology is also catching up in areas like immune pathogenesis, drug design and vaccine development. It is interesting to see how a practical problem sets priorities, attracts new workers and rapidly moves ahead. It is a bit disturbing that the questions involved are actually old ones, but that the fashions of science allowed work on those questions to decay once the questions had been posed. A defect in the field that was evidenced at this meeting was the lack of amateurs, people working in other fields who have thought about or done a few experiments with HIV. Howard Temin and I represented two of the more evident amateurs.

The major difference between this meeting and others in virology was the great importance of basic work being done in commercial settings. In a real sense, the search for drugs and vaccines is a partnership between industry and academic science. The negative side of that partnership is that when people from corporate settings present their work, one is always uncertain about whether the data presented are skewed to be self-serving and whether there is a complete openness and candor about what has been accomplished. The HIV field has suffered sufficiently from the pernicious effects of competition and doesn't need the further complication of competition for profits from corporations. Being realistic, however, we must at least partially accept this as a penalty to be paid for the great advantage of corporate involvement and we should recognize that competition is often a positive driving force in science. The major reason for raising this caution is the number of people who commented to me about their worries in this direction, suggesting that the problem requires open discussion and ways to minimize it should be found.

For all the progress that has been made, the AIDS problem worsens daily. One rough estimate is that during the time of this meeting as many as 50,000 new infections by HIV may have occurred worldwide. Such numbers involve guesswork because we do not have careful surveillance, especially in Africa, but the actual data presented from the military at this meeting shows that perhaps 15,000 new infections among Black Americans occurred between 1985-1986.

With the presidential election coming up, the AIDS problem is rapidly entering the realm of politics. During this meeting, the President of the United States made his first statement on AIDS. Congress is increasingly aware of the level of fear in the country and the need for political response.

The general population is beginning to understand the magnitude of the problem and the notion of risk group is rapidly changing to an understanding that there are risky behaviors indulged in by a significant fraction of the overall population. Some people are responding to this understanding by protecting themselves but others are, in the great tradition of McCarthyism, looking for scapegoats. This has lead to counterproductive proposals of massive screening and quarantine and to charges that the research community has not been aggressively following up every lead. One can only hope that cooler heads will prevail, because what is needed is careful thinking and hard work, not sacrificial lambs.

The AIDS problem requires that we work in the most optimum organizational frameworks at the fastest possible speed to bring the full strength of the scientific community to bear on the problem. We need to minimize secrecy and the destructive aspects of competition both in the academic and corporate worlds. It may not be too soon to turn back to the atomic bomb project of World War II and to abstract from it those organizational notions that are relevant to today's world. We certainly do not need the centralization that was required to maintain security during the Manhattan Project, but I think we can benefit from a more careful coordination of efforts and a deeper sense of commitment.

Index